Table of Contents

- Table of Contents i
- FREE GIFT! 16
- Introduction 17
- Paleo Recipes for Breakfast 18
  - Breakfast Tomato and Eggs 18
  - Breakfast Paleo Muffins 18
  - Paleo Banana Pancakes 19
  - Plantain Pancakes 19
  - Paleo Sweet Potato Waffles 20
  - Paleo Eggplant French Toast 20
  - Orange and Dates Granola 21
  - Paleo Breakfast Burrito 21
  - Spinach Frittata 22
  - Squash Blossom Frittata 22
  - Paleo Breakfast Burger 23
  - Paleo Maple Nut Porridge 23
  - Paleo Breakfast Sandwich 24
  - Paleo Turkey Breakfast Sandwich 24
  - Paleo Blueberry Smoothie 25
  - Paleo Green Smoothie 25
  - Paleo Red Breakfast Smoothie 26
  - Strawberry and Kiwi Breakfast Smoothie 26
  - Parsley and Pear Smoothie 27
  - Paleo Peach and Coconut Smoothie 27
  - Homemade Breakfast Granola 28
  - Cereal Bowl 28
  - Orange and Vanilla Breakfast Delight 29
  - Coconut and Almonds Granola 29
  - Special Burrito 30
  - Delicious Eggs and Artichokes 30
  - Italian Breakfast Eggs 31
  - Incredible Eggs and Ham 31
  - Delicious Kale Frittata 32
  - Bacon Muffins 32

Delicious Sausage Frittata	33
Spicy Eggs	33
Special Breakfast Pancakes	34
Different Breakfast Dish	34
Simple Burger	35
Delicious Sausage Balls	35
Delightful Wrapped Eggs	36
Special Blueberry Muffins	36
Amazing Pumpkin Muffins	37
Zucchini and Chocolate Muffins	37
Awesome Avocado Muffins	38
Simple Spinach Omelet	38
Apple Omelet	39
Veggie Omelet Cupcakes	39
Ham and Mushroom Breakfast	40
Breakfast Coconut Pancakes	40
Incredible Apple Pancakes	41
Tasty Porridge	41
Simple and Tasty Nuts Porridge	42
Portobello Sandwich	42
Bacon and Egg Breakfast Sandwich	43
Breakfast Sliders	43
Beef and Squash Skillet	44
Sweet Potato Breakfast	44
Pork Skillet	45
Chorizo Breakfast Skillet	45
Delicious Steak and Veggie Breakfast	46
Simple Breakfast Waffles	46
Delicious Chicken Waffles	47
Amazing Bacon Waffles	47
Paleo Soups and Stews Recipes	48
Special Paleo Soup	48
Tomato and Basil Soup	48
Paleo Chicken Soup	49
Delicious Cauliflower Soup	49
Paleo Beef Soup	50

Root Paleo Soup	50
Delightful Chicken Soup	51
Paleo Lemon and Garlic Soup	51
Rich Paleo Soup	52
Paleo Veggie Soup	52
Paleo Beef Stew	53
Paleo Slow Cooker Stew	53
Paleo Veggie and Chorizo Stew	54
Special Beef and Plantain Stew	54
Paleo Chicken Stew	55
Paleo Lamb and Coconut Stew	55
Paleo Veggie Stew	56
Paleo French Chicken Stew	56
Paleo Oxtail Stew	57
Paleo Eggplant Stew	57
Amazing Squash Soup	58
Simple Broccoli Soup	58
Delicious Gazpacho	59
Tasty Veggie Soup	59
Simple Chicken Soup	60
Tasty Green Soup	60
Delicious Mushroom Cream	61
Amazing Seafood Soup	61
Shrimp and Chicken Soup	62
Zucchini Soup	62
Coconut and Zucchini Soup	63
Delicious Cauliflower Cream	63
Nettles Soup	64
Sweet Potato Soup	64
Kale and Sausage Soup	65
Great Onion Soup	65
Delicious Clam Soup	66
Easy Asparagus Soup	66
Delicious Cucumber Soup	67
Tasty Brussels Sprouts Soup	67
Incredible Turkey Soup	68

- Special Celery Soup 68
- Delicious Beef Stew 69
- Mexican Stew 69
- Delightful Pork Stew 70
- Special and Tasty Beef Stew 70
- Tasty Chorizo Stew 71
- Hearty Meat Stew 71
- Exotic Beef Stew 72
- Beef and Sweet Potatoes Stew 72
- Simple Chicken Stew 73
- Slow Cooked Delicious Stew 73
- Special Stew 74
- Delicious Lamb Stew 74
- Roasted Veggie Stew 75
- French Chicken Stew 75
- African Stew 76
- Crazy Oxtail Stew 76
- Vietnamese Stew 77
- Special Eggplant Stew 77

Paleo Side Dish Recipes 78

- Paleo Roasted Carrots 78
- Paleo Zucchini and Leeks Side Dish 78
- Paleo Slow Cooked Mushrooms 79
- Paleo Mashed Cauliflower Dish 79
- Paleo Asparagus Side Dish 80
- Paleo Butternut Squash Side Dish 80
- Paleo Chard Side Dish 81
- Paleo Roasted Beets 81
- Paleo Roasted Brussels Sprouts 81
- Paleo Sweet Potatoes Dish 83
- Asparagus and Mushrooms Side Dish 83
- Paleo Mushrooms and Thyme Side Dish 84
- Paleo Roasted Cherry Tomatoes 84
- Paleo Sautéed Spinach Dish 85
- Paleo Mashed Carrots 85
- Paleo Roasted Bell Peppers 86

Paleo French Fries	86
Paleo Roasted Cabbage Side Dish	87
Delicious Roasted Okra	87
Paleo Grilled Artichokes	88
Delicious Mashed Sweet Potatoes	88
Amazing Roasted Beets	88
Simple Kale Dish	89
Delicious Pumpkin Fries	89
Delicious Pumpkin and Bok Choy	89
Creamy Mashed Pumpkin	90
Simple Pumpkin Salad	90
Amazing Turnips and Sauce	91
Great Fennel Side Dish	91
Plantain Fries	92
Roasted Broccoli	92
Incredible Side Salad	92
Simple Brussels Sprouts Side Dish	93
Tasty Veggie Mix	93
Tapioca Root Fries	93
Amazing Side Dish	94
Delicious Roasted Green Beans	94
Delicious Roasted Cauliflower	95
Special Plantain Mash	95
Amazing Poached Kohlrabi Dish	96
Delightful Spaghetti Squash	96
Incredibly Tasty Butternut Squash	97
Amazing Butternut Squash Mix	97
Great Stir Fried Side Dish	98
Flavored Taro Dish	98
Delicious Stuffed Artichokes	99
Ginger Cauliflower Rice	99
Basil Zucchini Spaghetti	100
Delicious Braised Cabbage Side Dish	100
Tasty Cauliflower and Leeks	101
Delicious Eggplant and Mushrooms	101
Special Mint Zucchini	102

Lovely Kale Dish 102

Kale, Mushrooms and Red Chard Side Dish 102

Tasty Kale and Beets 104

Amazing Spicy Sweet Potatoes 104

Delicious Broccoli and Tasty Hazelnuts 104

Tasty Squash and Cranberries 105

Incredible Chard 105

Dill Carrots 105

Paleo Snacks and Appetizers Recipes 106

Cauliflower Popcorn 106

Delicious Hummus 106

Simple Guacamole 107

Delightful and Special Hummus 107

Sun Dried Tomatoes Spread 108

Roasted Eggplant Spread 108

Delicious Stuffed Eggs 109

Egg Cups 109

Avocado Boats 110

Appetizer Salad 110

Special Mixed Snack 111

Butternut Squash Bites 111

Baked Zucchini Chips 112

Simple and Easy Pepperoni Bites 112

Amazing Party Meatballs 113

Incredible Chicken Strips 113

Simple Beef Jerky 114

Simple Chicken Skewers 114

Kale Chips and Tasty Dip 115

Rosemary Crackers 115

Delicious and Special Crackers 116

Simple Coconut Bars 116

Simple Nuts Snack 117

Carrot Balls 117

Wrapped Olives 118

Oyster Spread 118

Stuffed Mushrooms 119

Tasty Apricot Bites 119
Mushroom Boats 120
Special Mushroom and Broccoli Appetizer 120
Zucchini Rolls 121
Special Cauliflower Mini Hot Dogs 121
Watermelon Wraps 122
Cucumber Rolls 122
Crazy Chicken Appetizer 123
Fried Peppers 123
Spanish Appetizer Cakes 124
Chicken Bites 124
Scallops Bites 125
Delicious Cabbage Chips 125

Paleo Meat Recipes 126

Chicken Thighs with Tasty Butternut Squash 126
Paleo Turkey Casserole 126
Special Paleo Chicken and Veggies Stir Fry 127
Paleo Stuffed Quail 127
Paleo Roasted Duck Dish 128
Paleo Chicken Meatballs 128
Delicious Paleo Beef Casserole 129
Paleo Grilled Lamb Chops 129
Paleo Lamb Casserole 130
Paleo Lamb Chops with Mint Sauce 130
Paleo Beef Tenderloin with Special Sauce 131
Paleo Beef Stir Fry 131
Paleo Pork Dish with Delicious Blueberry Sauce 132
Tasty Paleo Pulled Pork 132
Paleo Barbeque Ribs 133
Special Paleo Pork Chops 133
Paleo Pork with Pear Salsa 134
Paleo Pork Tenderloin with Carrot Puree 134
Paleo Pork with Strawberry Sauce 135
Paleo Sausage Casserole 135
Amazing Souvlaki 136
Delicious Mexican Steaks 136

Different Grilled Steaks	138
Amazing Beef Lasagna	138
Steaks and Apricots	139
Delicious Filet Mignon and Special Sauce	139
Amazing Beef Kabobs	140
Delicious Steak	140
Great Beef Teriyaki	141
Delicious Beef and Wonderful Gravy	141
Steaks and Scallops	142
Sheppard's Pie	142
Amazing Lamb Chops	143
Carne Asada	143
Amazing Slow-Cooked Beef	144
Beef in Amazing Tomato Marinade	144
Amazing Lamb Chops and Mint Sauce	145
Amazing Roasted Lamb	145
Delicious Turkey Casserole	146
Indian Beef Patties	146
Different Beef Dish	147
Beef and Cabbage Delight	147
Simple Beef and Brussels Sprouts	148
Amazing Beef and Spinach	148
Incredible Beef and Basil	149
Summer Beef Skillet	149
Greek Style Beef Bowls	150
Beef Curry	150
Delicious Thai Curry	151
Hamburger Salad	151
Veal Rolls	152
Beef and Tasty Veggies	152
Steak and Amazing Blueberry Sauce	153
Beef and Bok Choy	153
Moroccan Lamb	154
Delicious Rosemary Lamb Chops	154
Lavender Lamb Chops	155
Lamb and Eggplant Puree	155

Thai Lamb Chops 156
Slow Cooked Lamb Shanks 156

Paleo Seafood and Fish Recipes 157

Amazing Paleo Shrimp Dish 157
Special Paleo Fish Dish 157
Paleo Glazed Salmon 158
Paleo Lobster with Sauce 158
Paleo Steamed Clams 159
Paleo Salmon Pie 159
Paleo Grilled Calamari 160
Paleo Shrimp and Zucchini Noodles 160
Paleo Scallops with Delicious Puree 161
Paleo Salmon with Avocado Sauce 161
Paleo Fish Tacos 162
Smoked Salmon and Fresh Veggies 162
Paleo Roasted Trout 163
Paleo Roasted Cod 163
Superb Tuna Dish 164
Paleo Salmon Tartar 164
Grilled Salmon with Peaches 165
Paleo Shrimp Burgers 165
Paleo Scallops Tartar 166
Paleo Shrimp Skewers 166
Salmon Skewers 167
Tuna and Chimichurri Sauce 167
Salmon and Chili Sauce 168
Infused Clams 168
Delightful Salmon Dish 169
Amazing Shrimp Dish 169
Delicious Scallops 170
Amazing Crab Cakes and Red Pepper Sauce 170
Delicious Grilled Oysters 171
Delicious Squid and Guacamole 171
Delicious Shrimp and Cauliflower Rice 172
Stuffed Salmon Fillets 172
Glazed Salmon 174

- Amazing Salmon and Spicy Slaw ... 174
- Spicy Shrimp ... 176
- Salmon and Lemon Relish ... 176
- Delicious Mussels Mix ... 177
- Amazing Mahi Mahi Dish ... 177
- Delicious Lobster and Sauce ... 178
- Grilled Salmon and Avocado Sauce ... 178
- Grilled Calamari ... 179
- Shrimp and Zucchini Noodles ... 179
- Wonderful Crusted Salmon ... 180
- Stuffed Calamari ... 180
- Amazing Salmon and Chives ... 181
- Roasted Cod ... 181
- Halibut and Tasty Salsa ... 182
- Special Salmon ... 182
- Cod and Herb Sauce ... 183
- Salmon and Tomato Pesto ... 183
- Salmon Delight ... 184
- Shrimp with Mango and Avocado Mix ... 184
- Thai Shrimp Delight ... 185
- Scallops Tartar ... 185
- Shrimp Cocktail ... 186
- Tilapia Surprise ... 186
- Tuna and Salsa ... 187
- Amazing Salmon Tartar ... 187
- Incredible Swordfish ... 188
- Crusted Snapper ... 188

Paleo Vegetables Recipes ... 189

- Paleo Falafel ... 189
- Paleo Daikon Rolls ... 189
- Paleo Cauliflower Pizza ... 190
- Paleo Endive Bites ... 190
- Paleo Veggies Dish with Tasty Sauce ... 191
- Paleo-Indian Pancakes ... 191
- Paleo Stuffed Mushrooms ... 192
- Stuffed Zucchinis ... 192

Paleo Stuffed Eggplant	193
Paleo Tomato and Mushroom Skewers	193
Amazing Paleo Potato Bites	194
Paleo Cucumber Salsa	194
Paleo Sweet Potatoes and Cabbage Bake	195
Paleo Kohlrabi Dish	195
Paleo Onion Rings	196
Paleo Baked Yuka with Tomato Sauce	196
Paleo Surprise Dinner Dish	197
Paleo Broccoli and Cauliflower Fritters	197
Paleo Spinach and Mushroom Dish	198
Paleo Celery Casserole	198
Rutabaga Noodles and Cherry Tomatoes	199
Simple Garlic Tomatoes	199
Tomato Quiche	200
Amazing Cherry Mix	200
Zucchini Noodles with Tomatoes and Spinach	201
Simple Roasted Tomatoes	201
Grilled Cherry Tomatoes	202
Veggies and Fish Mix	202
Spaghetti Squash and Tomatoes	204
Noodles and Capers Sauce	204
Zucchini Noodles and Tasty Pesto	205
Stuffed Portobello Mushrooms	205
Avocado Spread	206
Cucumber Noodles and Shrimp	206
Veggie Mix and Tasty Scallops	207
Cucumber Wraps	207
Delicious Stuffed Peppers	208
Mexican-Style Stuffed Peppers	208
Delicious Peppers Stuffed with Beef	209
Stuffed Poblanos	209
Delicious Stuffed Baby Peppers	210
Pork Stuffed Bell Peppers	210
Bell Peppers Stuffed with Tuna	211
Liver Stuffed Peppers	211

Baked Eggplant	212
Delicious Eggplant Dish	212
Delicious Eggplant Casserole	213
Eggplant and Garlic Sauce	213
Eggplant Hash	214
Eggplant Jam	214
Warm Watercress Mix	215
Watercress Soup	215
Delicious Artichokes Dish	216
Artichokes with Horseradish Sauce	216
Grilled Artichokes	217
Artichokes and Tomatoes Dip	217
Great Carrot Hash	218
Carrots and Lime Delight	218
Incredible Glazed Carrots	219
Delicious Purple Carrots	219
Paleo Salad Recipes	**220**
Paleo Egg Salad	220
Paleo Pear Salad with Tasty Dressing	220
Paleo Shrimp Salad	221
Paleo Eggplant and Tomato Salad	221
Paleo Potato Salad	222
Paleo Chicken Salad	222
Special Paleo Chicken Salad	223
Paleo Radish Salad	223
Brussels Sprouts Salad	224
Paleo Carrot and Cucumber Salad	224
Paleo Pomegranate Salad	225
Paleo Lobster Salad	225
Paleo Steak Salad	226
Paleo Summer Salad	226
Special Paleo Beef Salad	227
Warm Paleo Salad	227
Delicious Paleo Salad	228
Simple Scallops Salad	228
Paleo Pork Salad	229

Paleo Seafood Salad	229
Amazing Taco Salad	230
Delicious Summer Salad	230
Great Winter Salad	231
Kale and Carrots Salad	231
Simple Chicken Salad	232
Sweet Potato Salad	232
Rich Salad	233
Salmon Salad	233
Summer Salad	233
Tomato Salad	234
Broccoli Salad	234
Cabbage and Salmon Slaw	234
Watermelon Salad	235
Red Cabbage Salad	235
Avocado Salad	236
Quick and Tasty Salad	236
Tasty Sashimi Salad	236
Fresh Salad	237
Hearty Chicken Salad	237
Tomato and Chicken Salad	238
Kale and Avocado Salad	238
Chicken Salad and Raspberry Dressing	239
Delicious Dinner Salad	239
Broccoli and Carrots Salad	240
Salmon and Strawberry Salad	240
Incredible Autumn Salad	241
Beetroot Salad	242
Chorizo Salad	243
Shrimp and Radish Salad	243
Great Steak Salad	244
Russian Salad	244
Cucumber And Tomato Salad	245
Swiss Chard Salad	245
Figs and Cabbage Salad	246
Tasty Shrimp Cobb Salad	246

- Grilled Shrimp Salad 247
- Green Apple and Shrimp Salad 247
- Simple Cucumber Salad 248
- Cuban Radish Salad 248
- Radish and Eggs Salad 249

Paleo Dessert Recipes 250

- Paleo Hazelnut Balls 250
- Paleo Pumpkin Cookies 250
- Paleo Almond Bars 251
- Paleo Muffins 251
- Paleo Stuffed Apples 252
- Paleo Raspberry Popsicles 252
- Paleo Pumpkin Pudding 253
- Paleo Hazelnut Pancakes 253
- Simple Paleo Cherry Jam 254
- Paleo Coconut Macaroons 254
- Spring Cheesecake 255
- Poached Rhubarb 255
- Strawberry Cobbler 256
- Avocado Pudding 256
- Summer Sorbet 257
- Dessert Smoothie Bowl 257
- Spring Ice Cream 258
- Delicious Fruit Cream 258
- Chocolate Parfait 259
- Chocolate Butter Cups 259
- Caramel Ice Cream 260
- Chia Seeds Pudding 260
- Summer Lemon Fudge 261
- Summer Energy Bars 261
- Delicious Pomegranate Fudge 262
- Great and Intense Cheesecake 262
- Pumpkin Custard 263
- Berry and Cashew Cake 263
- Fruit Jelly 264
- Almond and Fig Dessert 264

Great Tomato Cake 265

Green Apple Smoothie 265

Grapefruit Granita 266

Mango Granita 266

Delicious Cherry Sorbet 267

Fruits Mix and Vinaigrette 267

Simple Passion Fruit Pudding 268

Summer Carrot Cake 268

Carrot Cupcakes 269

Special Cupcakes 269

Conclusion 270

Recipe Index 271

FREE GIFT!

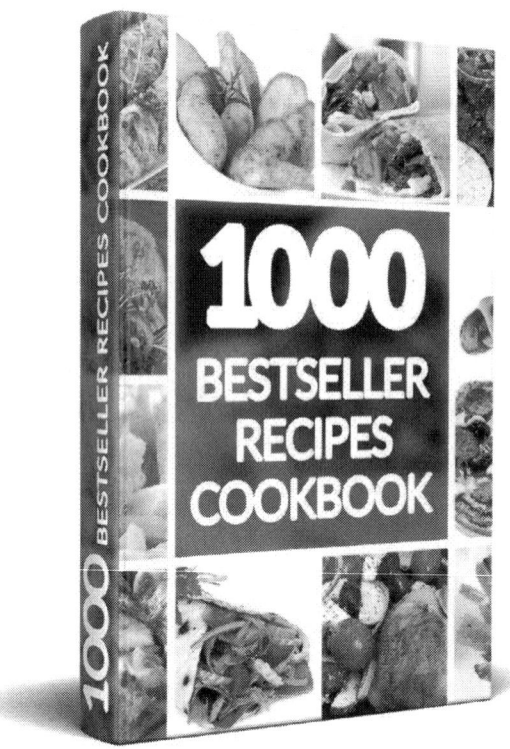

In order to thank you for buying my book I am glad to present you
- 1000 Bestseller Recipes Cookbook -

Please follow this link to get instant access to your Free Cookbook:
http://www.bookbuying.top/

Introduction

Why should you opt for a Paleo diet? Well, it's really simple! The Paleo diet is one of the healthiest diets ever. This great diet is the only one that can help you increase your energy levels, your strength, your overall health and that can help you lose weight at the same time! This diet brings many positive effects and it can really change your life for good!
This sound really great, doesn't it. Are you one of those people who feel they need to make such a change in their lives? Then, we are sure you are in the right place.

One of the best things about this diet is that it keeps you satisfied and happy all day long. You won't even feel you are on a diet.
Are you curious to find out what can you eat if you choose to follow a Paleo diet? Then check this out!

Professionals in the field recommend you to eat as many veggies and fruits as possible if you are on such a diet. Fruits and veggies are full of vitamins, minerals, antioxidants and nutrients. This is exactly what you need to stay healthy and lose some weight.
You can also consume a lot of seeds, nuts, red meat, poultry, fish and seafood but also healthy oils like avocado, coconut or olive oil.
On the other hand, you can't consume any grains, dairy, processed foods, sugar or starches.

If you make some adjustments in your lifestyle, you will soon see the difference.
You will impress everyone with your appearance and your health! Isn't that what we all want?
Then, don't wait too long!
Become a part of a huge community of people all over the world who already decided to start a Paleo diet!
Become one of the millions of healthier and happier people.

In order to help you get started, we've gathered the best Paleo dishes and we offer them to you!
Just check them out! These Paleo recipes are incredible and they will conquer your taste buds in no time!
We guarantee you!

Enjoy cooking and eating Paleo!

Paleo Recipes for Breakfast

Breakfast Tomato and Eggs

It's going to become one of your favorite paleo breakfasts in no time. It's really delicious!

Servings: 2
Preparation time: 10 minutes
Cooking time: 30 minutes

Ingredients:
- 2 eggs
- 2 tomatoes
- A pinch of black pepper
- 1 teaspoon parsley, finely chopped

Directions:
Cut tomatoes tops, scoop flesh and arrange them on a lined baking sheet. Crack an egg in each tomato. Season with salt and pepper. Introduce them in the oven at 350 degrees F and bake for 30 minutes. Take tomatoes out of the oven, divide between plates, season with pepper, sprinkle parsley at the end and serve. Enjoy!

Nutritional value: calories 186, protein 14, fat 10, sugar 6

Breakfast Paleo Muffins

It's a paleo breakfast that will provide you enough energy to face a busy day at work. Just try it!

Servings: 4
Preparation time: 10 minutes
Cooking time: 30 minutes

Ingredients:
- 1 cup kale, chopped
- ¼ cup chives, finely chopped
- ½ cup almond milk
- 6 eggs
- Black pepper to the taste
- Some coconut oil for greasing the muffin cups

Directions:
In a bowl, mix eggs with chives and kale and whisk very well. Add black pepper to the taste and almond milk and stir well. Divide this into 8 muffin cups after you've greased it with some coconut oil. Introduce this in preheated oven at 350 degrees F and bake for 30 minutes. Take muffins out of the oven, leave them to cool down, transfer them to plates and serve warm. Enjoy!

Nutritional value: calories 100, fat 5, protein 14, sugar 0

Paleo Banana Pancakes

These are so healthy and delicious! You will definitely enjoy making them, and you will love eating them!

Servings: 2
Preparation time: 10 minutes
Cooking time: 10 minutes

Ingredients:
- 4 eggs
- 2 bananas, peeled and chopped
- ¼ teaspoon baking powder
- Cooking spray

Directions:
In a bowl, mix eggs with chopped bananas and baking powder and whisk well. Transfer this to your food processor and blend very well. Heat up a pan over medium high heat after you've sprayed it with some cooking oil. Add some of the pancakes batter, spread in the pan, cook for 1 minute, flip and cook for 30 seconds and transfer to a plate. Repeat this with the rest of the batter, arrange pancakes on plates and serve. Enjoy!

Nutritional value: 120, fat 2, carbs 2, sugar 1, protein 4

Plantain Pancakes

These are not only very tasty! These paleo pancakes also look very good!

Servings: 1
Preparation time: 10 minutes
Cooking time: 10 minutes

Ingredients:
- 3 eggs
- ¼ cup coconut flour
- ¼ cup coconut water
- 1 teaspoon coconut oil
- ½ plantain, peeled and chopped
- ¼ teaspoon cream of tartar
- ¼ teaspoon baking soda
- ¼ teaspoon chai spice
- 1 tablespoon shaved coconut, toasted for serving
- 1 tablespoon coconut milk for serving

Directions:
In your food processor, mix eggs with coconut water and flour, plantain, cream of tartar, baking soda and chai spice and blend well. Heat up a pan with the coconut oil over medium heat, add ¼ cup pancake batter, spread evenly, cook until it becomes golden, flip pancake and cook for 1 more minute and transfer to a plate. Repeat this with the rest of the batter. Serve pancakes with shaved coconut and coconut milk. Enjoy!

Nutritional value: calories 372, fat 17, carbs 55, fiber 12, sugar 21, protein 23

Paleo Sweet Potato Waffles

You only need a few ingredients, and you have to follow some simple directions, and you will enjoy some delicious paleo waffles in no time!

Servings: 4
Preparation time: 10 minutes
Cooking time: 10 minutes

Ingredients:
- 2 sweet potatoes, peeled and finely grated
- 2 tablespoons melted coconut oil
- 3 eggs
- 1 teaspoon cinnamon powder
- ½ teaspoon nutmeg, ground
- Some apple sauce for serving

Directions:
In a bowl, mix eggs with sweet potatoes, coconut oil, cinnamon and nutmeg and whisk very well. Cook waffles in your waffle iron, arrange them on plates and serve with apple sauce drizzled on top. Enjoy!

Nutritional value: calories 227, fat 6, carbs 37, fiber 2, sugar 9, protein 6

Paleo Eggplant French Toast

You don't need to be an expert cook to make this amazing and delicious paleo breakfast! It's such and easy recipe!

Servings: 2
Preparation time: 5 minutes
Cooking time: 5 minutes

Ingredients:
- 1 eggplant, peeled and sliced
- 1 teaspoon vanilla extract
- 2 eggs
- Stevia to the taste
- 1 teaspoon coconut oil
- A pinch of cinnamon

Directions:
In a bowl, mix eggs with vanilla, stevia, and cinnamon and whisk well. Heat up a pan with the coconut oil over medium-high heat. Dip eggplant slices in eggs mix, add to heated pan and cook until they become golden on each side. Arrange them on plates and serve. Enjoy!

Nutritional value: calories 125, fat 5, protein 7.8, carbs 13, fiber 7.8

Orange and Dates Granola

We are so happy to share with you this incredible paleo breakfast granola! It's so great!

Servings: 6
Preparation time: 10 minutes
Cooking time: 15 minutes

Ingredients:
- 5 ounces dates, soaked in hot water
- Juice from 1 orange
- Grated rind of ½ orange
- 1 cup desiccated coconut
- ½ cup silvered almonds
- ½ cup pumpkin seeds
- ½ cup linseeds
- ½ cup sesame seeds
- Almond milk for serving

Directions:
In a bowl, mix almonds with orange rind, orange juice, linseeds, coconut, pumpkin and sesame seeds and stir well. Drain dates, add them to your food processor and blend well. Add this paste to almonds mix and stir well again. Spread this on a lined baking sheet, introduce in the oven at 350 degrees F and bake for 15 minutes, stirring every 4 minutes. Take granola out of the oven, leave aside to cool down a bit and then serve with almond milk. Enjoy!

Nutritional value: calories 208, protein 6, fiber 5, fat 9, sugar 0

Paleo Breakfast Burrito

It's more than you can imagine! It's such a great combination of ingredients! You'll see!

Servings: 4
Preparation time: 10 minutes
Cooking time: 7 minutes

Ingredients:
- 1 small yellow onion, finely chopped
- 4 eggs, egg yolks and whites separated
- ¼ cup canned green chilies, chopped
- 2 tomatoes, chopped
- 1 red bell pepper, cut into thin strips
- ¼ cup cilantro, finely chopped
- ½ cup chicken meat, already cooked and shredded
- Black pepper to the taste
- A drizzle of extra virgin olive oil
- 1 avocado, pitted, peeled and chopped
- Hot sauce for serving

Directions:
Put egg whites in a bowl, add some black pepper, whisk them well and leave them aside for now. Heat up a pan with a drizzle of oil over medium-high heat, add half of the egg whites, spread evenly, cook for 30 seconds, cover pan, cook fro 1 minute and then slide on a plate. Repeat this with the rest of the egg whites and leave the two "tortillas" aside. Heat up the same pan with another drizzle of oil over medium-high heat, add onions, stir and cook for 1 minute. Add red bell pepper, green chilies, tomato, meat and cilantro and stir. Add egg yolks to the pan and scramble the whole mix. Add avocado, stir, take off heat and spread evenly on the two egg whites "tortillas". Roll them, arrange on plates and serve with some hot sauce. Enjoy!

Nutritional value: calories 170, fat 5, carbs 1, sugar 0.6, fiber 0, protein 6

Spinach Frittata

There are many ingredients you can use to prepare a paleo frittata, but this is our favorite one!

Servings: 4
Preparation time: 10 minutes
Cooking time: 30 minutes

Ingredients:
- ½ pound sausage, ground
- 2 tablespoons ghee
- 1 cup mushrooms, thinly sliced
- 1 cup spinach leaves, chopped
- 10 eggs, whisked
- 1 small yellow onion, finely chopped
- Black pepper to the taste

Directions:
Heat up a pan with the ghee over medium-high heat, add onion and some black pepper, stir and cook until it browns. Add sausage, stir and also cook until it browns. Add spinach and mushrooms and cook for 4 minutes, stirring from time to time. Take the pan off the heat, add eggs, spread evenly, introduce frittata in the oven at 350 degrees F and bake for 20 minutes. Take frittata out of the oven, leave it aside for a few minutes to cool down, cut, arrange on plates and serve. Enjoy!

Nutritional value: calories 233, fat 13, carbs 4, fiber 1.2, sugar 1, protein 21

Squash Blossom Frittata

It's a special paleo breakfast that even the most pretentious people will adore!

Servings: 4
Preparation time: 10 minutes
Cooking time: 40 minutes

Ingredients:
- 10 eggs, whisked
- Black pepper to the taste
- ¼ cup coconut cream
- 1 yellow onion, finely chopped
- 1 leek, thinly sliced
- 2 scallions, thinly sliced
- 2 zucchinis, chopped
- 8 squash blossoms
- 2 tablespoons avocado oil

Directions:
In a bowl, mix eggs with coconut cream and black pepper to the taste and stir well. Heat up a pan with the oil over medium high heat, add leek and onions, stir and cook for 5 minutes. Add zucchini, stir and cook for 10 more minutes. Add eggs, spread, reduce heat to low, cook for 5 minutes. Sprinkle scallions and arrange squash blossoms on frittata, press blossoms into eggs, introduce everything in the oven at 350 degrees F and bake for 20 minutes. Take frittata out of the oven, leave it to cool down, cut, arrange on plates and serve it. Enjoy!

Nutritional value: calories 123, fat 8, protein 7, carbs 2, sugar 0

Paleo Breakfast Burger

Everybody loves a good and tasty burger, but this is much more! It's a paleo one!

Serving: 4
Preparation time: 10 minutes
Cooking time: 20 minutes

Ingredients:
- 5 eggs
- 1 pound ground beef meat
- ½ cup sausages, ground
- 8 slices bacon
- 3 sun-dried tomatoes, chopped
- 2 tablespoons almond meal
- 2 teaspoons basil leaves, chopped
- 1 teaspoon garlic, finely minced
- A drizzle of avocado oil
- Black pepper to the taste

Directions:
In a bowl, mix beef meat with 1 egg, almond meal, tomatoes, basil, pepper and garlic, stir well and form 4 burgers. Heat up a pan over medium high heat, add burgers, cook them 5 minutes on each side, transfer them to plates and leave aside for now. Heat up the same pan over medium-high heat, add sausages, stir, cook for 5 minutes and transfer them to a plate. Heat up the pan again, add bacon, cook for 4 minutes, drain excess grease and also leave aside on a plate. Fry the 4 eggs in a pan with a drizzle of oil over medium-high heat and place them on top of burgers. Add sausage and bacon and serve. Enjoy!

Nutritional value: calories 264, fat 12, carbs 5, fiber 0.3, sugar 0.7, protein 32

Paleo Maple Nut Porridge

If you want to eat something new and tasty, then you should really consider trying this porridge!

Servings: 2
Preparation time: 5 minutes
Cooking time: 5 minutes

Ingredients:
- 2 tablespoons coconut butter
- ½ cup pecans, soaked
- ¾ cup hot water
- 1 banana, peeled and chopped
- ½ teaspoon cinnamon
- 2 teaspoons maple syrup

Directions:
In your food processor, mix pecans with water, coconut butter, banana, cinnamon and maple syrup and blend well. Transfer this to a pan, heat up over medium heat until it thickens, pour into bowls and serve. Enjoy!

Nutritional value: calories 170, fat 9, carbs 20, fiber 6, protein 6

Paleo Breakfast Sandwich

This is great for breakfast, but you can also take it with you at work and eat it then!

Servings: 2
Preparation time: 10 minutes
Cooking time: 10 minutes

Ingredients:
- 3.5 ounces pumpkin flesh, peeled
- 4 slices paleo coconut bread
- 1 small avocado, pitted and peeled
- 1 carrot, finely grated
- 1 lettuce leaf, torn into 4 pieces

Directions:
Put pumpkin in a tray, introduce in the oven at 350 degrees F and bake for 10 minutes. Take pumpkin out of the oven, leave aside for 2-3 minutes, transfer to a bowl and mash it a bit. Put avocado in another bowl and also mash it with a fork. Spread avocado on 2 bread slices, add grated carrot, mashed pumpkin and 2 lettuce pieces on each and top them with the rest of the bread slices. Enjoy!

Nutritional value: calories 340, fat 7, protein 4, carbs 13, fiber 8, sugar 4

Paleo Turkey Breakfast Sandwich

No other sandwich will taste this good! Just wait and see!

Servings: 1
Preparation time: 5 minutes
Cooking time: 0

Ingredients:
- 2 ounces turkey meat, roasted and thinly sliced
- 2 tablespoons pecans, toasted and chopped
- 2 slices paleo coconut bread
- 2 tablespoons cranberry chutney
- ¼ cup arugula

Directions:
In a bowl, mix pecans with chutney and stir well. Spread this on bread slice, add turkey slices and arugula and top with the other bread slice. Serve right away. Enjoy!

Nutritional value: calories 540, fat 11, carbs 52, fiber 4, sugar 13, protein 32

Paleo Blueberry Smoothie

Why shouldn't you try a smoothie for breakfast? Here is one of our favorite ones!

Servings: 2
Preparation time: 5 minutes
Cooking time: 0

Ingredients:
- 2 cups blueberries
- 1 teaspoon lemon zest
- ½ cup coconut milk
- A pinch of cinnamon
- Water as needed

Directions:
In your kitchen blender, mix coconut milk with blueberries, lemon zest and a pinch of cinnamon and pulse a few times. Add water as needed to thin your smoothie and pulse a few more times. Transfer to a tall glass and serve. Enjoy!

Nutritional value: calories 177, fat 3, carbs 45, fiber 7, sugar 12, protein 3

Paleo Green Smoothie

Today it's time to try a green paleo smoothie for breakfast!

Serving: 3
Preparation time: 5 minutes
Cooking time: 0

Ingredients:
- 1 small cucumber, peeled and chopped
- 1 green apple, chopped
- Juice of ½ lemon
- Juice of ½ lime
- 1 tablespoon ginger, finely grated
- 1 tablespoon gelatin powder
- 1 cup kale, chopped
- 1 cup coconut water

Directions:
In your kitchen blender, mix the apple with cucumber, ginger, and kale and pulse a few times. Add lime and lemon juice, coconut water and gelatin powder and blend a few more times. Transfer to glasses and serve right away. Enjoy!

Nutritional value: calories 180, fat 1, carbs 42, fiber 7, sugar 0, protein 7

Paleo Red Breakfast Smoothie

It's a very healthy breakfast smoothie. You won't feel the need to eat anything else all day long!

Servings: 2
Preparation time: 5 minutes
Cooking time: 0

Ingredients:
- 1 small red bell pepper, seeded and roughly chopped
- 5 strawberries, cut in halves
- 1 tomato, cut into 4 wedges
- 1 cup red cabbage, chopped
- ½ cup raspberries
- 8 ounces water
- 2 ice cubes for serving

Directions:
In your food processor, mix cabbage with bell pepper, tomato, strawberries, and raspberries and pulse well until you obtain cream. Add water and pulse well a few more times. Transfer to glasses and serve with ice cubes. Enjoy!

Nutritional value: calories 189, fat 2, carbs 40, fiber 7, sugar 1, protein 5

Strawberry and Kiwi Breakfast Smoothie

It's a great summer breakfast idea, and it's 100% Paleo!

Servings: 2
Preparation time: 10 minutes
Cooking time: 0

Ingredients:
- 1 and ½ cups kiwi, chopped
- 1 and ½ cups frozen strawberries, chopped
- 8 mint leaves
- 2 cups crushed ice
- 2 ounces water

Directions:
In your blender, mix kiwi with strawberries and mint and pulse well. Add water and crushed ice and pulse again. Transfer to glasses and serve right away. Enjoy!

Nutritional value: calories 133, fat 1, carbs 34, fiber 4, sugar 9, protein 1.3

Parsley and Pear Smoothie

When it comes to smoothies, you have endless options! Here is another delicious one for you!

Servings: 6
Preparation time: 5 minutes
Cooking time: 0

Ingredients:
- 1 apple pear, chopped
- 1 bunch parsley, roughly chopped
- 1 small avocado, stoned and peeled
- 1 pear, peeled and chopped
- 1 green apple, chopped
- 1 Granny Smith apple, chopped
- 6 bananas, peeled and roughly chopped
- 2 plums, stoned
- 1 cup ice
- 1 cup water

Directions:
In your kitchen blender, mix parsley with avocado, apple pear, pear, green apple, Granny Smith apple, plums and bananas and blend very well. Add ice and water and blend again very well. Transfer to tall glasses and serve right away. Enjoy!

Nutritional value: calories 208, carbs 48, fiber 13, fat 3, protein 3, sugar 28

Paleo Peach and Coconut Smoothie

It's very delicious, creamy and easy to make! What more could you want?

Servings: 2
Preparation time: 5 minutes
Cooking time: 0

Ingredients:
- 1 cup ice
- 2 peaches, peeled and chopped
- Lemon zest to the taste
- 1 cup cold coconut milk
- 1 drop lemon essential oil

Directions:
In your kitchen blender, mix coconut milk with ice and peaches and pulse a few times. Add lemon zest to the taste and 1 drop lemon essential oil and pulse a few more time. Pour into glasses and serve right away. Enjoy!

Homemade Breakfast Granola

Don't be afraid! it's 100% Paleo!

Preparation time: 5 minutes
Cooking time: 50 minutes
Servings: 6

Ingredients:
- 2 teaspoons cinnamon powder
- 1 and ½ cups almond flour
- 2 teaspoons nutmeg, ground
- ½ cup coconut flakes
- 2 teaspoons vanilla extract
- ½ cup walnuts, chopped
- 1/3 cup coconut oil
- ¼ cup hemp hearts

Directions:
In a bowl, combine almond flour with coconut flakes, walnuts, cinnamon, nutmeg, vanilla, hemp, and walnuts, stir well and spread on a baking sheet. Bake in the oven at 275 degrees F and bake for 50 minutes, stirring every 10 minutes. Transfer to plates when the granola is cold and serve for breakfast. Enjoy!

Nutritional value: calories 250, fat 23, fiber 4, carbs 5, protein 6

Cereal Bowl

This is not some regular cereal bowl! Cereals are forbidden if you are on a Paleo Diet! This is something really tasty you can have for breakfast!

Preparation time: 10 minutes
Cooking time: 0 minutes
Servings: 2

Ingredients:
- 2 tablespoons pumpkin seeds
- 2 tablespoons almonds, chopped
- 1 tablespoon chia seeds
- A handful blueberries
- 1/3 cup water
- 1/3 cup almond milk

Directions:
Put half of the pumpkin seeds in your food processor and blend them. In 2 bowls, divide water, milk, the rest of the pumpkin seeds, chia seeds and almonds and stir. Add blended pumpkin seeds and stir gently everything.
Serve with blueberries on top. Enjoy!

Nutritional value: calories 150, fat 3, fiber 4, carbs 5, protein 6

Orange and Vanilla Breakfast Delight

This is something you need to make for breakfast soon because it's so tasty and easy to make!

Preparation time: 10 minutes
Cooking time: 0 minutes
Servings: 2

Ingredients:
- 2 cups coconut milk
- ½ cup chia seeds
- Juice from ¼ lemon
- Zest from 1 orange
- 1 tablespoon vanilla extract
- 1 tablespoon maple syrup

Directions:
Divide coconut milk, lemon juice, chia, orange zest, vanilla extract and maple syrup into 2 breakfast bowls. Stir well and keep in the fridge until you serve them. Enjoy!

Nutritional value: calories 200, fat 3, fiber 2, carbs 5, protein 4

Coconut and Almonds Granola

This is just delicious! It doesn't need any more introductions!

Preparation time: 10 minutes
Cooking time: 35 minutes
Servings: 4

Ingredients:
1. 3 cups coconut flakes
2. 1 and ½ cups almonds, chopped
3. ½ cup sesame seeds
4. ½ cup sunflower seeds
5. ½ teaspoon cinnamon, ground
6. 2 tablespoons chia seeds
7. ½ cup maple syrup
8. A pinch of cardamom
9. 1 teaspoon vanilla extract
10. 2 tablespoons olive oil

Directions:
In a bowl, mix almonds with sunflower seeds, sesame seeds, coconut, chia seeds, cardamom and cinnamon and stir. Meanwhile, heat up a small pot over medium heat, add oil, vanilla and maple syrup, stir well and cook for about 1 minute. Pour this over almonds mix, stir everything, spread on a baking sheet, bake in the oven at 300 degrees F for 25 minutes, stirring the mixture after 15 minutes. Leave your special granola to cool down before dividing it between plates and serving it. Enjoy!

Nutritional value: calories 270, fat 13, fiber 5, carbs 7, protein 8

Special Burrito

If you are on a Paleo diet, you should consider trying this special breakfast burrito!

Preparation time: 10 minutes
Cooking time: 15 minutes
Servings: 2
Ingredients:

- ¼ cup canned green chilies, chopped
- 1 small yellow onion, chopped
- 4 eggs, egg yolks and whites divided
- ¼ cup cilantro, chopped
- 1 red bell pepper, finely cut in strips
- 2 tomatoes, chopped
- ½ cup beef, ground and browned for 10 minutes
- 1 avocado, peeled, pitted and chopped
- Some hot sauce for serving
- A drizzle of olive oil

Directions:

Heat up a pan with a drizzle of olive oil over medium high heat, add half of the egg whites after you've whisked them in a bowl, spread evenly and cook for 1 minute. Flip them cook for 1 minute more, transfer to a plate and repeat the action with the rest of the egg whites. Heat up the same pan over medium high heat, add onions, stir and cook for 1 minute. Add chilies, bell pepper, tomato, meat, and cilantro, stir and cook for 5 minutes. Add egg yolks, stir well and cook until they are done. Arrange egg whites tortillas on 2 plates, divide eggs and meat mix between them, add some chopped avocado and hot sauce, roll and serve them for breakfast.

Nutritional value: calories 255, fat 23, fiber 3, carbs 7, protein 12

Delicious Eggs and Artichokes

This is really a special Paleo breakfast idea that everyone will appreciate for sure!

Preparation time: 20 minutes
Cooking time: 30 minutes
Servings: 2
Ingredients:

- 1 egg white
- 4 whole eggs
- ¾ cup balsamic vinegar
- 4 ounces bacon, chopped
- 4 artichoke hearts
- A pinch of sea salt
- Black pepper to the taste
- *For the sauce:*
- 1 tablespoon lemon juice
- ¾ cup ghee
- 4 egg yolks
- A pinch of paprika

Directions:

Put artichoke hearts in a bowl, add vinegar, toss a bit and leave aside for 20 minutes. Put the ghee in a pan and melt it over medium high heat. In a bowl, mix 4 egg yolks with paprika and lemon juice and stir well.
Put some water into a pot and bring to a simmer over medium heat. Put the bowl with the egg yolks on top of simmering water and stir constantly. Add melted ghee gradually, stir until sauce thickens and take off heat. Drain artichokes, place them on a lined baking sheet, brush tops with 1 egg white, add bacon on top and season with black pepper and a pinch of sea salt. Introduce them in the oven at 375 degrees F and bake for 20 minutes. Meanwhile, heat up a pot with water and bring to a simmer over medium high heat. Crack 4 eggs into simmering water but make sure you only crack one at a time. Poach eggs for 1 minute and transfer them to plates. Add artichokes and bacon on the side, drizzle the sauce you've made earlier on top and served.

Nutritional value: calories 270, fat 24, fiber 0, carbs 5, protein 16

Italian Breakfast Eggs

This time we suggest you try an Italian style Paleo breakfast!

Preparation time: 10 minutes
Cooking time: 15 minutes
Servings: 1

Ingredients:
- 2 eggs
- ¼ teaspoon rosemary, dried
- ½ cup cherry tomatoes halved
- 1 and ½ cups kale, chopped
- ½ teaspoon coconut oil
- 3 tablespoons water
- 1 teaspoon balsamic vinegar
- ¼ avocado, peeled and chopped

Directions:
Heat up a pan with the oil over medium high heat, add water, kale, rosemary, and tomatoes, stir, cover and cook for 4 minutes. Uncover pan, stir again and add eggs. Stir and scramble eggs for 3 minutes. Add vinegar, stir everything and transfer to a serving plate. Top with chopped avocado and serve. Enjoy!

Nutritional value: calories 185, fat 10, fiber 1, carbs 6, protein 7

Incredible Eggs and Ham

This is a Paleo breakfast that will impress you with its taste! And the best thing is that you only need few ingredients to make it!

Preparation time: 10 minutes
Cooking time: 15 minutes
Servings: 4

Ingredients:
- 4 eggs
- 10 ham slices
- 4 tablespoons scallions
- A pinch of black pepper
- A pinch of sweet paprika
- 1 tablespoon melted ghee

Directions:
Grease a muffin pan with melted ghee. Divide ham slices in each muffin mold to form your cups. In a bowl, mix eggs with scallions, pepper, and paprika and whisk well. Divide this mix on top of ham, introduce your ham cups in the oven at 400 degrees F and bake for 15 minutes. Leave cups to cool down before dividing on plates and serving. Enjoy!

Nutritional value: calories 250, fat 10, fiber 3, carbs 6, protein 12

Delicious Kale Frittata

This amazing frittata will light up your day! Trust us!

Preparation time: 10 minutes
Cooking time: 30 minutes
Servings: 4

Ingredients:
- 3 bacon slices, cooked and crumbled
- 1/3 cup yellow onion, chopped
- 1 tablespoon coconut oil
- ½ cup red bell pepper, chopped
- 2 cups kale, torn
- ½ cup almond milk
- 8 eggs
- A pinch of black pepper

Directions:
In a bowl, whisk eggs with some black pepper and almond milk. Heat up a pan with the oil over medium high heat, add bell pepper and onion, stir and cook for 3 minutes. Add kale, stir, cover pan and cook for 5 minutes more. Uncover your pan, add bacon and eggs, spread evenly around the pan and cook for 4 minutes. Introduce your pan in the oven at 350 degrees F and bake for 15 minutes. Take frittata out of the oven, leave it to cool down a bit before cutting and serving it for breakfast. Enjoy!

Nutritional value: calories 240, fat 13, fiber 2, carbs 5, protein 15

Bacon Muffins

These muffins are really easy to make! It's a great Paleo breakfast idea!

Preparation time: 10 minutes
Cooking time: 30 minutes
Servings: 4

Ingredients:
- 4 ounces bacon slices
- 3 garlic cloves, minced
- 1 small yellow onion, chopped
- 1 zucchini, thinly sliced
- A handful spinach, torn
- 6 canned and pickled artichoke hearts, chopped
- 8 eggs
- ¼ teaspoon paprika
- A pinch of black pepper
- A pinch of cayenne pepper
- ¼ cup coconut cream

Directions:
Heat up a pan over medium high heat, add bacon, stir, cook until it's crispy, transfer to paper towels, drain grease and leave aside for now. Heat up the same pan over medium heat again, add garlic and onion, stir and cook for 4 minutes. In a bowl, mix eggs with coconut cream, onions, garlic, paprika, black pepper and cayenne and whisk well. Add spinach, zucchini and artichoke pieces and stir everything. Divide crispy bacon slices in a muffin pan, add eggs mixture on top, introduce your muffins in the oven and bake at 400 degrees F for 20 minutes. Leave them to cool down before serving them for breakfast. Enjoy!

Nutritional value: calories 270, fat 12, fiber 4, carbs 6, protein 12

Delicious Sausage Frittata

This is very healthy and 100% Paleo! Try it soon!

Preparation time: 10 minutes
Cooking time: 30 minutes
Servings: 4

Ingredients:
- 10 eggs
- 2 tablespoons melted ghee
- 1 cup spinach, chopped
- ½ pound sausage, chopped
- 1 cup mushrooms, chopped
- 1 small yellow onion, chopped
- A pinch of sea salt
- Black pepper to the taste

Directions:
Heat up a pan with the ghee over medium high heat, add sausage pieces, stir and brown for a couple of minutes. Add onion, mushroom, spinach, a pinch of salt and black pepper to the taste, stir and cook for a few more minutes. Add whisked eggs, spread evenly and stir gently. Place in the oven at 350 degrees F and bake for 20 minutes. Leave your Paleo breakfast to cool down before slicing and serving it. Enjoy!

Nutritional value: calories 260, fat 8, fiber 2, carbs 4, protein 9

Spicy Eggs

These spicy eggs are really going to impress you!

Preparation time: 10 minutes
Cooking time: 25 minutes
Servings: 4

Ingredients:
- 4 bacon slices, cooked and crumbled
- 12 cherry tomatoes, halved
- ½ teaspoon turmeric
- ½ onion, chopped
- 5 eggs
- 2 Serrano peppers, chopped
- 1 green bell pepper, chopped
- Black pepper to the taste
- A pinch of sea salt

Directions:
In a bowl, whisk eggs with a pinch of salt, black pepper, Serrano peppers, green pepper, and turmeric. Heat up a pan over medium heat, add bacon, stir and cook for 3 minutes. Add onion, stir and cook for 2 minutes more. Add eggs and tomatoes, stir, cook for 6 minutes and then bake in the oven at 350 degrees F for 15 minutes. Leave your eggs to cool down before slicing and serving it. Enjoy!

Nutritional value: calories 240, fat 8, fiber 3, carbs 6, protein 8

Special Breakfast Pancakes

This breakfast will gain your attention really soon! It's so delicious!

Preparation time: 10 minutes
Cooking time: 30 minutes
Servings: 4

Ingredients:
- 12 bacon slices, chopped
- 8 eggs
- Black pepper to the taste
- 1 and ½ tablespoons coconut oil
- 10 grain-free pancakes

For the pancakes:
- 1 cup arrowroot
- ½ cup almond flour
- ½ cup coconut flour
- ½ teaspoon baking soda
- 1 teaspoon cinnamon
- 1 cup almond milk
- 2 eggs
- 1 teaspoon vanilla extract
- 3 tablespoons maple syrup
- 2 tablespoons coconut oil

Directions:
In a bowl, mix arrowroot with almond flour, coconut flour, baking soda and cinnamon and stir. Add almond milk, 2 eggs, vanilla extract and maple syrup and stir well until you obtain a smooth batter. Heat up a pan with 2 tablespoons coconut oil over medium high heat, pour some of the batter, spread in the pan, and cook for 1 minute, flip, cook for 2 minutes more and transfer pancake to a plate. Repeat with the rest of the batter. You will obtain 10 pancakes. Heat up a pan with ½ tablespoon coconut oil over medium high heat, add bacon, cook until it's crispy, transfer to paper towels, drain grease and leave it aside in a bowl for now. In another bowl, whisk 8 eggs with some black pepper. Heat up a pan with 1-tablespoon oil over medium high heat, add whisked eggs, cook until they are done and then mix them with cooked bacon. Stir everything well and take off heat. Divide this on your pancakes, roll them and serve for breakfast. Enjoy!

Nutritional value: calories 260, fat 7, fiber 4, carbs 5, protein 10

Different Breakfast Dish

We don't want to spoil your surprise! Just check out this recipe!

Preparation time: 10 minutes
Cooking time: 35 minutes
Servings: 8

Ingredients:
- 1 pound pork meat, ground
- 1 pound chorizo, ground
- A pinch of sea salt
- Black pepper to the taste
- 8 eggs
- 3 tablespoons ghee
- 1 avocado, pitted, peeled and chopped
- 1 tomato, chopped
- ½ cup red onion, chopped
- 2 tablespoons Paleo enchilada sauce

Directions:
In a bowl, mix pork with chorizo, a pinch of salt and black pepper and stir well. Spread this on a lined baking sheet, shape a circle out of it and spread enchilada sauce all over. Place in the oven and be at 350 degrees F for 25 minutes. Heat up a pan with the ghee over medium heat, add eggs, stir and scramble them. Spread them over pork mix and then add onion, tomato, and avocado. Divide between plates and serve. Enjoy!

Nutritional value: calories 345, fat 23, fiber 3, carbs 6, protein 23

Simple Burger

Try a Paleo burger for breakfast today!

Preparation time: 10 minutes
Cooking time: 20 minutes
Servings: 4

Ingredients:
- 8 bacon slices, chopped and cooked
- 5 eggs
- 1 pound beef, ground
- ½ cup sausage, ground
- 3 sun-dried tomatoes, chopped
- 2 tablespoons almond meal
- 2 teaspoons basil
- 2 tablespoons coconut oil
- 1 teaspoon garlic, minced

Directions:
In a bowl, mix beef with garlic, basil, tomatoes, almond meal and 1 egg, stir well and shape 4 burgers. Heat up a grill over medium high heat, add burgers, cook them for 5 minutes on each side, transfer to plates and leave them aside. Heat up a pan over medium high heat, add sausage, cook until it's done and divide into burgers. Add cooked bacon on top of sausages and leave aside for now. Heat up a pan with the coconut oil over medium high heat, crack one egg at a time, fry them well and divide them on burgers. Enjoy!

Nutritional value: calories 340, fat 20, fiber 3, carbs 7, protein 20

Delicious Sausage Balls

This special Paleo breakfast idea is meant to make your taste buds dance!

Preparation time: 10 minutes
Cooking time: 20 minutes
Servings: 8

Ingredients:
- 2 eggs
- 1 teaspoon baking soda
- 1 pound sausage, chopped
- ¼ cup coconut flour
- Black pepper to the taste
- 1 teaspoon smoked paprika

Directions:
In your food processor, mix sausage with eggs, baking soda, flour, pepper and paprika and pulse really well. Shape medium balls from this mix, arrange them on a lined baking sheet and bake them in the oven at 350 degrees F for 20 minutes. Divide them between plates and serve in the morning. Enjoy!

Nutritional value: calories 150, fat 7, fiber 3, carbs 4, protein 6

Delightful Wrapped Eggs

Just pay attention and learn how to make this tasty breakfast!

Preparation time: 10 minutes
Cooking time: 15 minutes
Servings: 2

Ingredients:
- 4 bacon slices
- 2 bacon slices, chopped
- 4 eggs
- ½ yellow onion, chopped
- 1 sweet potato, peeled and chopped
- 1 tablespoon olive oil
- A pinch of sea salt
- Black pepper to the taste

Directions:
Heat up a pan over medium high heat, add 4 bacon slices, cook until it's crispy, transfer to paper towels, drain grease and line 4 muffin molds with it. Crack an egg into each bacon cup, season with salt and pepper, place in the oven at 375 degrees F and bake for 15 minutes. Meanwhile, heat up a pan with the oil over medium high heat, add onion and sweet potato, stir and cook for a few minutes. Add the rest of the bacon, stir and cook for a few more minutes. Divide wrapped eggs on plates, add sweet potato mix on the side and serve. Enjoy!

Nutritional value: calories 200, fat 5, fiber 3, carbs 6, protein 5

Special Blueberry Muffins

Serve these in the morning with a glass of almond milk on the side!

Preparation time: 10 minutes
Cooking time: 25 minutes
Servings: 10

Ingredients:
- ½ teaspoon baking soda
- 2 and ½ cups almond flour
- 1 tablespoon vanilla extract
- ¼ cup coconut oil
- ¼ cup coconut milk
- 2 eggs
- ¼ cup maple syrup
- 1 tablespoon coconut flour
- 3 tablespoons cinnamon powder
- 1 cup blueberries

Directions:
In a bowl, mix almond flour with baking soda and coconut flour and stir. Add eggs, oil, coconut milk, cinnamon, maple syrup, vanilla and blueberries and stir everything using your mixer. Divide this into muffin cups, place in the oven at 350 degrees F and bake for 25 minutes. Leave your muffins to cool down a bit, divide between plates and serve them for breakfast. Enjoy!

Nutritional value: calories 240, fat 3, fiber 1, carbs 3, protein 1

Amazing Pumpkin Muffins

Serve these for breakfast tomorrow and take some at the office as well!

Preparation time: 10 minutes
Cooking time: 25 minutes
Servings: 10
Ingredients:
- 1 and ¼ cup almond meal
- 2 tablespoons flax meal
- 1 tablespoon flax seeds
- ¾ cup coconut flour
- 1 teaspoon baking soda
- 2 teaspoons pumpkin pie spice
- ½ teaspoon nutmeg, ground
- ½ teaspoon ginger powder
- 5 eggs
- ¼ cup coconut oil
- ¼ cup agave
- 1 cup pumpkin puree
- 1 cup blueberries
- 1 cup walnuts, chopped

Directions:
In a bowl, mix almond meal with flax meal, flax seeds, coconut flour, baking soda, nutmeg, ginger and pumpkin spice and stir. In another bowl, mix eggs with oil, agave, pumpkin puree, walnuts, and blueberries and whisk well. Combine the 2 mixtures and stir using your mixer. Divide this into a lined muffin tray, place in the oven at 350 degrees F and bake for 25 minutes. Leave your muffins to cool down, divide them between plates and serve. Enjoy!

Nutritional value: calories 240, fat 3, fiber 2, carbs 4, protein 6

Zucchini and Chocolate Muffins

We know this might sound a bit strange, but we can assure you they are the perfect Paleo breakfast idea!

Preparation time: 10 minutes
Cooking time: 30 minutes
Servings: 8
Ingredients:
- 4 eggs
- ¼ cup honey
- ¼ cup melted ghee
- ¼ cup coconut milk
- ¼ cup coconut flour
- ½ cup almond flour
- 1 teaspoon baking soda
- ¼ cup cocoa powder
- 1 zucchini, grated
- 4 ounces dark chocolate, chopped
- 1 teaspoon vanilla extract

Directions:
In a bowl, mix eggs with ghee and whisk using a mixer. Add coconut milk, honey, and vanilla and whisk well again. In another bowl, mix coconut flour with baking soda, almond flour, and cocoa powder and stir well. Combine the 2 mixtures and stir again. Add chocolate pieces and zucchini, stir gently, divide into a lined muffin tray and bake in the oven at 350 degrees F for 30 minutes. Serve your muffins cold. Enjoy!

Nutritional value: calories 230, fat 4, fiber 2, carbs 4, protein 6

Awesome Avocado Muffins

This is an incredible Paleo breakfast recipe even your kids will love!

Preparation time: 10 minutes
Cooking time: 30 minutes
Servings: 12

Ingredients:
- 6 thin bacon slices, chopped
- 1 yellow onion, chopped
- 4 avocados, pitted, peeled and chopped
- 4 eggs
- ½ cup coconut flour
- 1 cup coconut milk
- ½ teaspoon baking soda
- A pinch of sea salt
- Black pepper to the taste

Directions:
Heat up a pan over medium high heat, add bacon and onion, stir well and cook until they brown. Meanwhile, put avocado in a bowl and mash with a fork. Add eggs, a pinch of salt, black pepper, milk, baking soda and coconut flour and stir everything well. Add almost all of the bacon and onions, stir well again and divide into muffin pans. Sprinkle the rest of the bacon and onions on top, place in the oven at 350 degrees F and bake for 20 minutes. Leave your avocado muffins to cool down before dividing them on plates and serving. Enjoy!

Nutritional value: calories 240, fat 4, fiber 4, carbs 7, protein 3

Simple Spinach Omelet

You must try this Paleo omelet right away!

Preparation time: 10 minutes
Cooking time: 15 minutes
Servings: 4

Ingredients:
- 2 eggs, whisked
- 1 tablespoon ghee, melted
- A pinch of black pepper
- 1 handful baby spinach, torn
- 1 onion, chopped
- 4 thyme springs, chopped
- 3 garlic cloves, minced
- 1 red bell pepper, chopped
- 1 green bell pepper, chopped
- 3 tablespoon olive oil
- 1 cup cherry tomatoes, halved
- 1 red chili pepper, chopped

Directions:
Heat up a pan with the ghee over medium high heat, add eggs, black pepper, stir a bit, cook until eggs are done, add spinach, stir gently, cook for a few minutes and divide between plates. Heat up another pan with the oil over medium high heat, add onion, stir and cook for 3 minutes. Add garlic, stir and cook for 1 minute more. Add thyme, tomatoes, red, yellow pepper, and chili pepper, stir, cook for 5 minutes more and divide on top of the omelet. Serve hot. Enjoy!

Nutritional value: calories 200, fat 5, fiber 3, carbs 4, protein 4

Apple Omelet

You are going to love this amazing Paleo idea!

Preparation time: 10 minutes
Cooking time: 15 minutes
Servings: 1

Ingredients:
- 1 apple, peeled, cored and sliced
- 2 teaspoons ghee
- 3 teaspoons maple syrup
- ½ teaspoon cinnamon powder
- 2 eggs, whites, and yolks separated
- 2 tablespoons almond milk
- A pinch of sea salt
- Black pepper to the taste
- 2 tablespoons walnuts, toasted and chopped

Directions:
Heat up a pan with half of the ghee over medium high heat, add apple slices and cook them for about 5 minutes. Sprinkle them with cinnamon, drizzle maple syrup, stir gently, cook for 1 minute, transfer them to a plate and leave aside for now. In a bowl, whisk egg yolks with milk, a pinch of salt and black pepper and leave aside for now. In another bowl, whisk egg whites well using your mixer. Combine egg yolks with egg whites. Heat up a pan with the rest of the ghee over medium heat, add eggs mix, stir and cook for 3 minutes. Add apple slices, cover pan, cook eggs for 6 minutes more and transfer everything to a plate. Top with walnuts and serve. Enjoy!

Nutritional value: calories 150, fat 1, fiber 3, carbs 4, protein 12

Veggie Omelet Cupcakes

It's always great to learn great Paleo breakfast ideas! Here's another one!

Preparation time: 10 minutes
Cooking time: 20 minutes
Servings: 4

Ingredients:
- 4 bacon slices, chopped
- A handful spinach, chopped
- 1 white onion, chopped
- 1 red bell pepper, chopped
- 1 green bell pepper, chopped
- 1 yellow bell pepper, chopped
- 1 tomato, chopped
- 8 eggs
- A pinch of sea salt
- Black pepper to the taste

Directions:
Heat up a pan over medium high heat, add bacon, stir, cook until it's crispy, transfer to paper towels, drain grease and leave aside for now. Heat up the same pan with the bacon fat over medium high heat, add onion, stir and cook for 3 minutes. Add tomato, all bell peppers, a pinch of salt and black pepper, stir, cook for a couple more minutes and take off heat. In a bowl, whisk eggs with a pinch of salt and black pepper and mix with veggies and bacon. Stir, divide this into a lined muffin tray, place in the oven at 350 degrees F and bake for 17 minutes. Leave you special muffins to cool down, divide between plates and serve. Enjoy!

Nutritional value: calories 200, fat 4, fiber 2, carbs 5, protein 7

Ham and Mushroom Breakfast

This is much better than you could ever imagine!

Preparation time: 10 minutes
Cooking time: 10 minutes
Servings: 1

Ingredients:
- 2 tablespoons ghee
- ¼ cup coconut milk
- 3 eggs
- 3.5 ounces smoked ham, chopped
- 3 ounces mushrooms, sliced
- 1 cup arugula, torn
- A pinch of black pepper

Directions:
Heat up a pan with half of the ghee over medium heat, add mushrooms, stir and cook for 3 minutes. Add ham, stir, cook for 2-3 minutes more and transfer everything to a plate. In a bowl, mix eggs with coconut milk and black pepper and whisk well. Heat up the pan with the rest of the ghee over medium heat, add eggs, spread into the pan, cook for a couple of minutes, start stirring and cook until eggs are completely done. Transfer this to a serving bowl, add mushrooms mix on top and arugula. Toss everything to coat well and serve right away.

Nutritional value: calories 356, fat 23, fiber 2, carbs 6, protein 25

Breakfast Coconut Pancakes

These are simply delicious! Make these Paleo delights today!

Preparation time: 10 minutes
Cooking time: 10 minutes
Servings: 8

Ingredients:
- ¼ cup coconut milk
- ¼ cup coconut flour
- 1/8 teaspoon baking soda
- 3 eggs
- 2 tablespoons coconut oil
- ½ teaspoon vanilla extract
- 2 tablespoons honey
- Maple syrup for serving
- 2 tablespoons melted ghee

Directions:
In a bowl, whisk eggs with honey and coconut oil. Add vanilla, coconut milk, baking soda and coconut flour and stir very well. Heat up a pan with the ghee over medium heat, add some of the batter, spread into the pan, cook until it's golden, flip and cook on the other side as well. Repeat with the rest of the batter, divide your pancakes between plates and serve with maple syrup on top. Enjoy!

Nutritional value: calories 300, fat 5, fiber 2, carbs 4, protein 10

Incredible Apple Pancakes

These will make your day a lot better!

Preparation time: 10 minutes
Cooking time: 20 minutes
Servings: 18

Ingredients:
- 2 cups apples, peeled, cored and chopped
- 1 tablespoon coconut oil
- 4 eggs
- 2 teaspoons cinnamon powder
- 2 tablespoons honey
- 1 cup almond milk+ 3 tablespoons
- 1 teaspoon vanilla extract
- ½ cup coconut flour
- A pinch of nutmeg
- ½ teaspoon baking soda
- 3 tablespoons ghee
- 2 tablespoons maple syrup

Directions:
Heat up a pan with 1 tablespoon oil over medium heat, add apples and cinnamon, stir and cook for 5 minutes. In a bowl, whisk eggs with vanilla, 1 cup milk, honey, baking soda, coconut flour and nutmeg and whisk. Add apples and the rest of the almond milk and stir again well. Heat up a pan with the ghee over medium high heat, pour some of the pancake batter, spread, cook until it's done on one side, flip, cook on the other side as well and transfer to a plate. Repeat with the rest of the batter and serve your pancakes with maple syrup on top. Enjoy!

Nutritional value: calories 340, fat 14, fiber 4, carbs 7, protein 12

Tasty Porridge

This is one Paleo breakfast you won't forget!

Preparation time: 10 minutes
Cooking time: 6 minutes
Servings: 3

Ingredients:
- 1 big plantain, peeled and mashed
- ¼ cup flax meal
- 2 cups coconut milk
- ¾ cup almond meal
- 1 teaspoon cinnamon, powder
- A pinch of cloves, ground
- ½ teaspoon ginger powder
- A pinch of nutmeg, ground
- Maple syrup for serving
- Some unsweetened coconut flakes for serving

Directions:
In a small pan, mix plantain with flax meal, almond meal, coconut milk, cinnamon, cloves, ginger, and nutmeg, stir well, bring to a simmer over medium heat and cook for about 6 minutes. Divide your porridge into bowls, top with coconut flakes and maple syrup and serve. Enjoy!

Nutritional value: calories 140, fat 3, fiber 2, carbs 5, protein 6

Simple and Tasty Nuts Porridge

You better pay attention and learn how to make this great breakfast!

Preparation time: 10 minutes
Cooking time: 5 minutes
Servings: 2

Ingredients:
- ½ cup pecans, soaked overnight and drained
- ½ banana, mashed
- ¾ cup hot water
- 2 tablespoons coconut butter
- ½ teaspoon cinnamon
- 2 teaspoons maple syrup

Directions:
In a blender, mix pecans, with water, banana, coconut butter, cinnamon and maple syrup, pulse really well and transfer to a small pot. Heat everything up over medium heat, cook until it's creamy, transfer to serving bowls and serve. Enjoy!

Nutritional value: calories 150, fat 2, fiber 2, carbs 4, protein 6

Portobello Sandwich

This is the best Paleo sandwich!

Preparation time: 5 minutes
Cooking time: 10 minutes
Servings: 1

Ingredients:
- 2 Portobello mushroom caps
- Some lettuce leaves
- 2 avocado slices
- ½ pound bacon, chopped

Directions:
Heat up a pan over medium high heat, add bacon, cook until it's crispy, transfer to paper towels and drain grease. Heat up the pan with the bacon fat over medium high heat, add mushroom caps, cook for 2 minutes on each side and take off heat. Put 1 mushroom cap on a plate, add bacon, avocado slices, and lettuce leaves, top with the other mushroom cap and serve. Enjoy!

Nutritional value: calories 200, fat 4, fiber 2, carbs 4, protein 6

Bacon and Egg Breakfast Sandwich

You've got to try this tasty and special breakfast right away!

Preparation time: 10 minutes
Cooking time: 10 minutes
Servings: 2

Ingredients:
- 2 cups bell peppers, chopped
- ½ tablespoon avocado oil
- 3 eggs
- 4 bacon slices

Directions:
Heat up a pan with the oil over medium high heat, add bell peppers, stir and cook until they are soft. Heat up another pan over medium heat, add bacon, stir and cook until it's crispy. In a bowl, whisk eggs really well and add them to bell peppers. Cook until eggs are done for about 8 minutes. Divide half of the bacon slices between plates, add eggs, top with bacon slices and serve. Enjoy!

Nutritional value: calories 200, fat 4, fiber 3, carbs 6, protein 10

Breakfast Sliders

You must get your ingredients and make this tasty Paleo breakfast right away!

Preparation time: 10 minutes
Cooking time: 15 minutes
Servings: 3

Ingredients:
- 3 Portobello mushroom caps
- 4 bacon slices
- 3 eggs
- 4 ounces smoked salmon

Directions:
Heat up a pan over medium high heat, add bacon, cook until it's crispy, transfer to paper towels and drain grease. Heat up the pan with the bacon grease over medium heat and place egg rings in it. Crack and egg in each, cook them for 6 minutes and transfer them to a plate. Heat up the pan again over medium high heat, add mushroom caps, cook the for 5 minutes and transfer them to a platter. Top each mushroom cap with bacon, salmon, and eggs. Serve hot. Enjoy!

Nutritional value: calories 180, fat 3, fiber 5, carbs 7, protein 8

Beef and Squash Skillet

This is a very healthy Paleo breakfast mix! Try it today and see for yourself!

Preparation time: 10 minutes
Cooking time: 20 minutes
Servings: 3

Ingredients:
- 15 ounces beef, ground
- 2 tablespoons ghee
- 3 garlic cloves, minced
- 2 celery stalks, chopped
- 1 yellow onion, chopped
- A pinch of sea salt
- White pepper to the taste
- ½ teaspoon coriander, ground
- 1 teaspoon cumin, ground
- 1 teaspoon garam masala
- ½ butternut squash, chopped and already cooked
- 3 eggs
- 1 small avocado, peeled, pitted and chopped
- 15 ounces spinach

Directions:
Put spinach in a heatproof bowl, place in your microwave and cook for 1 minute. Squeeze spinach and leave it aside. Heat up a pan with the ghee over medium heat, add onion, garlic, celery, a pinch of salt and white pepper, stir and cook for 3 minutes. Add beef, cumin, garam masala, and coriander, stir and cook for a few minutes more. Add squash flesh and spinach, stir and make 3 holes in this mix. Crack an egg into each, cover pan, place in the oven at 375 degrees F and bake for 15 minutes. Divide this mix on plates and serve with avocado on top. Enjoy!

Nutritional value: calories 400, fat 23, fiber 7, carbs 8, protein 24

Sweet Potato Breakfast

This will be a real culinary treat for you and your loved ones!

Preparation time: 10 minutes
Cooking time: 15 minutes
Servings: 4

Ingredients:
- 2 Italian sausages, casings removed
- 4 tablespoons coconut oil
- 1 small green bell pepper, chopped
- ½ cup onion, chopped
- 2 garlic cloves, minced
- 2 cups sweet potato, chopped
- 1 avocado, peeled, pitted, cut into halves and thinly sliced
- 3 eggs
- 2 cups spinach

Directions:
Heat up a pan with the oil over medium high heat, add onion, stir and cook for 3 minutes. Add garlic and bell pepper, stir and cook for 1 minute. Add sausage meat, stir and brown for 4 minutes more. Add sweet potato, stir and cook for 4 minutes. Add spinach, stir and cook for 2 minutes. Make 3 holes in this mix, crack an egg in each, introduce pan in preheated broiler and cook for 3 minutes. Divide this tasty mix on plates, add avocado pieces on the side and serve. Enjoy!

Nutritional value: calories 200, fat 4, fiber 2, carbs 6, protein 9

Pork Skillet

This is a tasty, rich and textured breakfast idea!

Preparation time: 10 minutes
Cooking time: 20 minutes
Servings: 4

Ingredients:
- 8 ounces mushrooms, chopped
- 1 pound pork, ground
- 1 tablespoon olive oil
- Black pepper to the taste
- 2 zucchinis, cut in halves and then in half moons
- ½ teaspoon garlic powder
- ½ teaspoon basil, dried
- A pinch of sea salt
- 2 tablespoons Dijon mustard

Directions:
Heat up a pan with the oil over medium high heat, add mushrooms, stir and cook for 4 minutes. Add zucchinis, a pinch of salt and black pepper, stir and cook for 4 minutes more. Add pork, garlic powder and basil, stir and cook until meat is done. Add mustard, stir well, cook for a couple more minutes, divide between plates and serve. Enjoy!

Nutritional value: calories 200, fat 4, fiber 2, carbs 5, protein 12

Chorizo Breakfast Skillet

Here's another delicious and easy to make Paleo breakfast skillet!

Preparation time: 10 minutes
Cooking time: 30 minutes
Servings: 2

Ingredients:
- 1 small avocado, peeled, pitted and chopped
- ½ cup beef stock
- 1 pound chorizo, chopped
- 2 poblano peppers, chopped
- 1 cup kale, chopped
- 8 mushrooms, chopped
- ½ yellow onion, chopped
- 3 garlic cloves, minced
- ½ cup cilantro, chopped
- 4 bacon slices, chopped
- 4 eggs

Directions:
Heat up a pan over medium heat, add chorizo and bacon, stir and cook until they are browned. Add garlic, peppers, and onions, stir and cook for 6 minutes more. Add stock, mushrooms, and kale, stir and cook for 4 minutes more. Make holes in this mix, crack an egg in each, place in the oven at 350 degrees F and bake for 12 minutes. Divide this mix on plates, sprinkle cilantro and avocado on top and serve. Enjoy!

Nutritional value: calories 200, fat 6, fiber 3, carbs 6, protein 10

Delicious Steak and Veggie Breakfast

Serve this for breakfast, and you won't need anything else to eat all day!

Preparation time: 10 minutes
Cooking time: 25 minutes
Servings: 4

Ingredients:
- 2 sweet potatoes, chopped
- ¾ pound sirloin steak, cut into small pieces
- 1 yellow onion, chopped
- 1 green bell pepper, chopped
- 1 red bell pepper, chopped
- 2 tablespoons bacon fat
- Black pepper to the taste
- A pinch of sea salt
- 1 tomato, sliced
- 4 eggs

Directions:

Heat up a pan with half of the fat over medium high heat, add steak, cook for a few minutes until it browns and takes off heat. Heat up the same pan with the rest of the fat over medium high heat, add green and red peppers and onions, stir and cook for 5 minutes. Add sweet potatoes, stir and cook for 10 minutes more. Add steak pieces, stir well, make 4 holes, crack an egg in each, arrange tomato slices, sprinkle black pepper and a pinch of salt, place in the oven at 350 degrees F and bake for 12 minutes. Serve warm. Enjoy!

Nutritional value: calories 180, fat 4, fiber 3, carbs 6, protein 8

Simple Breakfast Waffles

These are exceptional! You should taste them!

Preparation time: 10 minutes
Cooking time: 10 minutes
Servings: 4

Ingredients:
- 2 eggs
- ½ cup almond milk
- 2 tablespoons coconut oil, melted
- ½ teaspoon cinnamon, ground
- 1 tablespoon baking powder
- 1 tablespoon coconut flour
- 2 tablespoons honey
- 1 and ½ cups almond flour
- ¼ cup tapioca flour
- 1 and ½ teaspoons vanilla extract
- Pure maple syrup for serving

Directions:

In your mixer bowl, combine coconut flour with almond flour, tapioca flour, baking powder and cinnamon and stir. Add egg yolks, almond milk, coconut oil, honey and vanilla extract and blend very well. In another bowl, whisk egg whites with your mixer. Add them to waffles mix and stir everything very well. Pour this into your waffle iron and make 8 waffles. Divide them on plates, top with maple syrup and serve. Enjoy!

Nutritional value: calories 160, fat 11, fiber 2, carbs 7, protein 6

Delicious Chicken Waffles

Can you believe such a thing? You can make Paleo chicken waffles! They are so delicious!

Preparation time: 10 minutes
Cooking time: 10 minutes
Servings: 4

Ingredients:
- 1 and ½ cups chicken, cooked and shredded
- ½ cup hot sauce
- 1 cup almond flour
- 2 green onions, chopped
- ½ cup tapioca flour
- 2 eggs
- 6 tablespoon coconut flour
- A pinch of cayenne pepper
- ¾ teaspoons baking soda
- 1 teaspoon garlic powder
- 1 cup coconut milk
- ¼ cup ghee+ some more for the waffle iron
- A pinch of sea salt

Directions:
In a bowl, mix almond flour with tapioca flour, coconut one, baking soda, garlic powder and a pinch of salt and stir well. Add chicken, hot sauce, green onions, eggs, milk and ¼ cup ghee and blend using your mixer. Pour some of the batter into your greased waffle iron, close the lid and make your waffle. Repeat with the rest of the batter, divide waffles between plates and serve them in the morning. Enjoy!

Nutritional value: calories 200, fat 11, fiber 1, carbs 7, protein 8

Amazing Bacon Waffles

These will really impress you!

Preparation time: 10 minutes
Cooking time: 30 minutes
Servings: 4

Ingredients:
1. 2 eggs
2. 6 bacon slices
3. ½ cup coconut milk
4. 1 teaspoon vanilla extract
5. 2 tablespoons maple syrup
6. ½ teaspoon baking soda
7. 1 and ¾ cups almond flour
8. 2 tablespoons ghee
9. Maple syrup for serving

Directions:
Place bacon slices on a lined baking sheet, place in the oven at 400 degrees F and bake for 20 minutes. Transfer bacon to paper towels, drain grease, crumble them and leave them aside. In a bowl, mix almond flour with baking soda. In another bowl, whisk eggs with vanilla extract, ghee, 2 tablespoons maple syrup and coconut milk.
Combine the wet and dry mixtures and stir well. Add crumbled bacon, stir again and pour some of the batter in your waffle iron. Close the lid, cook your waffle for 5 minutes and transfer it to a plate. Repeat with the rest of the batter, divide waffles between plates and serve them with maple syrup on top. Enjoy!

Nutritional value: calories 200, fat 12, fiber 4, carbs 7, protein 10

Paleo Soups and Stews Recipes

Special Paleo Soup

It's simply perfect! Make it today and enjoy its wonderful taste!

Servings: 6
Preparation time: 15 minutes
Cooking time: 40 minutes

Ingredients:
- 1 yellow onion, finely chopped
- 1 tablespoon avocado oil
- 3 thyme springs, chopped
- 3 garlic cloves, finely minced
- 28 ounces canned tomatoes, chopped
- 6 ounces tomato paste
- ¼ cup water
- 1 pound sausage, chopped
- 14 ounces beef stock
- 6 mushrooms, chopped
- 1 small red bell pepper, chopped
- 5 ounces pepperoni
- 2.5 ounces black olives, chopped
- A pinch of red pepper flakes

Directions:
Heat up a pot with the oil over medium high heat and melt it. Add half of the onion, garlic, and thyme, stir and cook for 5 minutes. Add tomatoes, tomato paste and water, stir, bring to a boil, reduce heat to medium-low and simmer for 20 minutes. Pour this into your blender, pulse well and leave aside for now. Heat up a pot over medium-high heat, add sausage, stir and cook for a few minutes, breaking into small pieces with a fork. Add the rest of the onion, mushrooms and the bell pepper, stir and cook for 5 minutes. Add tomato soup you've blended and beef stock, stir and cook for 5 more minutes. Heat up a pan over medium high heat, add pepperoni slices, stir and cook until they brown. Pour soup into bowls, top with red pepper flakes, olives, and pepperoni. Enjoy!

Nutritional value: calories 224, fat 16, carbs 8, fiber 3, sugar 5.5, protein 7

Tomato and Basil Soup

It's just what you need on a cold day!

Servings: 4
Preparation time: 10 minutes
Cooking time: 35 minutes

Ingredients:
- 56 ounces canned tomatoes, crushed
- 2 cups tomato juice
- 2 cups chicken stock
- ¼ pound coconut butter
- 14 basil leaves, torn
- 1 cup coconut milk
- Salt and black pepper to the taste

Directions:
Put tomatoes, tomato juice and stock in a pot, heat up over medium-high heat, bring to a boil, reduce heat, stir and simmer for 30 minutes. Pour this into your blender, add basil, pulse very well and return to pot. Heat up soup again, add butter and coconut milk, stir and cook on low heat for a few more minutes. Add salt and pepper to the taste, stir well, pour into soup bowls and serve. Enjoy!

Nutritional value: calories 170, fat 10, carbs 14, protein 2, sugar 1

Paleo Chicken Soup

It's such an incredible soup! It tastes wonderful, and it looks so good!

Servings: 4
Preparation time: 15 minutes
Cooking time: 60 minutes

Ingredients:
- 2 teaspoons coconut oil
- 3 carrots, chopped
- 1 yellow onion, chopped
- 1 zucchini, chopped
- 12 ounces canned mushrooms, chopped
- ¼ butternut squash, cubed
- 4 cups chicken meat, already cooked and shredded
- 2 teaspoons rosemary, dried
- 1 teaspoon thyme, dried
- 1 tablespoon apple cider vinegar
- 1 teaspoon cumin
- 2 and ½ cups chicken stock
- A pinch of sea salt
- Black pepper to the taste

Directions:
Heat up a pot with the coconut oil over medium heat, add carrots and onion, stir and cook for 5 minutes. Add zucchini, mushrooms, and squash, stir and cook for 5 more minutes. Add chicken meat, rosemary, thyme, vinegar, cumin and chicken stock, stir, bring to a boil, reduce heat to medium-low and simmer for 40 minutes. Add a pinch of salt and pepper to the taste, stir again, take off heat and pour into soup bowls. Enjoy!

Nutritional value: calories 390, fat 2, carbs 34, protein 6, sugar 0, fiber 4

Delicious Cauliflower Soup

It's delicious and very hearty! You need to purchase all the ingredients and make it today!

Servings: 6
Preparation time: 10 minutes
Cooking time: 60 minutes

Ingredients:
- 1 yellow onion, finely chopped
- 2 tablespoons extra virgin olive oil
- 2 pounds cauliflower florets
- A pinch of sea salt
- Black pepper to the taste
- 20 saffron threads
- 2 garlic cloves, minced
- 5 cups veggie stock

Directions:
Heat up a pot with the oil over medium heat, add onion and garlic, stir and cook for 10 minutes. Add cauliflower, a pinch of sea salt and pepper to the taste, stir and cook for 12 more minutes. Add stock, stir, bring to a boil, reduce heat to medium and simmer for 25 minutes. Take soup off the heat, add saffron, cover pot and leave it aside for 20 minutes. Transfer soup to your blender and pulse very well. Pour into soup bowls and serve right away. Enjoy!

Nutritional value: calories 170, fat 11, carbs 5, fiber 2, sugar 0.1, protein 7

Paleo Beef Soup

Your family will enjoy eating this flavored soup! You will love it too!

Servings: 6
Preparation time: 10 minutes
Cooking time: 1 hour

Ingredients:
- 1 pound organic beef, ground
- 1 pound sausage, sliced
- 4 cups beef stock
- 30 ounces canned tomatoes, diced
- 1 green bell pepper, chopped
- 3 zucchinis, chopped
- 1 cup celery, chopped
- 1 teaspoon Italian seasoning
- ½ yellow onion, chopped
- ½ teaspoon oregano, dried
- ½ teaspoon basil, dried
- ¼ teaspoon garlic powder
- A pinch of sea salt
- Black pepper to the taste

Directions:
Heat up a pot over medium heat, add sausage and beef, stir, cook until it browns and drains excess fat. Add tomatoes, zucchini, bell pepper, celery, onion, Italian seasoning, basil, oregano, garlic powder, sea salt, pepper to the taste and the stock, stir, bring to a boil, reduce heat to medium-low and simmer for 1 hour. Pour into soup bowls and serve right away. Enjoy!

Nutritional value: calories 370, fat 17, carbs 35, fiber 10, protein 25

Root Paleo Soup

The root veggies you'll use for this soup taste wonderful! The soup is perfect!

Servings: 8
Preparation time: 10 minutes
Cooking time: 1 hour and 30 minutes

Ingredients:
- 1 sweet onion, chopped
- 2 tablespoons ghee
- 5 carrots, chopped
- 3 parsnips, chopped
- 3 beets, chopped
- 3 bacon slices
- 1-quart chicken stock
- A pinch of sea salt
- Black pepper to the taste
- 2 quarts water
- ½ teaspoon chili flakes
- 1 tablespoons mixed thyme and rosemary

Directions:
Heat up a Dutch oven with the ghee over medium-high heat, add onion, stir and cook for 5 minutes. Add carrots, parsnips, beets, bacon, chicken stock and water and stir. Also add sea salt, pepper to the taste, chili flakes, thyme, and rosemary, stir again, bring to a boil, reduce heat to medium-low and simmer for 1 hour and 30 minutes. Pour into soup bowls and serve hot. Enjoy!

Nutritional value: calories 180, fat 2, carbs 4, fiber 1, sugar 0.5, protein 3.5

Delightful Chicken Soup

This amazing paleo chicken soup is such an elegant option for a fancy lunch!

Servings: 6
Preparation time: 15 minutes
Cooking time: 30 minutes

Ingredients:
- 2 celery stalks, chopped
- ½ cup coconut oil
- 2 carrots, chopped
- ½ cup arrowroot
- 6 cups chicken stock
- 1 teaspoon dry parsley
- ½ cup water
- 1 bay leaf
- A pinch of sea salt
- Black pepper to the taste
- ½ teaspoon dry thyme
- 1 and ½ cups coconut milk
- 3 cups organic chicken meat, already cooked and cubed

Directions:
Heat up a soup pot with the oil over medium-high heat, add carrots and celery, stir and cook for 10 minutes. Add stock, stir and bring to a boil. In a bowl, mix arrowroot with ½ cup water and whisk well. Add this to soup and also add parsley, sea salt, pepper to the taste, bay leaf and thyme. Stir and cook everything for 15 minutes. Add chicken meat and coconut milk, stir, cook 1 more minute, take off heat, pour into soup bowls and serve. Enjoy!

Nutritional value: calories 412, fat 31, carbs 8, fiber 2, protein 27, sugar 4

Paleo Lemon and Garlic Soup

This is an exotic style soup! It's also very easy to make!

Servings: 4
Preparation time: 10 minutes
Cooking time: 10 minutes

Ingredients:
- 6 cups shellfish stock
- 1 tablespoons garlic, finely minced
- 1 tablespoon coconut oil, melted
- 2 eggs
- ½ cup lemon juice
- A pinch of sea salt
- White pepper to the taste
- 1 tablespoon arrowroot powder
- Cilantro, finely chopped for serving

Directions:
Heat up a pot with the oil over medium high heat, add garlic, stir and cook for 2 minutes. Add stock but reserve ½ cup, stir and bring to a simmer. Meanwhile, in a bowl, mix eggs with sea salt, pepper, reserved stock, lemon juice and arrowroot and whisk very well. Pour this into soup, stir and cook for a few minutes. Ladle into bowls and serve with chopped cilantro on top. Enjoy!

Nutritional value: calories 135, fat 3, carbs 12, fiber 1, protein 8, sugar 0

Rich Paleo Soup

It's a very rich soup with such a strong color! Taste it today!

Servings: 3
Preparation time: 10 minutes
Cooking time: 0

Ingredients:
- 1 avocado, pitted and chopped
- 1 cucumber, chopped
- 2 bunches spinach
- 1 and ½ cups watermelon, chopped
- 1 bunch cilantro, roughly chopped
- Juice from 2 lemons
- ½ cup coconut aminos
- ½ cup lime juice

Directions:
In your kitchen blender, mix cucumber with avocado and pulse well. Add cilantro, spinach, and watermelon and blend again well. Add lemon and lime juice and coconut amino and pulse a few more times. Transfer to soup bowls and enjoy!

Nutritional value: calories 100, fat 7, carbs 6.5, fiber 3.5, sugar 2.4, protein 2.3

Paleo Veggie Soup

This is a true winter soup, very flavored and textured!

Servings: 4
Preparation time: 10 minutes
Cooking time: 45 minutes

Ingredients:
- 2 sweet potatoes, peeled and chopped
- 2 yellow onions, cut into eighths
- 2 pounds carrots, diced
- 4 tablespoons coconut oil
- 1 head garlic, cloves peeled
- A pinch of sea salt
- Black pepper to the taste
- 2 cups chicken stock
- 3 tablespoons maple syrup

Directions:
Put onions, carrots, sweet potatoes and garlic in a baking dish, add coconut oil, a pinch of sea salt and pepper to the taste, toss to coat, introduce in the oven at 425 degrees F and bake for 35 minutes. Take veggies out of the oven, transfer to a pot, add chicken stock and heat everything up on the stove on medium-high heat. Bring soup to a boil, reduce heat to medium, cover and simmer for 10 minutes. Transfer soup to your blender, add more pepper and the maple syrup, pulse well to obtain a cream, pour into soup bowls and serve. Enjoy!

Nutritional value: calories 130, fat 3, carbs 12, fiber 3.5, sugar 6, protein 3

Paleo Beef Stew

It's a very tasty stew! The meat is so tender and succulent! It's divine!

Servings: 4
Preparation time: 10 minutes
Cooking time: 2 hours
Ingredients:

- 2 pounds beef fillet, cubed
- 1 red chili, seeded and chopped
- 1 brown onion, finely chopped
- 1 teaspoon ghee
- 2 tablespoons extra virgin olive oil
- A pinch of sea salt
- Black pepper to the taste
- 2/3 teaspoon nutmeg
- 2 tablespoon Worcestershire sauce, gluten free
- 1 garlic clove, minced
- ½ cup dried mushrooms
- ½ cup white wine
- ½ tablespoon dry sherry
- 1 teaspoon rosemary, dry
- 4 thyme springs
- ¼ teaspoon fennel seeds
- 1-star anise
- 2 celery stick, chopped
- 2 carrots, thinly sliced
- 1-quart beef stock
- 6 button mushrooms, chopped
- 2 tablespoons almond flour
- 1 sweet potato, chopped

Directions:

Heat up a pot with the ghee and the olive oil over medium-high heat, add onion, chili, some sea salt and pepper, stir and cook for 2-3 minutes. Add meat, stir and brown it for 5 minutes. Add Worcestershire sauce, wine, sherry, dried mushrooms, garlic, stock, thyme, fennel, rosemary, nutmeg, and star anise, stir, bring to a boil, cover, reduce heat to low and cook for 1 hour and 10 minutes. Add celery, carrots, fresh mushrooms, potato, stir, cover and cook for 15 minutes. Increase heat to medium, uncover the pot and cook the stew for 15 minutes. In a bowl, mix the flour with a cup of liquid from the stew, stir well, pour over stew and cook for 15 more minutes. Transfer to bowls and serve hot. Enjoy!

Nutritional value: calories 313, fat 8, carbs 21, fiber 3, sugar 7, protein 38

Paleo Slow Cooker Stew

This is an Irish style stew! It's a comforting stew and the fact that it's made in a slow cooker makes it even better!

Servings: 6
Preparation time: 1 day
Cooking time: 8 hours
Ingredients:

- 2 pounds beef stew meat, cubed
- 3 cups dark beer
- 7 garlic cloves, finely minced
- A pinch of sea salt
- Black pepper to the taste
- 4 carrots, chopped
- 1 cup coconut flour
- 2 yellow onions, finely chopped
- ½ head cabbage, finely chopped
- 30 ounces canned tomatoes, diced
- 2 cups reserved beef marinade
- 3 cups beef stock

Directions:

In a bowl, mix beef with beer and 3 garlic cloves, toss to coat and keep in the fridge for 1 day.
In a bowl, mix coconut flour with a pinch of sea salt and pepper to the taste and stir.
Drain meat and reserve the 2 cups of the marinade.
Add meat to tapioca bowls and toss to coat.
Heat up a pan over medium-high heat, add meat, stir and brown it for 2-3 minutes.
Transfer meat to your slow cooker.
Add reserved marinade, carrots, cabbage, onions, tomatoes, 4 garlic cloves, beef stock, salt and pepper to the taste, cover pot and cook stew on Low for 8 hours.
Uncover pot, transfer stew to bowls and serve.

Nutritional value: calories 247, fat 4.5, carbs 25, fiber 4.2, sugar 4, protein 24.2

Paleo Veggie and Chorizo Stew

If you are looking for a colored dish, full of intense flavors, then you must give this stew a chance!

Servings: 3
Preparation time: 10 minutes
Cooking time: 30 minutes

Ingredients:

- 1 yellow onion, chopped
- 1 tablespoon coconut oil
- 2 chorizo sausages, skinless and thinly sliced
- 1 red bell pepper, chopped
- 1 carrot, thinly sliced
- 1 celery stick, chopped
- 1 tomato, chopped
- 2 garlic cloves, finely minced
- 2 cups chicken broth
- 1 tablespoon lemon juice
- Black pepper to the taste
- 1 zucchini, chopped
- A handful parsley leaves, finely chopped

Directions:
Heat up a pan with the oil over medium-high heat, add chorizo, onion, celery and carrot, stir and cook for 3 minutes. Add red bell pepper, tomatoes and garlic, stir and cook 1 minute. Add lemon juice, stock and pepper, stir, bring to a boil, cover pan, reduce heat to medium and cook for 10 minutes. Add zucchini, stir, cover again and cook for 10 more minutes. Uncover pan, cook the stew for 2 minutes more stirring often. Add parsley, stir, take off heat, transfer to dishes and serve. Enjoy!

Nutritional value: calories 420, fat 12, carbs 45, fiber 11, sugar 5, protein 33.2

Special Beef and Plantain Stew

It's a fantastic idea for lunch or even for dinner! Try it right away!

Servings: 4
Preparation time: 10 minutes
Cooking time: 5 hours

Ingredients:

- 6 plantains, skinless and cubed
- 2 pounds beef meat, cubed
- 3 cups collard greens, chopped
- A pinch of sea salt
- Black pepper to the taste
- 3 cups water
- ½ cup sweet paprika
- 3 tablespoons allspice
- ¼ cup garlic powder
- 1 teaspoon chili powder
- 1 teaspoon cayenne pepper

Directions:
In your slow cooker, mix beef with plantains, collard greens, water, paprika, garlic powder, allspice, chili powder, cayenne, a pinch of salt and pepper to the taste. Stir, cover pot and cook on High for 5 hours. Uncover slow cooker, leave stew to cool down for a few minutes, transfer to bowls and serve. Enjoy!

Nutritional value: calories 410, fat 11, carbs 39, fiber 10, protein 34, sugar 5

Paleo Chicken Stew

Do you need a new idea for dinner tonight? Well, here is what we recommend you to try!

Servings: 6
Preparation time: 15 minutes
Cooking time: 8 hours

Ingredients:
- 5 garlic cloves, finely chopped
- 2 celery stalks, chopped
- 2 yellow onions, chopped
- 2 carrots, chopped
- 30 ounces canned pumpkin puree
- 2 quarts chicken stock
- 2 cups chicken meat, chopped
- ¼ cup coconut flour
- Black pepper to the taste
- ½ pound baby spinach
- ¼ teaspoon cayenne pepper

Directions:
In your slow cooker, mix chicken meat with onions, carrots, celery, garlic, pumpkin puree, chicken stock, black pepper, flour and cayenne, stir well, cover and cook on low for 7 hours and 50 minutes. Uncover slow cooker, add spinach, cover again and cook for 10 more minutes. Transfer to bowls and serve hot. Enjoy!

Nutritional value: calories 244, fat 2, carbs 38, fiber 6, sugar 4, protein 20

Paleo Lamb and Coconut Stew

It's an Indian style stew you should make for you and your loved ones as soon as possible!

Servings: 4
Preparation time: 15 minutes
Cooking time: 1 hour and 50 minutes

Ingredients:
- 1 and ½ pounds lamb meat, diced
- 1 tablespoon coconut oil
- ½ red chili, seedless and chopped
- 1 brown onion, chopped
- 3 garlic cloves, minced
- 2 celery sticks, chopped
- 2 and ½ teaspoons garam masala powder
- 1 teaspoon fennel seeds
- A pinch of sea salt
- Black pepper to the taste
- 1 and ¼ teaspoons turmeric
- 1 and ½ teaspoons ghee
- 14 ounces canned coconut milk
- 1 cup water
- 1 tablespoon lemon juice
- 2 carrots, chopped
- A handful parsley leaves, finely chopped

Directions:
Heat up a pan with the oil over medium-high heat, add lamb, stir and brown for 4 minutes. Add celery, chili and onion, stir and cook 1 minute. Reduce heat to medium, add garam masala, garlic, ghee, fennel, and turmeric, stir and cook 1 minute. Add a pinch of sea salt, pepper to the taste, tomato paste, coconut milk and water, stir, bring to a boil, reduce heat to low, cover and cook for 1 hour. Add carrots and cook for 40 minutes more, stirring from time to time. Add lemon juice and parsley, stir, take off heat, transfer to bowls and serve. Enjoy!

Nutritional value: calories 450, fat 31, carbs 40, fiber 1, sugar 2, protein 50

Paleo Veggie Stew

It's a delicious spring dish that proves you don't need meat every day!

Servings: 6
Preparation time: 10 minutes
Cooking time: 1 hour

Ingredients:

- 4 pounds mixed root vegetables (parsnips, carrots, rutabagas, beets, celery root, turnips), chopped
- 6 tablespoons extra virgin olive oil
- 1 garlic head, cloves separated and peeled
- ½ cup yellow onion, chopped
- Black pepper to the taste
- 28 ounces canned tomatoes, peeled and chopped
- 1 tablespoon tomato paste
- 2 cups kale leaves, torn
- 1 teaspoon oregano, dried
- Tabasco sauce for serving

Directions:

In a baking dish, mix all root vegetables with black pepper, half of the oil and garlic, toss to coat, introduce in the oven at 450 degrees G and roast them for 45 minutes. Heat up a pot with the rest of the oil over medium-high heat, add onions and cook for 2-3 minutes stirring often. Add tomato paste, stir and cook 1 more minute. Add tomatoes and their liquid, some salt and pepper and the oregano, stir, bring to a simmer, reduce heat to low and cook until veggies become roasted. Take root veggies out of the oven, add them to the pot and stir. Add kale, stir and cook for 5 minutes. Add Tabasco sauce to the taste, stir, transfer to bowls and serve. Enjoy!

Nutritional value: calories 150, fat 7, carbs 17.2, fiber 3.7, sugar 5, protein 2.4

Paleo French Chicken Stew

This chicken stew smells unbelievable, and it tastes even better!

Servings: 4
Preparation time: 15 minutes
Cooking time: 2 hours

Ingredients:

- 10 garlic cloves, peeled
- 30 black olives, pitted
- 2 pounds chicken pieces
- 2 cups chicken stock
- 28 ounces canned tomatoes, chopped
- 2 tablespoon rosemary, chopped
- 2 tablespoons parsley leaves, chopped
- 2 tablespoons basil leaves, chopped
- A pinch of sea salt
- Black pepper to the taste
- A drizzle of extra virgin olive oil

Directions:

Heat up a pot with some olive oil over medium-high heat, add chicken pieces, a pinch of sea salt, and pepper to the taste and cook for 4 minutes, stirring often. Add garlic, stir and brown for 2 minutes. Add chicken stock, tomatoes, olives, thyme, and rosemary, stir, cover pot and bake in the oven at 325 degrees F for 1 hour. Add parsley and basil, stir, introduce in the oven again and bake for 45 more minutes. Leave stew to cool down for a few minutes, transfer to plates and serve. Enjoy!

Nutritional value: calories 300, fat 48, carbs 16, sugar 0, protein 61

Paleo Oxtail Stew

You've never tried something similar! It's insanely good!

Servings: 8
Preparation time: 15 minutes
Cooking time: 6 hours

Ingredients:
- 4 and ½ pounds oxtail, cut into medium chunks
- A drizzle of extra virgin olive oil
- 1 tablespoons extra virgin olive oil
- 2 leeks, chopped
- 4 carrots, chopped
- 2 celery sticks, chopped
- 4 thyme springs, chopped
- 4 rosemary springs, chopped
- 4 cloves
- 4 bay leaves
- Black pepper to the taste
- 2 tablespoons coconut flour
- 28 ounces canned plum tomatoes, chopped
- 9 ounces red wine
- 1-quart beef stock

Directions:
In a roasting pan, mix oxtail with black pepper and a drizzle of oil. Toss to coat, introduce in the oven at 425 degrees F and bake for 20 minutes. Heat up a pot with 1 tablespoon oil over medium heat, add leeks, celery, and carrots, stir and cook for 4 minutes. Add thyme, rosemary and bay leaves, stir and cook everything for 20 minutes. Take oxtail out of the oven and leave aside for a few minutes. Add flour and cloves to veggies and stir. Also add tomatoes, wine, oxtail and its juices and stock, stir, increase heat to high and bring to a boil. Introduce pot in the oven at 325 degrees F and bake for 5 hours. Take stew out of the oven, leave aside for 10 minutes, take oxtail out of the pot and discard bones. Return meat to pot, add more pepper to the taste, stir, transfer to plates and serve. Enjoy!

Nutritional value: calories 523, fat 38, carbs 12, sugar 6.5, fiber 2.6, protein 28

Paleo Eggplant Stew

It's time to teach you how to make the best paleo eggplant stew! Pay attention!

Servings: 3
Preparation time: 10 minutes
Cooking time: 30 minutes

Ingredients:
- 1 eggplant, chopped
- 1 yellow onion, chopped
- 2 tomatoes, chopped
- 1 teaspoon cumin powder
- A pinch of sea salt
- Black pepper to the taste
- 1 cup tomato paste
- A pinch of cayenne pepper
- ½ cup water

Directions:
Heat up a pan over medium-high heat, add water, tomato paste, a pinch of salt and pepper, cayenne and cumin and stir well. Add the eggplant, tomato, and onion, stir, bring to a boil, reduce heat to medium and cook for 30 minutes. Take stew off heat, add a black pepper if needed, transfer to plates and serve. Enjoy!

Nutritional value: calories 82, fat 0, carbs 16, fiber 1, sugar 0.5, protein 5

Amazing Squash Soup

This will gain your heart for sure! It's amazing and very delicious!

Preparation time: 10 minutes
Cooking time: 50 minutes
Servings: 4

Ingredients:
- 1 butternut squash, cut in halves lengthwise and deseeded
- 14 ounces coconut milk
- A pinch of sea salt
- Black pepper to the taste
- A handful parsley, chopped
- A pinch of nutmeg, ground

Directions:
Place butternut squash halves on a lined baking sheet, place in the oven at 350 degrees F and bake for 45 minutes. Leave squash to cool down, scoop flesh and transfer it to pot. Add half of the coconut milk and blend everything using an immersion blender. Heat this soup up over medium-low heat, add the rest of the coconut milk, a pinch of sea salt, black pepper to the taste, nutmeg and parsley, blend using your immersion blender for a few seconds, cook for about 4 minutes, divide into soup bowls and serve. Enjoy!

Nutritional value: calories 144, fat 10, fiber 2, carbs 7, protein 2

Simple Broccoli Soup

This is an easy and very tasty soup you can make today!

Preparation time: 10 minutes
Cooking time: 20 minutes
Servings: 4

Ingredients:
- 1 yellow onion, chopped
- 2 tablespoons olive oil
- 1 celery stick, chopped
- Zest from ½ lemon
- 1-quart veggie stock
- 17 ounces water
- 1 teaspoon cumin, ground
- 1 broccoli head, florets separated
- Black pepper to the taste
- 3 garlic cloves, minced
- 2 bay leaves
- Juice of ½ lemon
- A pinch of sea salt

For the pesto:
- ½ cup almonds, chopped
- 1 garlic clove
- 2 tablespoons lemon juice
- 2 tablespoons olive oil
- 4 tablespoons green olives, pitted and chopped

Directions:
Heat up a pot with 2 tablespoons olive oil over medium high heat, add onion, lemon zest and a pinch of salt, stir and cook for 3 minutes. Add celery and 3 garlic cloves, stir and cook for 1 minute more. Add stock, cumin, water, and black pepper, stir, cover, bring to a boil and simmer for 10 minutes. Add bay leaves and broccoli, stir, cover again and cook for 6 minutes more. Take soup off the heat, discard bay leaves, transfer to your blender and pulse really well. Add juice from ½ lemon, pulse again, return to the pot and heat up again over medium-low heat. Meanwhile, in your food processor, blend well almond with 1 garlic clove, 2 tablespoon lemon juice, 2 tablespoons olive oil and green olives. Divide soup into bowls, top with the pesto you've just made and serve hot. Enjoy!

Nutritional value: calories 139, fat 2, fiber 1, carbs 4, protein 1

Delicious Gazpacho

This Paleo soup is perfect for a hot summer day!

Preparation time: 10 minutes
Cooking time: 2 minutes
Servings: 4

Ingredients:
- 8 tomatoes
- 1 red onion, chopped
- 1 cucumber, peeled and chopped
- 1 red bell pepper, chopped
- 1 green bell pepper, chopped
- 1 red chili pepper, chopped
- 3 garlic cloves
- 1 cup tomato juice
- 1 cup water
- 2 tablespoon apple cider vinegar
- Zest from ½ orange
- ¾ cup olive oil
- A pinch of sea salt
- Black pepper to the taste

Directions:
Put some water in a pot and bring to a boil over medium high heat. Add tomatoes, leave them in boiling water for 2 minutes, drain and rinse them. Peel, chop and put them in your food processor. Add red onion, cucumber, red bell pepper, green bell pepper, chili pepper, garlic, tomato juice, water, vinegar, orange zest, olive oil, a pinch of salt and black pepper to the taste and pulse really well until you obtain cream. Ladle into soup bowls and serve cold. Enjoy!

Nutritional value: calories 140, fat 1, fiber 1, carbs 3, protein 2

Tasty Veggie Soup

We suggest you try a tasty Paleo veggie soup today! You will love it!

Preparation time: 10 minutes
Cooking time: 15 minutes
Servings: 4

Ingredients:
- 1 yellow onion, chopped
- 2 carrots, chopped
- 6 mushrooms, chopped
- 1 red chili pepper, chopped
- 2 celery sticks, chopped
- 1 tablespoon coconut oil
- A pinch of sea salt
- Black pepper to the taste
- A handful dried porcini mushrooms
- 4 garlic cloves, minced
- 4 ounces kale, chopped
- 1 cup canned tomatoes, chopped
- 1 zucchini, chopped
- 1-quart veggie stock
- 1 bay leaf
- Some lemon zest, grated for serving
- A handful parsley, chopped for serving

Directions:
Set your instant pot on Sauté mode, add oil and heat it up. Add celery, carrots, onion, a pinch of salt and black pepper, stir and cook for 2 minutes. Add chili pepper, garlic, dried mushrooms, and mushrooms, stir and cook for 2 minutes. Add tomatoes, stock, bay leaf, kale and zucchinis, stir, cover pot and cook on High for 10 minutes. Release pressure, stir soup again, ladle into bowls, top with lemon zest and parsley and serve. Enjoy!

Nutritional value: calories 150, fat 2, fiber 2, carbs 4, protein 6

Simple Chicken Soup

It's very easy to make this tasty soup, and it will taste delicious!

Preparation time: 10 minutes
Cooking time: 15 minutes
Servings: 2

Ingredients:
- 1 red bell pepper, chopped
- 1 teaspoon coconut oil
- 1 yellow onion, chopped
- ¼ cup pickled jalapeno peppers, chopped
- 2 garlic cloves, minced
- 1 tablespoon ghee
- 1 teaspoon cumin, ground
- 1 teaspoon coriander, ground
- 1 teaspoon oregano, dried
- 1 and ½ cups chicken breast, cooked and shredded
- 2 and ½ cups chicken stock
- 2 cups kale, torn
- Zest from 1 lime, grated
- Juice from 1 lime
- A pinch of sea salt
- 15 ounces canned tomatoes, chopped
- 2 tablespoons spring onions, chopped
- 3 tablespoons pumpkin seeds, chopped
- 1 avocado, peeled, pitted and sliced
- 1 teaspoon sweet paprika
- 3 tablespoons coriander, chopped

Directions:
Heat up a pot with the oil over medium heat, add onion, stir and cook for 2 minutes. Add red bell peppers, stir and cook for 1 minute. Add garlic, jalapenos, oregano, cumin, coriander, and ghee, stir and cook for 1 minute more. Add tomatoes, kale, chicken, lime zest, stock, lime juice and a pinch of salt, stir, bring to a boil, cook for 5 minutes and take off heat. Heat up a pan over medium heat, add pumpkin seeds, toast them for 2 minutes and take off heat. Ladle soup into bowls, top with pumpkin seeds, green onion, paprika, chopped coriander and avocado and serve. Enjoy!

Nutritional value: calories 170, fat 2, fiber 3, carbs 4, protein 7

Tasty Green Soup

This green soup is so healthy and 100% Paleo!

Preparation time: 10 minutes
Cooking time: 25 minutes
Servings: 6

Ingredients:
- 2 leeks, chopped
- 2 tablespoons ghee
- 4 celery sticks, chopped
- 4 garlic cloves, minced
- 2 broccoli heads, florets separated
- 1 small cauliflower head, florets separated
- 2 handfuls spinach, chopped
- 8 cups veggie stock
- 1 handful parsley, chopped
- 1 tablespoon coconut cream
- A pinch of nutmeg, ground
- Black pepper to the taste

Directions:
Heat up a pot with the ghee over medium heat, add garlic and leeks, stir and cook for 3 minutes. Add broccoli, celery and cauliflower, stir and cook for 5 minutes, Add stock, bring to a boil, cover pot and cook for 15 minutes. Add parsley and spinach, stir and blend using an immersion blender. Add black pepper and nutmeg, stir, ladle soup into bowls and serve with some coconut cream on top. Enjoy!

Nutritional value: calories 103, fat 4, fiber 3, carbs 10, protein 4

Delicious Mushroom Cream

This amazing Paleo soup will impress everyone! Try it!

Preparation time: 10 minutes
Cooking time: 20 minutes
Servings: 4

Ingredients:

- 1 ounce dried porcini mushrooms
- 1 leek, chopped
- 2 tablespoons olive oil
- 1 celery stick, chopped
- 3 garlic cloves, chopped
- 14 brown mushrooms, chopped
- 1 tablespoon thyme, chopped
- 3 cups veggie stock
- 1 sweet potato, peeled and chopped
- 2 bay leaves
- ½ teaspoon Dijon mustard
- 1 teaspoon lemon zest, grated
- ½ teaspoon black pepper
- 1 tablespoon lemon juice
- 3 tablespoons sunflower seed butter

Directions:

Put dried mushrooms in a small bowl, cover with boiling water, leave aside for 10 minutes, strain, reserve water and chop them. Heat up a pot with the oil over medium heat, add celery and leek, stir and cook for 5 minutes. Add mushrooms, thyme, garlic and sweet potatoes, stir and cook for 1 minute. Add dried mushrooms and half of their liquid, stock, bay leaves, mustard, black pepper and lemon zest, stir, cover pot and simmer soup over medium heat for 15 minutes. Discard bay leaves, use an immersion blender to make your mushroom cream, add lemon juice and sunflower seed butter, stir well, ladle into bowls and serve. Enjoy!

Nutritional value: calories 100, fat 2, fiber 1, carbs 4, protein 3

Amazing Seafood Soup

You've never tried something like this before! We can assure you!

Preparation time: 2 hours and 10 minutes
Cooking time: 30 minutes
Servings: 4

Ingredients:

- 1 pound cod fillets, cubed
- 10 garlic cloves, minced
- 3 tablespoons olive oil
- 1 tablespoon lemon juice
- ¼ cup parsley, chopped
- 1 yellow onion, chopped
- 2 tomatoes, chopped
- 1 tablespoon tomato paste
- 2 bay leaves
- 2 and ½ cups water
- A pinch of sea salt
- Black pepper to the taste
- 1 pound shrimp, peeled and deveined
- 10 cherry tomatoes, halved
- 1 pound mussels, scrubbed

Directions:

In a bowl, mix 6 garlic cloves with 2 tablespoons oil, parsley and lemon juice and stir. Add fish cubes, toss to coat, cover bowl and keep in the fridge for 2 hours. Heat up a pot with the rest of the oil over medium high heat, add onion, stir and cook for 2 minutes. Add the rest of the garlic, stir and cook for 1 minute.
Add tomatoes, tomato paste, bay leaves, water, salt, pepper and marinated fish, stir, bring to a simmer and cook for 10 minutes. Add shrimp, cherry tomatoes and mussels, stir and cook for 6 minutes more. Discard unopened mussels, ladle soup into bowls and serve. Enjoy!

Nutritional value: calories 160, fat 2, fiber 2, carbs 4, protein 7

Shrimp and Chicken Soup

The combination is really delicious! Trust us!

Preparation time: 10 minutes
Cooking time: 30 minutes
Servings: 4

Ingredients:
- 5 tablespoons curry paste
- 1 tablespoon coconut oil
- 1 big chicken breast, cut into thin strips
- 4 tablespoons coconut aminos
- 2 cups chicken stock
- Juice from 1 lime
- 1 and ½ cups coconut milk
- 1 pound shrimp, peeled and deveined
- ½ cup coconut cream
- A small broccoli head, florets separated
- 5 Chinese broccoli leaves, chopped
- 1 zucchini, chopped
- 1 carrot, chopped
- 1 cucumber, chopped
- Some chopped cilantro, chopped for serving

Directions:
Heat up a pot with the oil over medium heat, add curry paste, stir and cook for 1 minute. Add chicken, stir and cook for 1 minute more. Add stock and lime juice, stir and cook for 2 minutes. Add coconut cream, aminos and coconut milk, stir and cook for 10 minutes. Add broccoli leaves, broccoli florets and carrots, stir and cook for 3 minutes. Add shrimp and zucchini, stir and cook for 2 minutes. Ladle into bowls, top with cilantro and cucumber pieces and serve. Enjoy!

Nutritional value: calories 160, fat 3, fiber 2, carbs 6, protein 8

Zucchini Soup

You will probably think that this is a very simple soup, but we want you to know that it's so yummy and amazing!

Preparation time: 10 minutes
Cooking time: 20 minutes
Servings: 4

Ingredients:
- 1 onion, chopped
- 3 zucchinis, cut into medium chunks
- 2 tablespoons coconut milk
- 2 garlic cloves, minced
- 4 cups chicken stock
- 2 tablespoons coconut oil
- A pinch of sea salt
- Black pepper to the taste

Directions:
Heat up a pot with the oil over medium heat, add zucchinis, garlic, and onion, stir and cook for 5 minutes. Add stock, salt, pepper, stir, bring to a boil, cover pot, simmer soup for 20 minutes and take off heat. Add coconut milk, blend using an immersion blender, ladle into bowls and serve. Enjoy!

Nutritional value: calories 160, fat 2, fiber 2, carbs 4, protein 7

Coconut and Zucchini Soup

It's an elegant and delightful Paleo soup!

Preparation time: 10 minutes
Cooking time: 15 minutes
Servings: 2

Ingredients:
- 1 brown onion, chopped
- 1 tablespoon coconut oil
- 2 zucchinis, cubed
- A pinch of sea salt
- White pepper to the taste
- 2 teaspoons turmeric powder
- 3 garlic cloves, chopped
- 1 teaspoon curry powder
- 1 cup coconut milk
- 1 cup veggie stock
- 2 tablespoons lime juice
- Some chopped cilantro for serving

Directions:
Heat up a pot with the oil over medium heat, add onion, stir and cook for 4 minutes. Add garlic, salt, pepper, and zucchinis, stir and cook for 1 minute. Add turmeric and curry powder, stir well and cook for 1 minute more. Add coconut milk and stock, stir, bring to a boil, cover pot and simmer soup for 10 minutes. Add lime juice and cilantro, stir, ladle into bowls and serve. Enjoy!

Nutritional value: calories 140, fat 1, fiber 1, carbs 2, protein 1

Delicious Cauliflower Cream

This is one of the most textured and delicious soups you'll ever taste!

Preparation time: 10 minutes
Cooking time: 20 minutes
Servings: 2

Ingredients:
- 1 yellow onion, chopped
- 2 tablespoons olive oil
- 1 cauliflower head, florets separated and chopped
- 3 cups veggie stock
- 3 garlic cloves, minced
- Black pepper to the taste
- A pinch of sea salt
- ¾ cup bacon, chopped
- 1 teaspoon coconut oil
- 1 egg
- 2 tablespoons cilantro, chopped

Directions:
Heat up a pot with the olive oil over medium heat, add onion, stir and cook for 4 minutes. Add stock, cauliflower and garlic, stir and bring to a boil. Reduce heat to medium-low, season with a pinch of salt and black pepper to the taste, cover pot and simmer soup for 10 minutes. Meanwhile, heat up a pan with the coconut oil over medium heat, add bacon, cook until it's crispy, transfer to paper towels, drain grease and leave aside for now. Meanwhile, put water in a pot and bring to a boil. Place a bowl on top of boiling water, crack the egg into the bowl, whisk it for 3 minutes and take off heat. Take your cauliflower soup off the heat, blend it using an immersion blender, add whisked egg and blend some more. Ladle into bowls, sprinkle crumbled bacon and cilantro on top and serve.

Nutritional value: calories 200, fat 3, fiber 2, carbs 4, protein 7

Nettles Soup

You must really give this soup a chance! Try it!

Preparation time: 10 minutes
Cooking time: 20 minutes
Servings: 3

Ingredients:
- 1 tablespoon coconut oil
- 1 cup sweet potato, chopped
- 1 yellow onion, chopped
- ½ broccoli head, florets separated
- ½ cauliflower head, florets separated
- 1 bay leaf
- 3 garlic cloves, minced
- Zest from 1 lemon, grated
- 1 teaspoon Dijon mustard
- 3 and ½ cups veggie stock
- Black pepper to the taste
- A pinch of sea salt
- 4 cups nettles
- Juice of 1 lemon
- 5 thyme springs, leaves separated
- 4 bacon slices, cooked and crumbled
- ½ cup coconut cream

Directions:
Heat up a pot with the coconut oil over medium heat, add sweet potato, onion, broccoli, and cauliflower, stir and cook for 6 minutes. Add bay leaf, garlic, veggie stock, lemon zest, salt, pepper, and mustard, stir and bring to a boil. Reduce heat, cover pot and cook for 10 minutes. Meanwhile, put water in a pot and bring to a boil. Cut nettles leaves with scissors, add leaves to water, leave there for 2 minutes, drain them and transfer them to the pot with the soup. Cook for 3 minutes more, add lemon juice, blend using an immersion blender and then heat up the soup again. Add thyme and coconut cream, stir, cook for 1 minute and ladle into soup bowls. Top with bacon and serve. Enjoy!

Nutritional value: calories 170, fat 2, fiber 2, carbs 2, protein 8

Sweet Potato Soup

Sweet potatoes are allowed on a Paleo diet! So, make this soup today for you and your loved ones!

Preparation time: 10 minutes
Cooking time: 25 minutes
Servings: 2

Ingredients:
- 4 tablespoons olive oil
- 5 garlic cloves, minced
- 1 sweet potato, chopped
- 4 lemon peels
- ½ teaspoon cumin seeds
- Black pepper to the taste
- 14 ounces veggie stock
- A pinch of sea salt
- 4 tablespoons pine nuts

Directions:
Heat up a pot with the oil over medium heat, add garlic, stir and cook for 4 minutes. Add lemon peel, sweet potato, stock, cumin, a pinch of salt and black pepper to the taste, stir, bring to a boil and cook for 15 minutes. Heat up a pan over medium high heat, add pine nuts, stir and cook for 4 minutes. Discard lemon peel from soup, blend it using an immersion blender and mix with half of the pine nuts. Blend again, ladle into bowls and sprinkle the rest of the pine nuts on top. Enjoy!

Nutritional value: calories 150, fat 2, fiber 2, carbs 7, protein 3

Kale and Sausage Soup

This is a Portuguese style Paleo soup! It's very tasty!

Preparation time: 10 minutes
Cooking time: 35 minutes
Servings: 4

Ingredients:
- 1 yellow onion, chopped
- 16 ounces sausage, chopped
- 3 sweet potatoes, chopped
- 4 cups chicken stock
- 1 pound kale, chopped
- A pinch of sea salt and black pepper

Directions:
Heat up a pot over medium heat, add sausage, stir, brown on both sides and transfer to a bowl. Heat up the pot again over medium heat, add onion, stir and cook for 5 minutes. Add stock and sweet potatoes, stir, bring to a simmer and cook for 20 minutes. Use an immersion blender to blend your soup, add kale, a pinch of salt and black pepper and simmer everything for 2 minutes more. Ladle soup into bowls, top with sausage pieces and serve. Enjoy!

Nutritional value: calories 200, fat 2, fiber 2, carbs 6, protein 8

Great Onion Soup

This is a special and elegant French style soup you should try!

Preparation time: 10 minutes
Cooking time: 3 hours
Servings: 4

Ingredients:
- 2 tablespoons avocado oil
- 5 yellow onions, cut into halves and then slice
- Black pepper to the taste
- 5 cups beef stock
- 3 thyme springs
- 1 tablespoon tomato paste

Directions:
Heat up a pot with the oil over medium high heat, add onions and thyme, stir, reduce heat to low, cover and cook for 30 minutes. Uncover the pot and cook onions for 1 hour and 30 minutes more stirring often. Add tomato paste and stock, stir and simmer soup for 1 hour more. Ladle soup into bowls and serve. Enjoy!

Nutritional value: calories 200, fat 4, fiber 4, carbs 6, protein 8

Delicious Clam Soup

Try something really exciting and delicious!

Preparation time: 10 minutes
Cooking time: 30 minutes
Servings: 6

Ingredients:
- 1 small cauliflower head, florets separated
- 2 tablespoons coconut oil
- 2 cups chicken stock
- 2 carrots, chopped
- 1 onion, chopped
- 2 sweet potatoes, chopped
- 20 ounces canned clams
- 1 celery rib, chopped
- 1 cup coconut milk
- A pinch of sea salt
- Black pepper to the taste

Directions:
Heat up a pot with half of the oil over medium high heat, add half of the onion, cauliflower, and stock, stir, bring to a boil and cook for 10 minutes. Use an immersion blender to make cream, transfer this to a bowl and leave aside for now. Heat up the same pot with the rest of the oil over medium high heat, add the rest of the onion, celery, carrot, a pinch of sea salt and black pepper to the taste, stir and cook for 10 minutes. Add potato, 2 cups of the cauliflower cream , stir, bring to a boil and simmer for 10 minutes. Add coconut milk, clams and the rest of the cauliflower cream, stir and cook for 2 minutes more. Ladle into soup bowls and serve. Enjoy!

Nutritional value: calories 250, fat 13, fiber 3, carbs 6, protein 12

Easy Asparagus Soup

An asparagus soup is a real Paleo treat! You'll see!

Preparation time: 10 minutes
Cooking time: 25 minutes
Servings: 3

Ingredients:
- 1 celery stick, chopped
- 1 zucchini, chopped
- 1 yellow onion, chopped
- 2 pounds asparagus, trimmed and roughly chopped
- 2 garlic cloves, minced
- Grated lemon peel from ½ lemon
- Black pepper to the taste
- 2 cups water
- 1 tablespoon olive oil

Directions:
Place asparagus, zucchini, celery, onion, lemon peel and garlic on a lined baking sheet, drizzle the oil, season with black pepper, place in the oven at 400 degrees F and bake for 25 minutes. Transfer these to a food processor, add the water and pulse really well. Transfer soup to a pot and heat up over medium high heat. Ladle into bowls and serve right away. Enjoy!

Nutritional value: calories 160, fat 3, fiber 2, carbs 6, protein 6

Delicious Cucumber Soup

This is a very special Paleo soup you can serve on a hot summer day!

Preparation time: 2 hours and 10 minutes
Cooking time: 0 minutes
Servings: 2

Ingredients:
- 2 cucumbers, chopped
- 1 cup coconut cream
- 1 garlic clove, minced
- 1 tablespoon olive oil
- 3 tablespoons lemon juice
- A pinch of sea salt
- Black pepper to the taste

Directions:
In your food processor, blend cucumber with a pinch of sea salt and black pepper, coconut cream, garlic, oil and lemon juice and pulse really well. Divide into soup bowls and serve cold. Enjoy!

Nutritional value: calories 120, fat 1, fiber 1, carbs 3, protein 1

Tasty Brussels Sprouts Soup

This is light, tasty and super easy to make! What more could you want?

Preparation time: 10 minutes
Cooking time: 20 minutes
Servings: 4

Ingredients:
- 2 tablespoons olive oil
- 1 yellow onion, chopped
- 2 pounds Brussels sprouts, trimmed and halved
- 4 cups chicken stock
- ¼ cup coconut cream
- A pinch of black pepper

Directions:
Heat up a pot with the oil over medium high heat, add onion, stir and cook for 3 minutes. Add Brussels sprouts, stir and cook for 2 minutes. Add stock and black pepper, stir, bring to a simmer and cook for 20 minutes. Use an immersion blender to make your cream, add coconut cream, stir well and ladle into bowls. Serve right away and serve. Enjoy!

Nutritional value: calories 200, fat 11, fiber 3, carbs 6, protein 11

Incredible Turkey Soup

Try this delicious Paleo soup! You won't regret it!

Preparation time: 10 minutes
Cooking time: 30 minutes
Servings: 4

Ingredients:
- 3 and ½ cups chicken stock
- 3 tablespoons coconut oil
- 1 cup coconut cream
- 3 celery stalks, chopped
- 2 carrots, chopped
- 1 sweet potato, peeled and cubed
- 2 cups turkey meat, cooked and shredded
- 1 yellow onion, chopped
- 1 tablespoon sage, chopped
- 1 teaspoon thyme, dried
- A handful parsley, chopped
- Black pepper to the taste
- A pinch of sea salt

Directions:
Heat up a pot with the oil over medium heat, add celery, onions, sweet potato and carrots, stir and cook for 5 minutes. Add stock, a pinch of salt, black pepper to the taste, stir, bring to a simmer and cook for 20 minutes. Add turkey, coconut cream, sage, parsley and thyme, stir, cook for 2 minutes more, ladle into bowls and serve. Enjoy!

Nutritional value: calories 180, fat 3, fiber 2, carbs 3, protein 5

Special Celery Soup

This celery soup will be the best one ever tasted!

Preparation time: 10 minutes
Cooking time: 20 minutes
Servings: 2

Ingredients:
- 2 tablespoons cashews, chopped
- 17 ounces veggie stock
- A pinch of sea salt
- Black pepper to the taste
- 1 and ½ tablespoons olive oil
- 1 yellow onion, chopped
- 13 ounces celery, chopped

Directions:
Heat up a pot with the oil over medium high heat, add onion and celery, stir and cook for 5 minutes. Add stock, a pinch of salt and black pepper to the taste, stir, bring to a simmer and cook for 10 minutes. Add cashews, stir and cook for 5 minutes more. Transfer this to your blender, pulse really well until you obtain cream, divide into bowls and serve. Enjoy!

Nutritional value: calories 150, fat 2, fiber 2, carbs 4, protein 7

Delicious Beef Stew

It's the perfect meal for a cold winter day!

Preparation time: 10 minutes
Cooking time: 2 hours
Servings: 4

Ingredients:

- 2 pounds organic beef steak, cubed
- 1 tablespoon coconut oil
- A pinch of sea salt
- Black pepper to the taste
- 1 red chili pepper, chopped
- 1 yellow onion, chopped
- 1 tablespoon coconut aminos
- ½ cup white wine
- 1 tablespoon lemon juice
- A pinch of nutmeg, ground
- 2 garlic cloves, minced
- 1 teaspoon thyme, dried
- ¼ teaspoon fennel seeds
- 1-star anise
- 1 teaspoon rosemary, dried
- 4 cups beef stock
- 2 carrots, chopped
- 2 celery, sticks, chopped
- 1 and ½ tablespoons arrowroot flour
- 1 sweet potato, chopped
- 6 white mushrooms, chopped

Directions:

Heat up a pot with the oil over medium heat, add onion, stir and cook for 5 minutes. Add a pinch of sea salt, black pepper to the taste and the chili pepper, stir and cook for 1-2 minutes more. Add beef, stir and cook for 5 minutes. Add coconut aminos, wine, lemon juice, garlic, thyme, rosemary, fennel, nutmeg, star anise and stock, stir and bring to a boil. Cover the pot, cook for 1 hour and 15 minutes and then mix with celery, sweet potato, carrots, and mushrooms. Stir, cover pot again and cook for 10 minutes more. Uncover pot, stir and cook everything for 15 minutes. In a bowl, mix 2 tablespoons cooking liquid from the pot with the arrowroot flour and stir very well. Add this to the stew, stir, cook for a couple more minutes, divide into bowls and serve.

Nutritional value: calories 313, fat 7, fiber 3, carbs 10, protein 23

Mexican Stew

Try a different Paleo stew today! We recommend this great Mexican style one!

Preparation time: 10 minutes
Cooking time: 50 minutes
Servings: 4

Ingredients:

- 1 pound beef meat, cubed
- 2 tablespoons avocado oil
- 1 tablespoon garlic, minced
- 1 brown onion, chopped
- 1 bay leaf
- 1 Serrano pepper, chopped
- 1 teaspoon chili powder
- 1 teaspoon cumin, ground
- 1 teaspoon paprika
- Black pepper to the taste
- ½ teaspoon oregano, dried
- ½ teaspoon chipotle powder
- 1 cup chicken stock
- 1 tablespoon tapioca flour
- ½ cup tomato sauce

Directions:

Set you pressure cooker on Sauté mode, add oil, heat it up, add beef, stir and brown for a few minutes on each side. Add garlic, Serrano pepper, onion, bay leaf, black pepper, paprika, chili powder, cumin, oregano and chipotle powder, stir and cook for 4 minutes more. Add stock, tapioca flour and tomato sauce, stir, cover pot and cook on High for 35 minutes. Release the pressure, uncover, stir you stew one more time and serve right away. Enjoy!

Nutritional value: calories 300, fat 12, fiber 3, carbs 6, protein 17

Delightful Pork Stew

A slow cooked Paleo stew is sometimes all you need!

Preparation time: 10 minutes
Cooking time: 8 hours
Servings: 8

Ingredients:
- 2 pounds pork loin, cubed and marinated in some beer in the fridge for 1 day
- 1 tablespoon coconut oil
- 3 garlic cloves, minced
- 1 cup arrowroot flour
- 6 carrots, chopped
- Black pepper to the taste
- A pinch of sea salt
- 2 yellow onions, chopped
- 1 small cabbage head, finely chopped
- 5 small sweet potatoes, chopped
- 30 ounces canned tomatoes, chopped
- 3 cups beef stock

Directions:
In a bowl mix arrowroot flour with marinated pork cubes and rub them well. Heat up a pan with the oil over medium high heat, add pork cubes, brown them on all sides and transfer to your slow cooker. Add garlic, carrots, a pinch of salt, black pepper, onion, cabbage, sweet potatoes, tomatoes and stock, stir, cover pot and cook your stew on Low for 8 hours. Uncover pot, stir stew again, divide into bowls and serve. Enjoy!

Nutritional value: calories 260, fat 6, fiber 4, carbs 7, protein 14

Special and Tasty Beef Stew

This is a special and rather different stew we suggest you try soon!

Preparation time: 10 minutes
Cooking time: 2 hours and 30 minutes
Servings: 4

Ingredients:
- 2 pounds beef meat, cubed
- 3 yellow onions, chopped
- Black pepper to the taste
- 2 tablespoons Moroccan spices
- 1/3 cup ghee
- 2 cups beef stock
- 3 garlic cloves, minced
- 1 lemon, sliced
- Juice of 1 lemon
- Zest from 1 lemon, grated
- 1 butternut squash, peeled, seeded and cubed
- 1 bunch cilantro, chopped

Directions:
Heat up a Dutch oven with the ghee over medium heat, add beef, onions, spices, black pepper, garlic, lemon slices, lemon juice and zest and stock, stir, place in the oven at 300 degrees F and cook for 2 hours. Add cilantro and squash, stir and cook in the oven for 30 minutes more. Divide into bowls and serve. Enjoy!

Nutritional value: calories 300, fat 12, fiber 3, carbs 6, protein 17

Tasty Chorizo Stew

You have got to try this tasty stew!

Preparation time: 10 minutes
Cooking time: 30 minutes
Servings: 3

Ingredients:
- 1 carrot, chopped
- 1 yellow onion, chopped
- 1 tablespoon coconut oil
- 2 chorizo sausages, chopped
- 1 red bell pepper, chopped
- 1 celery stick, chopped
- 2 sweet potatoes, chopped
- 2 garlic cloves, minced
- 1 tomato, chopped
- 2 cups chicken stock
- A handful parsley, chopped
- 1 zucchini, chopped
- 1 tablespoon lemon juice
- A pinch of sea salt
- Black pepper to the taste

Directions:
Heat up a pan with the oil over medium high heat, add carrot, onion, chorizo, and celery, stir and cook for 3 minutes. Add sweet potatoes, garlic, tomato, and red bell pepper, stir and cook for 1 minute more. Add lemon juice, a pinch of salt, black pepper, and stock, stir, cover, bring to a simmer and cook for 10 minutes. Add zucchini, stir and cook for 12 minutes more. Add parsley, stir well, divide into bowls and serve. Enjoy!

Nutritional value: calories 270, fat 8, fiber 3, carbs 5, protein 8

Hearty Meat Stew

This Paleo combination between beef, pork, and lamb is extraordinaire!

Preparation time: 10 minutes
Cooking time: 4 hours
Servings: 8

Ingredients:
- 2 leeks, chopped
- 2 yellow onions, chopped
- 2 bay leaves
- 1 carrot, chopped
- 3 garlic cloves, minced
- 1 and ½ teaspoons thyme, chopped
- 3 cups veggie stock
- 1 tablespoon lemon juice
- 3 tablespoons parsley, chopped
- Black pepper to the taste
- A pinch of sea salt
- 1 pound beef chuck, cubed
- 1 pound pork butt, cubed
- 1 pound lamb shoulder, cubed
- 3 sweet potatoes, cubed
- 1 tablespoon coconut oil
- 3 bacon slices

Directions:
In a Dutch oven, mix leeks with onions, bay leaves, carrot, garlic, thyme, parsley, lemon juice, beef, pork, lamb, a pinch of salt and black pepper to the taste and toss to coat Add oil, potatoes and top with bacon, place in the oven at 350 degrees F and bake for 4 hours. Divide into bowls and serve. Enjoy!

Nutritional value: calories 340, fat 9, fiber 5, carbs 7, protein 15

Exotic Beef Stew

This is so unique and delicious! We love it!

Preparation time: 10 minutes
Cooking time: 8 hours
Servings: 4

Ingredients:
- 2 and ½ pounds beef chuck, cubed
- 3 cups collard greens
- 3 cups water
- 5 green plantains, peeled and cubed
- 3 tablespoons allspice
- ¼ cup garlic powder
- 1/3 cup sweet paprika
- 1 teaspoon cayenne pepper
- 1 teaspoon chili powder

Directions:
In your slow cooker, mix beef with greens, plantains, water, allspice, garlic powder, paprika, cayenne and chili powder, stir well, cover and cook on Low for 8 hours. Keep stirring from time to time. Divide into bowls and serve. Enjoy!

Nutritional value: calories 250, fat 4, fiber 3, carbs 5, protein 9

Beef and Sweet Potatoes Stew

Get ready for a delightful meal! This is the best sweet potatoes and beef stew!

Preparation time: 10 minutes
Cooking time: 35 minutes
Servings: 4

Ingredients:
- 1 red onion, chopped
- 1 tablespoon balsamic vinegar
- 2 tablespoons coconut oil
- A pinch of sea salt
- 1 pound beef, ground
- ¼ cup pine nuts
- 3 garlic cloves, minced
- 2/3 teaspoon ginger, grated
- 1 teaspoon coriander seeds
- 1 teaspoon cumin, ground
- 1 teaspoon paprika
- 3 cups sweet potatoes, peeled and cubed
- 1 and ½ cups veggie stock
- 1 carrot, chopped
- 2/3 cup canned tomatoes, chopped
- ¼ cup parsley, chopped
- Zest from 1 lemon, grated

Directions:
Heat up a pot with the oil over medium heat, add onion and a pinch of salt, stir and cook for 10 minutes. Add vinegar, stir and cook for 1 minute more. Heat up another pan over medium heat, add pine nuts, stir, toast for 2 minutes and transfer to a bowl. Add ginger and meat to onions, stir and cook for 2 minutes. Add garlic, coriander, cumin, and paprika, stir and cook for 2 minutes. Add pine nuts, stock, carrot, tomatoes and lemon zest, stir, cover and cook for 20 minutes. Add parsley, stir, cook for 2 minutes more, divide into bowls and serve. Enjoy!

Nutritional value: calories 200, fat 5, fiber 3, carbs 6, protein 10

Simple Chicken Stew

It's really simple and super delicious!

Preparation time: 10 minutes
Cooking time: 8 hours
Servings: 6

Ingredients:
- 2 carrots, chopped
- 5 garlic cloves, minced
- 2 celery sticks, chopped
- 2 onions, chopped
- 2 sweet potatoes, cubed
- 30 ounces canned pumpkin puree
- 2 quarts chicken stock
- 2 cups chicken meat, skinless, boneless and shredded
- A pinch of sea salt
- Black pepper to the taste
- ¼ teaspoon cayenne pepper
- ¼ cup arrowroot powder
- ½ pound baby spinach

Directions:
In your slow cooker, mix carrots with garlic, celery, onion, sweet potatoes, pumpkin puree, chicken, stock, salt, pepper, cayenne and arrowroot powder, stir, cover and cook on Low for 7 hours and 40 minutes. Uncover slow cooker, add spinach, cover again and cook on Low for 20 minutes more. Divide into bowls and serve. Enjoy!

Nutritional value: calories 280, fat 3, fiber 3, carbs 6, protein 7

Slow Cooked Delicious Stew

It's a slowly cooked delight for you to enjoy on a cold winter day!

Preparation time: 10 minutes
Cooking time: 7 hours
Servings: 4

Ingredients:
- 2 tablespoons olive oil
- 8 carrots, chopped
- 2 parsnips, chopped
- 1 and ½ pounds beef meat, cubed
- 2 bay leaves
- ½ teaspoon peppercorns
- 1 yellow onion, chopped
- ¼ cup tapioca flour
- 1 tablespoon thyme, chopped
- 2 tablespoons water
- 4 cups beef stock
- A pinch of sea salt
- Black pepper to the taste

Directions:
Heat up a pan with the oil over medium high heat, add beef, stir, brown for 4 minutes on all sides and transfer to your slow cooker. Add peppercorns, parsnips, carrots, onion, bay leaves, thyme, stock, a pinch of salt and black pepper, stir, cover and cook on High for 6 hours and 30 minutes. Uncover slow cooker, add tapioca mixed with the water, stir, cover again and cook on High for 30 minutes more. Uncover pot again, discard bay leaves, divide stew into bowls and serve. Enjoy!

Nutritional value: calories 200, fat 5, fiber 3, carbs 4, protein 8

Special Stew

This is a very special and yummy stew you can try today!

Preparation time: 10 minutes
Cooking time: 8 hours
Servings: 6

Ingredients:
- 1 cup carrots, chopped
- 1 cup celery, chopped
- 2 cups onions, chopped
- 3 pounds osso buco, bones in
- 4 garlic cloves, minced
- 6 teaspoons baharat
- A pinch of black pepper
- 2 cups beef stock
- A handful parsley, chopped
- 1 kale, chopped

Directions:
In your slow cooker, mix osso buco with carrots, celery, onions, garlic, baharat, black pepper and stock, stir, cover and cook on Low for 7 hours and 30 minutes. Uncover your slow cooker, add kale and parsley, cover again and cook for 30 minutes more. Divide stew into bowls and serve. Enjoy!

Nutritional value: 340, fat 2, fiber 3, carbs 4, protein 10

Delicious Lamb Stew

This is really something delicious and special! You should get all the ingredients and make it today!

Preparation time: 10 minutes
Cooking time: 1 hour and 50 minutes
Servings: 4

Ingredients:
- 1 and ½ pounds lamb meat, cubed
- 1 tablespoon coconut oil
- 1 small red chili pepper, chopped
- 1 yellow onion, chopped
- 3 garlic cloves, minced
- 2 celery sticks, chopped
- 2 and ½ teaspoons garam masala
- 1 teaspoon fennel seeds
- 1 and ¼ teaspoons turmeric
- 1 and ½ cups coconut milk
- 1 and ½ teaspoons ghee
- 1 and ½ tablespoons tomato paste
- 2 carrots, chopped
- 1 cup water
- A pinch of sea salt
- 1 tablespoon lemon juice
- Chopped parsley for serving

Directions:
Heat up a pot with the oil over medium high heat, add lamb, stir and cook for 4 minutes. Add celery, chili and onion, stir and cook for 1 minute. Reduce heat to medium, add turmeric, garam masala, garlic, ghee and fennel seeds, stir and cook for 2 minutes more. Add tomato paste, coconut milk, water and a pinch of sea salt, stir, bring to a boil, cover and cook for 1 hour. Add carrots, stir, cover pot again and cook for 40 minutes more. Add lemon juice and parsley, stir, divide into bowls and serve hot. Enjoy!

Nutritional value: calories 360, fat 7, fiber 2, carbs 8, protein 20

Roasted Veggie Stew

This is very flavored! It's a delicious Paleo stew we recommend you to try soon!

Preparation time: 10 minutes
Cooking time: 1 hour
Servings: 6

Ingredients:
- 1 garlic head, cloves peeled
- 4 pounds mixed parsnips, carrots, turnips and celery root, peeled and roughly chopped
- ½ cup yellow onion, chopped
- 6 tablespoons olive oil
- 1 tablespoon tomato paste
- 28 ounces canned tomatoes, chopped
- A pinch of sea salt
- Black pepper to the taste
- 2 cups kale, chopped
- 1 teaspoon oregano, dried

Directions:
In a big baking dish, mix root veggies with garlic cloves, half of the oil, a pinch of salt and pepper, toss to coat, place in the oven at 450 degrees F and roast for 45 minutes. Heat up a pan with the rest of the oil over medium high heat, add onion, stir and cook for 3 minutes. Add tomato paste, stir and cook for 1 minute. Add canned tomatoes, oregano and some black pepper, stir, bring to a simmer and cook for a few minute more. Take veggies out of the oven and add them to the pot with the tomatoes. Also, add kale, stir and cook everything for 5 minutes. Divide into bowls and serve. Enjoy!

Nutritional value: calories 200, fat 3, fiber 3, carbs 5, protein 5

French Chicken Stew

This is a Paleo stew you will love and try again for sure!

Preparation time: 10 minutes
Cooking time: 2 hours
Servings: 4

Ingredients:
- 10 garlic cloves
- 2 pounds chicken pieces
- 30 ounces canned tomatoes, chopped
- 30 black olives, pitted and chopped
- 2 cups chicken stock
- 2 tablespoons parsley, chopped
- 2 tablespoons thyme, chopped
- 2 tablespoons basil, chopped
- 2 tablespoons coconut oil
- A pinch of sea salt
- Black pepper to the taste
- 2 tablespoons rosemary, chopped

Directions:
Heat up a pot with the oil over medium high heat, add chicken pieces, season with a pinch of salt and black pepper to the taste, stir and brown them for 2 minutes on each side. Add garlic, stock, thyme, tomatoes, olives, rosemary, basil and parsley, stir, cover, place in the oven at 325 degrees F and bake for 2 hours. Divide into bowls and serve. Enjoy!

Nutritional value: calories 240, fat 10, fiber 4, carbs 6, protein 24

African Stew

Have you ever heard about this great Paleo chicken stew? This is really delicious!

Preparation time: 10 minutes
Cooking time: 45 minutes
Servings: 4

Ingredients:
- 4 chicken thighs
- 1 small brown onion, chopped
- ½ tablespoon coconut oil
- A pinch of sea salt
- Black pepper to the taste
- 1 tablespoon ginger, grated
- 1 tablespoon garlic, minced
- ½ teaspoon paprika
- ½ tablespoon coriander
- ½ teaspoon chili powder
- 2 cloves
- 2 bay leaves
- 1 and ½ cups canned tomatoes, chopped
- 2 and ½ tablespoons cashew butter
- ¼ cup water
- 1 tablespoon parsley, chopped
- ¼ teaspoon vanilla extract

Directions:
Heat up a pan with the oil over medium high heat, add chicken pieces, season with a pinch of salt and black pepper to the taste, stir, brown for 4 minutes on each side and transfer them to a bowl. Heat up the same pan over medium heat, add ginger and onion, stir and cook for 6 minutes. Add garlic, paprika, coriander, bay leaves, cloves and chili powder, stir and cook for 1 minute. Add water, tomatoes and chicken pieces, stir, cover, bring to a boil and simmer for 25 minutes. Take chicken out of the pot, add cashew butter and vanilla, stir and cook for 2 minutes more. Divide chicken into bowls, add stew on top, sprinkle parsley and serve hot. Enjoy!

Nutritional value: calories 200, fat 4, fiber 2, carbs 5, protein 8

Crazy Oxtail Stew

This is insane! It's one of the best and most delicious Paleo stews you'll ever taste!

Preparation time: 10 minutes
Cooking time: 6 hours
Servings: 8
Ingredients:
- 5 pounds oxtail, cut into medium chunks
- 2 celery stick, chopped
- 2 leeks, chopped
- A pinch of sea salt
- Black pepper to the taste
- 2 tablespoons avocado oil
- 3 thyme springs
- 4 carrots, chopped
- 3 rosemary springs
- 2 tablespoons coconut flour
- 4 cloves
- 4 bay leaves
- 28 ounces canned tomatoes, chopped
- 1-quart beef stock

Directions:
Place oxtail in a roasting pan, season with a pinch of salt and black pepper, drizzle half of the avocado oil, rub well, place in the oven at 425 degrees F and roast for 20 minutes. Heat up a pan with the rest of the oil over medium heat, add leeks, carrots, celery, thyme, rosemary, and bay leaf, stir and cook for 20 minutes. Add coconut flour, cloves, tomatoes and stock and stir. Add oxtail, stir, cover pan and cook on low heat for 5 hours. Take oxtail out of the pot, discard bones, return them to the pot, stir, divide into bowls and serve. Enjoy!

Nutritional value: calories 435, fat 23, fiber 3, carbs 7, protein 30

Vietnamese Stew

This is much more delicious than you can imagine!

Preparation time: 30 minutes
Cooking time: 3 hours
Servings: 6

Ingredients:
- 1 lemongrass stalk, chopped
- 2 and ½ pounds organic beef brisket, cut into medium chunks
- 1 and ½ teaspoons curry powder
- 2 and ½ tablespoons ginger, grated
- 2 tablespoons unsweetened applesauce
- 3 tablespoons ghee
- 1 bay leaf
- 1 yellow onion, chopped
- 2-star anise
- 2 cups canned tomatoes, chopped
- 3 cups water
- 1 pound carrots, chopped
- ¼ cup cilantro, chopped
- A pinch of sea salt
- Black pepper to the taste

Directions:
In a bowl, mix applesauce with lemongrass, curry powder, bay leaf, ginger and beef, toss to coat well and leave aside for 30 minutes. Heat up a pot with the ghee over medium high heat, add beef, stir, brown on all sides and transfer to a plate. Add marinade to browned beef and toss again. Return pot to medium heat, add onion, stir and cook for a few minutes. Add a pinch of salt, black pepper and tomatoes, stir and cook for 15 minutes. Add beef and its marinade and star anise, stir and cook for 5 minutes. Add carrots and water, stir, bring to a boil, cover, place in the oven at 300 degrees and bake for 2 hours and 30 minutes. Discard bay leaf and star anise, stir the stew, divide into bowls, sprinkle cilantro on top and serve. Enjoy!

Nutritional value: calories 300, fat 4, fiber 3, carbs 6, protein 12

Special Eggplant Stew

It's a great and fresh Paleo combination you must try!

Preparation time: 10 minutes
Cooking time: 25 minutes
Servings: 3

Ingredients:
- 2 big tomatoes, chopped
- 1 eggplant, chopped
- 1 cup tomato paste
- 1 yellow onion, chopped
- A pinch of cayenne pepper
- 1 teaspoon cumin powder
- A pinch pink salt
- ½ cup water

Directions:
Put the water in a small pot and heat up over medium heat. Add tomato paste, cayenne and a pinch of salt and stir well. Add tomatoes, eggplant and onion, stir and bring to a simmer. Cover the pot and cook the stew for 25 minutes. Divide into bowls and serve. Enjoy!

Nutritional value: calories 170, fat 2, fiber 3, carbs 4, protein 6

Paleo Side Dish Recipes

Paleo Roasted Carrots

All you have to do is to serve this with a roasted beef or pork dish! It's the perfect side dish!

Servings: 4
Preparation time: 10 minutes
Cooking time: 30 minutes

Ingredients:

- 1 and ½ pounds young carrots (yellow, purple and red ones)
- 2 tablespoons balsamic vinegar
- 2 garlic cloves, finely minced
- 2 tablespoons coconut oil, melted
- A pinch of sea salt
- 1 tablespoon honey
- Black pepper to the taste
- A handful parsley leaves, finely chopped

Directions:
In a bowl, mix vinegar with oil, honey, garlic, a pinch of salt, and pepper to the taste and stir very well. Add carrots and toss to coat. Transfer this to a baking dish, introduce in the oven at 400 degrees F and bake for 30 minutes. Take carrots out of the oven, sprinkle parsley on top, toss gently and serve right away as a side dish. Enjoy!

Nutritional value: calories 40, carbs 20, protein 2, fat 6, sugar 1, fiber 1

Paleo Zucchini and Leeks Side Dish

You can use this as a side dish for chicken or fish, but you can also serve it with a hearty stew!

Servings: 4
Preparation time: 10 minutes
Cooking time: 10 minutes

Ingredients:

- 2 leeks, sliced lengthwise
- ¼ cup extra virgin olive oil
- 1/3 cup walnuts, toasted and chopped
- ¼ cup cilantro, chopped
- ¼ cup parsley, chopped
- A pinch of sea salt
- Black pepper to the taste
- Juice of 1 lemon
- 2 garlic cloves, minced
- 2 zucchinis, sliced

Directions:
Season leeks and zucchinis with a pinch of sea salt and pepper to the taste, arrange them on heated grill over medium-high heat and cook them for 8 minutes, flipping them from time to time. Transfer veggies to a bowl, add walnuts, parsley, oil, cilantro, garlic and lemon. Toss to coat and serve as a side dish. Enjoy!

Nutritional value: calories 120, fat 20, carbs 12, sugar 0, fiber 1, protein 4

Paleo Slow Cooked Mushrooms

This tasty side dish goes with a roasted chicken! It's rich and flavored!

Servings: 4
Preparation time: 10 minutes
Cooking time: 4 hours

Ingredients:
- 4 garlic cloves, finely minced
- ¼ teaspoon thyme, dried
- ½ teaspoon basil, dried
- ½ teaspoon oregano, dried
- 24 ounces cremini mushrooms
- 1 bay leaf
- 2 tablespoons parsley leaves, chopped
- ¼ cup coconut milk
- 1 cup veggie stock
- 2 tablespoons ghee
- Black pepper to the taste
- A pinch of sea salt

Directions:
In your slow cooker, mix mushrooms with garlic, basil, oregano, thyme, parsley, and bay leaf. Add coconut milk, ghee, veggie stock, salt and pepper, stir, cover pot and cook on Low for 4 hours. Uncover pot, discard bay leaf, transfer to plates and serve as a side dish. Enjoy!

Nutritional value: calories 100, fat 10, carbs 6, sugar 1, fiber 1, protein 5

Paleo Mashed Cauliflower Dish

This is a side dish that combines perfectly with a beef steak. It's a hearty side dish that will make you so happy!

Servings: 4
Preparation time: 15 minutes
Cooking time: 20 minutes

Ingredients:
- 4 bacon slices, already cooked and crumbled
- 2 garlic cloves, finely chopped
- 6 cups cauliflower florets
- 2 green onions, thinly sliced
- A pinch of sea salt
- Black pepper to the taste
- 3 tablespoons ghee

Directions:
Put water in a pot, place on stove over medium-high heat and bring to a boil. Add cauliflower, cook for 20 minutes, drain water and leave cauliflower in the pot. Add a pinch of salt, pepper to the taste and the ghee and mash everything using a hand mixer. Transfer to plates, sprinkle crumbled bacon and chopped green onions on top and serve as a side dish. Enjoy!

Nutritional value: calories 70, fat 15, carbs 9, sugar 2, fiber 3, protein 7

Paleo Asparagus Side Dish

This healthy side dish goes with delicious pork tenderloin! Try it!

Servings: 4
Preparation time: 10 minutes
Cooking time: 10 minutes

Ingredients:
- ¼ cup caramelized pecans, chopped
- 4 bacon slices, already cooked and crumbled
- 1 and ½ pounds asparagus
- A pinch of sea salt
- Black pepper to the taste
- 2 garlic cloves, minced
- 1 shallot, finely chopped
- ½ teaspoon red chili flakes
- 2 teaspoons mustard
- 1 teaspoon maple syrup
- 2 tablespoons ghee
- 2 teaspoons balsamic vinegar

Directions:
In a bowl, mix vinegar with mustard, maple syrup, sea salt, and pepper to the taste and stir well. Heat up a pan with the ghee over medium high heat, add garlic, shallots and pepper flakes, stir and cook for 2 minutes. Add asparagus, stir and cook for 5 minutes. Add vinegar mix and more pepper, toss to coat and cook for 3 minutes more. Transfer to plates, top with bacon and pecans and serve as a side dish. Enjoy!

Nutritional value: calories 80, fat 4, carbs 4, fiber 2, sugar 0, protein 2

Paleo Butternut Squash Side Dish

This goes with beef or pork dish! It's so simple to make it and so tasty!

Servings: 4
Preparation time: 10 minutes
Cooking time: 40 minutes

Ingredients:
- 2 tablespoons coconut oil
- 1 butternut squash, peeled and chopped
- 3 garlic cloves, finely minced
- 1 tablespoon thyme, chopped
- A pinch of sea salt
- Black pepper to the taste

Directions:
Heat up a pan with the oil over medium-high heat, add garlic, squash, and thyme, stir and cook for 5-6 minutes. Spread well in the pan and cook for another 5 minutes. Reduce heat, cover pan and cook for 10 more minutes, stirring from time to time. Add a pinch of salt and pepper to the taste, stir again, take off heat, transfer to plates and serve as a side dish. Enjoy!

Nutritional value: calories 83, fat 2.4, carbs 16, fiber 3, sugar 3, protein 1.4

Paleo Chard Side Dish

This sautéed side dish is perfect for a chicken or beef main course!

Servings: 2
Preparation time: 10 minutes
Cooking time: 10 minutes
Ingredients:

- ½ cup cashews, chopped
- 1 bunch chard, cut into thin strips
- A pinch of sea salt
- Black pepper to the taste
- 1 tablespoon coconut oil

Directions:
Heat up a pan with the oil over medium heat, add chard and cashews, stir and cook for 10 minutes. Add a pinch of salt and pepper to the taste, stir, cook for 1 minute more, take off heat, transfer to plates and serve as a side dish. Enjoy!
Nutritional value: calories 60, fat 0.3, carbs 2, fiber 1, protein 2, sugar 0

Paleo Roasted Beets

Check out this delicious paleo side dish! Combine it with pork or beef!

Servings: 4
Preparation time: 10 minutes
Cooking time: 1 hour

Ingredients:

- 2 tablespoons extra virgin olive oil
- 6 beets, cut into quarters and then thinly sliced
- A pinch of sea salt
- Black pepper to the taste
- ½ cup balsamic vinegar
- 1 teaspoon orange zest
- 2 teaspoons maple syrup

Directions:
Arrange beets on a lined baking sheet, add a pinch of salt and pepper and the olive oil, toss to coat well, introduce in preheated oven at 325 degrees F and roast for 45 minutes. Heat up a pan over medium heat, add vinegar and maple syrup, stir well, cook until vinegar is reduced and take off heat. Take beets out of the oven, leave them to cool down a bit, transfer to plates, drizzle the glaze on top, sprinkle orange zest and serve right away as a side dish. Enjoy!
Nutritional value: calories 80, fat 1, carbs 8, fiber 2, sugar 7, protein 2

Paleo Roasted Brussels Sprouts

This is a very colored and interesting side dish that will be a perfect addition to a meat-based main course!

Servings: 6
Preparation time: 10 minutes
Cooking time: 30 minutes
Ingredients:

- 1 and ½ pounds Brussels sprouts, cut in halves
- A pinch of sea salt
- Black pepper to the taste
- 1 teaspoon garlic powder
- 2/3 cups pecans, chopped
- 1 cup pomegranate seeds
- 2 tablespoons extra virgin olive oil

Directions:
In a bowl, mix oil with a pinch of sea salt, pepper and garlic powder and stir well. Add Brussels sprouts and pecans and toss to coat. Spread this in lined baking dish, introduce in the oven at 400 degrees F and bake for 30 minutes. Take sprouts out of the oven, transfer to plates, top with pomegranate seeds and serve as a side dish. Enjoy!

Nutritional value: calories 100, fat 1, carbs 10, fiber 4, sugar 1, protein 4

Paleo Sweet Potatoes Dish

You should try this as a side dish for a chicken or pork main course! Trust us!

Servings: 4
Preparation time: 10 minutes
Cooking time: 45 minutes

Ingredients:
- 3 sweet potatoes, pricked with a fork and ends cut off
- A pinch of sea salt
- ½ cup coconut milk
- ¼ cup coconut, toasted and shredded
- 2 tablespoons cilantro, chopped
- Seeds from 1 pomegranate
- 1 lime, cut into wedges

Directions:
Arrange potatoes on a lined baking sheet, introduce in the oven at 400 degrees F and bake for 45 minutes. Take sweet potatoes out of the oven, leave them to cool down, peel and mash them with a fork and put in a bowl. Add a pinch of sea salt, shredded coconut, coconut milk and pomegranate seeds and stir well. Transfer to plates and serve as a side dish. Enjoy!

Nutritional value: calories 160, fat 1, carbs 20, fiber 4, sugar 2, protein 5

Asparagus and Mushrooms Side Dish

You can serve this both with pork or a main fish course! It's really tasty!

Servings: 4
Preparation time: 10 minutes
Cooking time: 10 minutes

Ingredients:
- 1 pound asparagus, trimmed
- A pinch of sea salt
- Black pepper to the taste
- 8 green onions, thinly sliced
- 2 tablespoons coconut oil
- 2 tablespoons red wine vinegar
- 2 tablespoons hazelnuts, toasted and chopped
- 1 pound mushrooms, chopped

Directions:
In a bowl, mix vinegar with a pinch of sea salt, pepper to the taste and half of the oil and whisk well. Put some water in a pot, bring to a boil over medium heat, add asparagus, cook for 3 minutes, drain and transfer to a bowl filled with cold water. Heat up a pan with the rest of the oil over medium-high heat, add mushrooms and cook them for 4-5 minutes stirring from time to time. Add onions, stir and cook for 1 minute. Add drained asparagus, stir, cook 3 more minutes and take off heat. Add vinegar mix, stir and transfer to plates. Sprinkle hazelnuts at the end and serve as a side dish! Enjoy!

Nutritional value: calories 70, fat 2.5, carbs 7, fiber 3.2, sugar 2, protein 5

Paleo Mushrooms and Thyme Side Dish

It's a flavored side dish full of fresh and intense tastes! Why shouldn't you try it today?

Servings: 4
Preparation time: 10 minutes
Cooking time: 25 minutes

Ingredients:
- 4 garlic cloves, finely chopped
- 2 tablespoons extra virgin olive oil
- 8 thyme springs
- 16 ounces mushrooms
- A pinch of sea salt
- White pepper to the taste

Directions:
Grease a baking dish with some of the oil and spread thyme on the bottom. Add mushrooms, garlic, season them with a pinch of salt and pepper to the taste and drizzle the rest of the olive oil all over. Introduce dish in the oven at 375 degrees F and bake for 25 minutes. Take mushrooms out of the oven, divide between plates, pour pan sauces over them and serve as a side dish. Enjoy!

Nutritional value: calories 131, fat 7, carbs 10, fiber 3, sugar 2. protein 8.1

Paleo Roasted Cherry Tomatoes

This is a great side dish that looks just wonderful!

Servings: 4
Preparation time: 5 minutes
Cooking time: 20 minutes

Ingredients:
- 2 tablespoons extra virgin olive oil
- 20 ounces colored cherry tomatoes, cut in halves
- 6 garlic cloves, finely minced
- A pinch of sea salt
- Black pepper to the taste
- 1 tablespoon basil leaves, finely chopped

Directions:
In a large bowl, mix tomatoes with a pinch of sea salt, pepper to the taste, olive oil, garlic and basil and toss to coat. Spread these on a lined baking dish, introduce in the oven at 375 degrees F and bake for 20 minutes. Take tomatoes out of the oven, leave them to cool down, divide to plates and serve as a side dish for a frittata for example. Enjoy!

Nutritional value: calories 35, fat 2.4, carbs 2, fiber 0.4, sugar 0, protein 0.4

Paleo Sautéed Spinach Dish

This side dish goes with a chicken or fish main course! It is so tasty!

Servings: 3
Preparation time: 10 minutes
Cooking time: 33 minutes

Ingredients:
- 3 cups spinach, torn
- 3 yellow onions, sliced
- 3 garlic cloves, finely minced
- A pinch of sea salt
- Black pepper to the taste
- 10 mushrooms, sliced
- 1 tablespoon coconut oil
- 1 tablespoon balsamic vinegar
- 1 tablespoon ghee

Directions:
Heat up a pan with the oil and ghee over medium-high heat, add garlic and onions, stir and cook for 10 minutes. Reduce temperature to low and cook onions for 20 minutes, stirring from time to time. Add vinegar, mushrooms, salt and pepper, stir and cook for 10 minutes. Add spinach, stir, cook for 3 minutes more, take off heat, divide among plates and serve. Enjoy!

Nutritional value: calories 89, fat 7, carbs 3.7, fiber 1.4, sugar 0.3, protein 2

Paleo Mashed Carrots

There are many interesting and delicious side dishes out there, but this is one of the most amazing ones!

Servings: 4
Preparation time: 6 minutes
Cooking time: 20 minutes

Ingredients:
- 1 pound rutabaga, peeled and chopped
- A pinch of sea salt
- Black pepper to the taste
- 4 tablespoons ghee
- 1 pound carrots, chopped
- 1 tablespoon parsley, chopped

Directions:
Put rutabaga and carrots in a pot, add water to cover, place on stove, bring to a boil over medium-high heat, reduce temperature, cover pot and cook for 20 minutes. Drain carrots and rutabaga, transfer them to a bowl, mash with a potato masher, mix with ghee, a pinch of salt and pepper to the taste, stir well and divide among plates. Sprinkle parsley on top and serve as a side dish. Enjoy!

Nutritional value: calories 100, fat 1, carbs 11, fiber 3.5, sugar 3, fiber 1.4

Paleo Roasted Bell Peppers

Are you having some trouble finding a new paleo side dish for the main fish course? Why don't you try this one?

Servings: 4
Preparation time: 10 minutes
Cooking time: 1 hour

Ingredients:
- 6 bell peppers (green, yellow and red)
- 1 garlic clove, finely minced
- 2 tablespoon capers
- 2 tablespoons extra virgin olive oil
- ¼ cup red wine vinegar
- A pinch of sea salt
- Black pepper to the taste
- 2 tablespoons parsley, finely chopped

Directions:
Arrange bell peppers on a lined baking sheet, introduce them in the oven at 400 degrees F and bake for 40 minutes. Transfer bell peppers to a bowl, cover and leave them aside for 15 minutes. Peel bell peppers, discard seeds, cut into strips and transfer them to a bowl. Add a pinch of sea salt and pepper to the taste, vinegar, oil, garlic, capers and parsley and toss to coat. Divide between plates and serve as a side dish. Enjoy!

Nutritional value: calories 98, fat 1, carbs 10, fiber 3, sugar 2, protein 2

Paleo French Fries

Who doesn't love French fries? That's why we recommend you the paleo version of French fries!

Servings: 3
Preparation time: 10 minutes
Cooking time: 30 minutes

Ingredients:
- 2 pounds sweet potatoes, cut into wedges
- A pinch of sea salt
- Black pepper to the taste
- ¼ cup ghee
- 3 teaspoons thyme and rosemary, dried

Directions:
In a bowl, mix potato wedges with ghee, a pinch of salt and pepper to the taste and dried herbs and toss to coat. Spread potatoes on a lined baking sheet and bake in the oven at 425 degrees F for 25 minutes. Take potatoes out of the oven, leave them aside for 5 minutes, divide between plates and serve as a side dish. Enjoy!

Nutritional value: calories 120, carbs 12, fiber 4, sugar 1, protein 12

Paleo Roasted Cabbage Side Dish

It really goes with the main pork course! It's one of the best cabbage side dishes ever!

Servings: 4
Preparation time: 10 minutes
Cooking time: 30 minutes

Ingredients:
- 1 green cabbage head, cut into medium wedges
- A pinch of sea salt
- Black pepper to the taste
- A pinch of red chili flakes
- A pinch of garlic powder
- 2 tablespoons extra virgin olive oil
- Juice from 2 lemons

Directions:
Brush cabbage wedges with olive oil, season with a pinch of sea salt and pepper to the taste, sprinkle garlic powder and pepper flakes and arrange them on a lined baking sheet. Introduce in preheated oven at 450 degrees F and bake for 15 minutes. Flip cabbage wedges, bake for 15 more minutes, take out of the oven and divide them between plates. Serve as a side dish with lemon juice squeezed on top. Enjoy!

Nutritional value: calories 67, fat 6, carbs 1, fiber 2, protein 0, sugar 0

Delicious Roasted Okra

It's a great and delicious addition to any main course! It will fascinate you!

Servings: 3
Preparation time: 10 minutes
Cooking time: 25 minutes

Ingredients:
- 18 okra pods, sliced
- A pinch of sea salt
- Black pepper to the taste
- Sweet paprika to the taste
- 1 tablespoon extra virgin olive oil

Directions:
Put okra in a baking dish, season with, paprika, a pinch of salt, and pepper to the taste and drizzle olive oil. Introduce in preheated oven at 425 degrees F and bake for 15 minutes. Take okra out of the oven, leave them to cool down, divide between plates and serve as a side dish. Enjoy!

Nutritional value: calories 76, fat 0.8, carbs 16, fiber 7.3, sugar 2.7, protein 4.6

Paleo Grilled Artichokes

This is a very healthy paleo side dish! Try it soon for you and all your loved ones! You will enjoy it for sure!

Servings: 4
Preparation time: 10 minutes
Cooking time: 30 minutes

Ingredients:
- Juice of 1 lemon
- A pinch of sea salt
- Black pepper to the taste
- 2 artichokes, trimmed and cut into halves lengthwise
- 4 garlic cloves, chopped
- ¾ cup extra virgin olive oil

Directions:
Put water in a bowl, add half of the lemon juice and artichoke halves and leave aside for now. Put water in a bowl, place on stove over medium high heat, bring to a boil, add artichokes, cook for 15 minutes and drain them. Put artichokes in a bowl, add the rest of the lemon juice, the oil, a pinch of salt, black pepper to the taste and garlic and toss to coat. Drain artichokes and reserve lemon dressing, arrange them on preheated grill over medium-high heat, grill them for 10 minutes and transfer them to a plate. Serve as a side dish with the reserved dressing drizzled on top. Enjoy!

Nutritional value: calories 119, fat 3.8, carbs 23, fiber 11.4, protein 6.1

Delicious Mashed Sweet Potatoes

This is a simple and very tasty Paleo side dish you can try whenever you want!

Preparation time: 10 minutes
Cooking time: 1 hour and 15 minutes
Servings: 6

Ingredients:
- ¼ cup coconut oil
- 3 pounds sweet potatoes
- A pinch of sea salt
- Black pepper to the taste

Directions:
Wash sweet potatoes and arrange them on a lined baking sheet. Place in the oven at 375 degrees F and bake them for 1 hour. Leave potatoes to cool down, peel and transfer flesh to a baking dish. Mash them well, add oil and stir very well. Also, add a pinch of salt and black pepper to the taste, stir well again and bake in the oven at 375 degrees F for 15 minutes more. Divide between plates and serve as a side dish. Enjoy!

Nutritional value: calories 240, fat 1, fiber 4, carbs 6, protein 4

Amazing Roasted Beets

This is really impressive and delicious!

Preparation time: 10 minutes
Cooking time: 1 hour
Servings: 4

Ingredients:
- 2 tablespoons balsamic vinegar
- 8 beets, cut in quarters
- 1 tablespoon melted coconut oil
- ¼ teaspoon truffle salt

Directions:
In a bowl, mix beets with vinegar, oil and truffle salt, toss to coat well and spread them on a lined baking sheet. Introduce beets in the oven at 350 degrees F and roast them for 1 hour. Divide beets between plates and serve them. Enjoy!

Nutritional value: calories 150, fat 3, fiber 3, carbs 5, protein 10

Simple Kale Dish

This is very nutritious, and everyone should try it every once in a while.

Preparation time: 10 minutes
Cooking time: 8 minutes
Servings: 4
Ingredients:
- 3 ounces bacon, chopped
- 1 bunch kale, roughly chopped
- ½ cup veggie stock
- 1 tablespoon lemon juice
- 1 garlic clove, minced
- Black pepper to the taste

Directions:
Put bacon in a pan and heat it up over medium high heat. Cook for 3 minutes, stirring all the time. Add kale, stock, and black pepper to the taste, stir and cook for 4 minutes. Add lemon juice and garlic, stir, cook for 1 minute more, divide between plates and serve as a side dish. Enjoy!
Nutritional value: calories 150, fat 5, fiber 2, carbs 4, protein 3

Delicious Pumpkin Fries

If you are on a Paleo diet, you should really try this dish!

Preparation time: 10 minutes
Cooking time: 35 minutes
Servings: 4
Ingredients:
- 1 big pumpkin, peeled and cut in medium fries
- 1 tablespoon sriracha sauce
- 1 tablespoon maple syrup
- 1 tablespoon coconut oil, melted

Directions:
Drizzle the oil on a lined baking sheet, add pumpkin fries and toss them well. Add maple syrup and sriracha, toss to coat well again, place in the oven at 400 degrees F and bake for 35 minutes. Divide pumpkin fries between plates and serve them as a Paleo side dish. Enjoy!
Nutritional value: calories 60, fat 2, fiber 1, carbs 1, protein 1

Delicious Pumpkin and Bok Choy

This Paleo side dish is going to make you ask for more! It's really great!

Preparation time: 10 minutes
Cooking time: 15 minutes
Servings: 4
Ingredients:
- 2 teaspoons sesame oil
- 2 tablespoons olive oil
- 3 tablespoons coconut aminos
- 1 inch ginger, grated
- A pinch of red pepper flakes
- 4 bok choy heads, cut in quarters
- 2 garlic cloves, minced
- 1 small pumpkin, peeled, seeded and thinly sliced
- 1 tablespoon sesame seeds, toasted

Directions:
Heat up a pan with the sesame and olive oil over medium heat, add coconut aminos, garlic, pepper flakes and ginger, stir, cook for 1 minute and take off heat. Heat up another pan, add some water, bring to a simmer over medium high heat, add pumpkin pieces, cover and cook them for 10 minutes. Drain pumpkin slices really well and transfer them to a platter. Add bok choy to the pan with the water, heat it up again over medium high heat, cover and cook for 5 minutes. Drain this as well and add to the same platter with the pumpkin. Add sesame oil mix from the pan, add sesame seeds as well, toss everything and serve as a side dish. Enjoy!
Nutritional value: calories 160, fat 2, fiber 2, carbs 4, protein 5

Creamy Mashed Pumpkin

This rich and very creamy Paleo side dish is just what you were looking for!

Preparation time: 10 minutes
Cooking time: 45 minutes
Servings: 4

Ingredients:
- 1 teaspoon cinnamon powder
- 1 cup unsweetened coconut, shredded
- 1 pumpkin, peeled, seeded and cubed
- ½ cup coconut oil
- A pinch of white pepper
- A pinch of sea salt

Directions:
Put water in a pot, add pumpkin cubes, heat up over medium high heat, cover and cook for 30 minutes. Drain water, add a pinch of salt and pepper, oil and coconut to the pan, stir and cook everything for 3 minutes more. Mash using a potato masher, add cinnamon, stir well, cook for 2 minutes more, divide between plates and serve. Enjoy!

Nutritional value: calories 100, fat 2, fiber 2, carbs 3, protein 3

Simple Pumpkin Salad

This is a fresh and tasty side salad you just need to try!

Preparation time: 10 minutes
Cooking time: 30 minutes
Servings: 6

Ingredients:
- 1 tablespoon honey + 2 teaspoons honey
- 2 tablespoons olive oil + 2 teaspoons olive oil
- 21 ounces pumpkin, peeled, seeded and cut into medium pieces
- 2 teaspoons sesame seeds
- 1 tablespoon lemon juice
- 2 teaspoons mustard
- 4 ounces baby spinach
- 2 tablespoons pine nuts, toasted
- A pinch of sea salt
- Black pepper to the taste

Directions:
In a bowl, mix pumpkin with a pinch of salt, black pepper, 2 teaspoons oil and 2 teaspoons honey, toss to coat well, spread on a lined baking sheet, place in the oven at 400 degrees F and bake for 25 minutes. Leave pumpkin pieces to cool down a bit, add sesame seeds, toss to coat, place in the oven again and bake for 5 minutes more. In a bowl, mix lemon juice with 1 tablespoon honey, 2 tablespoon oil and mustard and stir well. Leave pumpkin to completely cool down and transfer it to a salad bowl. Add baby spinach and pine nuts and stir. Add salad dressing you've made, toss to coat well, divide between plates and serve as a side salad. Enjoy!

Nutritional value: calories 220, fat 10, fiber 2, carbs 7, protein 6

Amazing Turnips and Sauce

This incredible turnips dish is superb!

Preparation time: 10 minutes
Cooking time: 15 minutes
Servings: 4

Ingredients:
- 1 tablespoon lemon juice
- Zest from 2 oranges
- 16 ounces turnips, thinly sliced
- 3 tablespoons coconut oil
- 1 tablespoon rosemary, chopped
- A pinch of sea salt
- Black pepper to the taste

Directions:
Heat up a pan with the oil over medium high heat, add turnips, stir and cook for 4 minutes. Add lemon juice, a pinch of salt, black pepper, and rosemary, stir and cook for 10 minutes more. Take off heat, add orange zest, stir, divide between plates and serve. Enjoy!

Nutritional value: calories 90, fat 1, fiber 2, carbs 3, protein 4

Great Fennel Side Dish

This is so flavored and rich! Enjoy it as a Paleo side anytime!

Preparation time: 10 minutes
Cooking time: 0 minutes
Servings: 4

Ingredients:
- 3 tablespoons lemon juice
- 1 pound fennel, chopped
- A pinch of sea salt
- 2 tablespoons olive oil
- A pinch of black pepper

Directions:
In a salad bowl, mix fennel with a pinch of salt and black pepper and stir. In another bowl, mix oil with a pinch of salt, pepper and lemon juice and whisk well. Add this to the salad bowl, toss to coat well and divide between plates. Serve as a Paleo side. Enjoy!

Nutritional value: calories 100, fat 1, fiber 1, carbs 1, protein 3

Plantain Fries

You've got to try this amazing and very simple side today!

Preparation time: 10 minutes
Cooking time: 10 minutes
Servings: 4

Ingredients:
- ½ cup duck fat
- 2 green plantains, peeled and sliced
- A pinch of sea salt
- Black pepper to the taste

Directions:
Heat up a pan with the duck fat over medium high heat, season plantain slices with a pinch of salt and black pepper, add half of them to the pan, cook for 5 minutes and transfer to paper towels. Fry the second batch of plantain slices, drain grease as well, divide them between plates and serve them as a side. Enjoy!

Nutritional value: calories 120, fat 2, fiber 2, carbs 4, protein 3

Roasted Broccoli

This is very healthy and extremely easy to make at home!

Preparation time: 10 minutes
Cooking time: 30 minutes
Servings: 4

Ingredients:
- 8 garlic cloves, minced
- ¼ cup avocado oil
- 8 cups broccoli florets
- Zest from 1 lemon, grated
- ¼ cup parsley, chopped
- Black pepper to the taste
- A pinch of sea salt

Directions:
In a bowl, mix broccoli with salt, pepper, oil, garlic and lemon zest, toss to coat, spread on a lined baking sheet, place in the oven at 450 degrees F and bake for 30 minutes. Take baked broccoli out of the oven, divide between plates, sprinkle parsley on top and serve as a side. Enjoy!

Nutritional value: calories 120, fat 1, fiber 2, carbs 3, protein 6

Incredible Side Salad

This is all you need! It's a great Paleo side dish!

Preparation time: 10 minutes
Cooking time: 0 minutes
Servings: 2

Ingredients:
- 2 cups arugula
- 1 tablespoon olive oil
- 1 tablespoon balsamic vinegar
- 2 cups kale, torn
- 3 tablespoons red onion, chopped
- 4 kumquats, sliced
- 1 small avocado, pitted, peeled and cubed
- 3 figs, chopped
- ½ cup walnuts, chopped

Directions:
In a bowl, mix vinegar with the oil, whisk well and leave aside for now. In a salad bowl, mix arugula with kale, onion, kumquats, avocado, figs, and walnuts and stir. Add salad dressing, toss to coat and serve. Enjoy!

Nutritional value: calories 100, fat 1, fiber 0, carbs 0, protein 4

Simple Brussels Sprouts Side Dish

Brussels sprouts are always a great option for a Paleo side dish!

Preparation time: 10 minutes
Cooking time: 30 minutes
Servings: 4

Ingredients:
- ¼ cup avocado oil
- 4 pounds Brussels sprouts, cut in quarters
- A pinch of sea salt
- Black pepper to the taste

Directions:
In a bowl, mix Brussels sprouts with oil, salt, and pepper, toss to coat well, spread on a lined baking sheet, place in the oven at 375 degrees F and bake for 30 minutes. Divide between plates and serve as a Paleo side dish! Enjoy!

Nutritional value: calories 120, fat 1, fiber 1, carbs 2, protein 5

Tasty Veggie Mix

Try this colored and rich Paleo side today!

Preparation time: 10 minutes
Cooking time: 1 hour and 30 minutes
Servings: 8

Ingredients:
- 1 pound yellow squash, peeled and chopped
- 1 yellow onion, chopped
- 3 tablespoons olive oil
- 2 garlic cloves, minced
- 2 cups chicken stock
- 4 pounds mixed sweet potatoes, parsnips and carrots, chopped
- 1 cup white wine
- A pinch of black pepper

Directions:
Heat up a pan with half of the oil over medium high heat, add onion, stir, cook for 10 minutes and transfer to a baking dish. Add the rest of the oil to the pan and heat up again over medium heat. Add squash, stir and cook for 10 minutes more. Add garlic, stir and cook for 2 minutes. Add stock, wine and a pinch of black pepper, stir, cook for 10 minutes more, transfer to a blender and pulse really well. Spread this over sautéed onions from the baking dish, also add mixed veggies, toss a bit, place in the oven at 400 degrees F and bake for 1 hour. Divide between plates and serve warm as a side dish. Enjoy!

Nutritional value: calories 230, fat 4, fiber 4, carbs 6, protein 12

Tapioca Root Fries

If you are a fan of French fries but you are on a Paleo diet, then you should try these fries instead!

Preparation time: 10 minutes
Cooking time: 1 hour
Servings: 4

Ingredients:
- 2 and ½ pound tapioca root, cut in medium fries
- ½ cup duck fat, soft
- Black pepper to the taste
- A pinch of smoked paprika

Directions:
Put some water in a pot and bring to a boil over medium high heat. Add tapioca fries, boil for 10 minutes and drain them well. Spread them on a lined baking sheet, add black pepper, paprika, and duck fat, toss everything to coat well, place in the oven at 375 degrees F and bake for 45 minutes. Leave your tapioca fries to cool down a bit, divide them between plates and serve as a side. Enjoy!

Nutritional value: calories 120, fat 2, fiber 2, carbs 4, protein 10

Amazing Side Dish

This is a unique and delicious Paleo side dish that everyone will like for sure!

Preparation time: 10 minutes
Cooking time: 1 hour
Servings: 4

Ingredients:
- 6 cups cauliflower florets
- 1 and ½ pounds turnips, thinly sliced
- 1 egg
- 2 cups chicken stock
- ¼ cup avocado oil
- A pinch of sea salt
- Black pepper to the taste

Directions:
Put stock in a pot, bring to a simmer over medium high heat, add cauliflower, stir, cover and cook for 15 minutes. Transfer this to your food processor and blend well. Add oil and blend well again. In a bowl, whisk the egg with 1 tablespoon of the cauliflower mix. Add this to cauliflower and pulse again well. Add a pinch of salt and pepper and stir again. Arrange turnips slices into a baking dish, pour the cauliflower purée over them, place in the oven at 375 degrees F and bake for 30 minutes. Divide between plates and serve. Enjoy!

Nutritional value: calories 230, fat 3, fiber 2, carbs 4, protein 6

Delicious Roasted Green Beans

Green beans are always an excellent choice for a side dish!

Preparation time: 10 minutes
Cooking time: 20 minutes
Servings: 4

Ingredients:
- 1 and ½ pounds green beans
- 2 tablespoons lemon juice
- A pinch of sea salt
- 3 tablespoons avocado oil

Directions:
In a bowl, mix green beans with a pinch of salt, oil and lemon juice, toss to coat well, spread on a lined baking sheet, place in the oven at 450 degrees F and roast for 20 minutes. Leave green beans to cool down a bit, divide them between plates and serve. Enjoy!

Nutritional value: calories 100, fat 3, fiber 1, carbs 4, protein 9

Delicious Roasted Cauliflower

You should always try new things! This Paleo side dish is one of them!

Preparation time: 10 minutes
Cooking time: 30 minutes
Servings: 4

Ingredients:
- 1 cauliflower head, florets separated
- ¼ cup coconut oil, melted
- ¼ cup parsley, chopped
- 2 teaspoons lemon zest, grated
- A pinch of sea salt and black pepper
- 10 garlic cloves, minced

Directions:
Spread cauliflower florets on a lined baking sheet, add oil and toss to coat. Add a pinch of salt and black pepper, garlic, and lemon zest, toss again to coat well, place in the oven at 450 degrees F and bake for 30 minutes. Take cauliflower out of the oven, sprinkle parsley on top, stir gently, divide between plates and serve. Enjoy!

Nutritional value: calories 100, fat 1, fiber 2, carbs 4, protein 12

Special Plantain Mash

As you can see, you have a lot of options when it comes to Paleo sides!

Preparation time: 10 minutes
Cooking time: 30 minutes
Servings: 4

Ingredients:
- 6 ounces bacon, chopped
- 3 green bananas, peeled, cut in halves lengthwise and cut in semi-circles
- 4 garlic cloves, minced
- 1 yellow onion, chopped
- 2 tablespoons coconut oil
- A pinch of sea salt

Directions:
Put water in a pot, bring to a boil over medium high heat, add plantain slices, cover and cook them for 20 minutes. Drain plantains and leave them aside for now. Heat up a pan over medium high heat, add bacon, stir and cook for 5 minutes. Add garlic and onion, stir, cook for 5 minutes more, drain excess grease and transfer everything to a blender. Add plantains and 2 tablespoons oil and pulse really well. Add a pinch of sea salt, blend again, divide between plates and serve. Enjoy!

Nutritional value: calories 200, fat 1, fiber 4, carbs 6, protein 2

Amazing Poached Kohlrabi Dish

This is just amazing! Try it right away!

Preparation time: 10 minutes
Cooking time: 17 minutes
Servings: 3

Ingredients:
- 4 tablespoons ghee
- 3 kohlrabi, peeled and cubed
- 1 tablespoon sage, chopped
- A pinch of sea salt and black pepper

Directions:
Heat up a pan with the ghee over medium high heat, add kohlrabi, a pinch of salt and black pepper, stir and cook for 15 minutes. Add sage, stir again, cook for 2 minutes more, divide between plates and serve. Enjoy!

Nutritional value: calories 120, fat 2, fiber 1, carbs 2, protein 5

Delightful Spaghetti Squash

This light Paleo side dish is just so tasty!

Preparation time: 10 minutes
Cooking time: 55 minutes
Servings: 4

Ingredients:
- 1 spaghetti squash, cut in halves and seeded
- 12 sage leaves
- 3 tablespoons ghee
- A pinch of sea salt
- Black pepper to the taste

Directions:
Place spaghetti squash on a lined baking sheet, place in the oven at 375 degrees F and bake for 40 minutes. Take spaghetti squash out of the oven and scoop strings of flesh. Heat up a pan with the ghee over medium heat, add sage, cook for 5 minutes and transfer them to paper towels. Heat up the pan again over medium heat, add spaghetti squash, a pinch of sea salt and black pepper to the taste, stir and cook for 3 minutes. Crumble sage leaves, add them to spaghetti, stir, divide between plates and serve as a side. Enjoy!

Nutritional value: calories 100, fat 6, fiber 2, carbs 6, protein 2

Incredibly Tasty Butternut Squash

This tastes delicious, and it looks great too!

Preparation time: 10 minutes
Cooking time: 35 minutes
Servings: 6

Ingredients:
- 2 tablespoons coconut oil, melted
- 2 pounds butternut squash, peeled, seeded and cubed
- 2 teaspoons thyme, chopped
- A pinch of black pepper

Directions
In a bowl, mix squash cubes with oil, thyme, and pepper and toss to coat well. Spread this on a lined baking sheet, place in the oven at 425 degrees F and bake for 35 minutes, stirring every once in a while. Leave roasted squash pieces to cool down, divide between plates and serve as a Paleo side. Enjoy!

Nutritional value: calories 100, fat 1, fiber 2, carbs 3, protein 6

Amazing Butternut Squash Mix

This is a genius Paleo side dish!

Preparation time: 10 minutes
Cooking time: 30 minutes
Servings: 4

Ingredients:
- ½ teaspoon cinnamon powder
- 2 tablespoons red palm oil
- 2 apples, peeled, cored and cubed
- 1 green plantain, peeled and cubed
- 1 and ½ pounds butternut squash, peeled, seeded and cubed

Directions:
In a baking dish, mix apples with plantain, squash, cinnamon, and oil, toss to coat, place in the oven at 350 degrees F and roast for 30 minutes. Leave this mix to cool down a bit before dividing on plates and serving. Enjoy!

Nutritional value: calories 100, fat 2, fiber 2, carbs 4, protein 10

Great Stir Fried Side Dish

Get all the ingredients and make this tasty Paleo side today!

Preparation time: 10 minutes
Cooking time: 15 minutes
Servings: 4

Ingredients:
- 1 teaspoon ginger, grated
- 1 pound white mushrooms, sliced
- 1 bunch turnip greens, trimmed
- 2 garlic cloves, minced
- Black pepper to the taste
- A pinch of sea salt
- ½ cup raw almonds
- ¼ cup lime juice
- 2 tablespoons coconut oil, melted
- 1 tablespoon coconut aminos
- 2 teaspoons arrowroot flour

Directions:
Heat up a pan with the oil over medium high heat, add mushrooms and turnips greens, stir and cook for 2 minutes. Add ginger and garlic, stir and cook for 2 minutes more. Add lime juice, almonds, arrowroot, coconut aminos, a pinch of salt and black pepper, stir and cook for 10 minutes more. Stir your mix again, divide it between plates and serve. Enjoy!

Nutritional value: calories 120, fat 2, fiber 2, carbs 4, protein 5

Flavored Taro Dish

This is one of the best side dishes ever!

Preparation time: 10 minutes
Cooking time: 25 minutes
Servings: 4

Ingredients:
- 2 teaspoons rosemary, dried
- 2 pounds taro
- 3 tablespoons coconut oil
- ½ teaspoon garlic powder
- A pinch of sea salt
- Black pepper to the taste

Directions:
Put taro in a steamer, steam for 15 minutes, leave them to cool down, peel them and cut into quarters. Heat up a pan with the oil over medium high heat, add taro, rosemary, garlic powder, salt, and pepper, toss to coat and place in preheated broiler. Broil for 10 minutes, divide between plates and serve as a Paleo side dish. Enjoy!

Nutritional value: calories 120, fat 3, fiber 2, carbs 4, protein 7

Delicious Stuffed Artichokes

Serve with a tasty steak and that's it!

Preparation time: 10 minutes
Cooking time: 1 hour and 10 minutes
Servings: 4

Ingredients:
- 4 artichokes, stems cut off and hearts chopped
- 3 garlic cloves, minced
- 2 cups spinach, chopped
- 1 tablespoon coconut oil
- 1 yellow onion, chopped
- 4 ounces bacon, chopped, cooked and crumbled
- A pinch of black pepper

Directions:
Put artichokes in a pot, add water to cover, bring to a boil over medium heat, cook for 30 minutes, drain them and leave them aside to cool down. Heat up a pan with the oil over medium high heat, add onion, stir and cook for 10 minutes. Add spinach, stir, cook for 3 minutes, take off heat and leave aside to cool down. Put cooked bacon in your food processor, add artichoke insides as well and pulse really well. Add this to spinach and onion mix and stir well everything. Place artichoke cups on a lined baking sheet, stuff them with spinach mix, place in the oven at 375 degrees F and bake for 30 minutes. Arrange them on plates and serve as a side with a juicy steak. Enjoy!

Nutritional value: calories 200, fat 3, fiber 2, carbs 6, protein 8

Ginger Cauliflower Rice

This is the perfect side dish for a meat-based main course!

Preparation time: 10 minutes
Cooking time: 10 minutes
Servings: 4

Ingredients:
- 5 cups cauliflower florets
- 3 tablespoons coconut oil
- 4 ginger slices, grated
- 1 tablespoon coconut vinegar
- 3 garlic cloves, minced
- 1 tablespoon chives, minced
- A pinch of sea salt
- Black pepper to the taste

Directions:
Put cauliflower florets in a food processor and pulse well. Heat up a pan with the oil over medium high heat, add ginger, stir and cook for 3 minutes. Add cauliflower and garlic, stir and cook for 7 minutes. Add a pinch of salt, black pepper, vinegar, and chives, stir, cook for a few seconds more, divide between plates and serve. Enjoy!

Nutritional value: calories 100, fat 2, fiber 5, carbs 6, protein 8

Basil Zucchini Spaghetti

This is a great side dish for a succulent beef dish!

Preparation time: 1 hour and 10 minutes
Cooking time: 10 minutes
Servings: 4

Ingredients:
- 1/3 cup bacon grease
- 4 zucchinis, cut with a spiralizer
- ¼ cup basil, chopped
- A pinch of sea salt
- Black pepper to the taste
- ½ cup walnuts, chopped
- 2 garlic cloves, minced

Directions:
In a bowl, mix zucchini spaghetti with a pinch of salt and pepper, toss to coat, leave aside for 1 hour, drain well, rinse, drain again and put in a bowl. Heat up a pan with the bacon grease over medium high heat, add zucchini spaghetti and garlic, stir and cook for 5 minutes. Add basil and walnuts and some black pepper, stir and cook for 3 minutes more. Divide between plates and serve. Enjoy!

Nutritional value: calories 240, fat 1, fiber 4, carbs 7, protein 13

Delicious Braised Cabbage Side Dish

Are you looking for a hearty Paleo side dish? Maybe this is what you need!

Preparation time: 10 minutes
Cooking time: 20 minutes
Servings: 4

Ingredients:
- 1 small cabbage head, shredded
- 2 tablespoons water
- 6 ounces bacon, chopped
- A pinch of black pepper
- A pinch of sweet paprika
- 1 tablespoon dill, chopped

Directions:
Put bacon in a pan and heat up over medium high heat. Stir and cook for 8 minutes. Add cabbage and 1 tablespoon water, stir and cook for 5 minutes. Add the rest of the water, black pepper, paprika, and dill, stir and cook for 5 minutes more. Divide between plates and serve as a side dish! Enjoy!

Nutritional value: calories 90, fat 2, fiber 2, carbs 8, protein 6

Tasty Cauliflower and Leeks

This is a really tasty combination, and we can assure you it's really easy to make!

Preparation time: 10 minutes
Cooking time: 20 minutes
Servings: 4

Ingredients:
- 1 and ½ cups leeks, chopped
- 1 and ½ cups cauliflower florets
- 2 garlic cloves, minced
- 1 and ½ cups artichoke hearts
- 2 tablespoons bacon grease
- Black pepper to the taste

Directions:
Heat up a pan with the bacon grease over medium high heat, add garlic, leeks, cauliflower florets and artichoke hearts, stir and cook for 20 minutes. Add black pepper, stir, divide between plates and serve. Enjoy!

Nutritional value: calories 110, fat 2, fiber 2, carbs 6, protein 3

Delicious Eggplant and Mushrooms

This Paleo side dish is really exceptional!

Preparation time: 1 hour and 10 minutes
Cooking time: 30 minutes
Servings: 4

Ingredients:
- 2 pounds oyster mushrooms, chopped
- 6 ounces bacon, chopped
- 1 yellow onion, chopped
- 2 eggplants, cubed
- 3 celery stalks, chopped
- 1 tablespoon parsley, chopped
- A pinch of sea salt
- Black pepper to the taste
- 1 tablespoon savory, dried
- 3 tablespoons coconut oil

Directions:
Put eggplant pieces in a bowl, add a pinch of salt and black pepper, toss a bit, leave aside for 1 hour, drain well and leave aside in a bowl. Heat up a pan with the oil over medium high heat, add onion, stir and cook for 4 minutes. Add bacon, stir and cook for 4 more minutes. Add eggplant pieces, mushrooms, celery, savory and black pepper to the taste, stir and cook for 15 minutes. Add parsley, stir again, cook for a couple more minutes, divide between plates and serve. Enjoy!

Directions: calories 200, fat 3, fiber 3, carbs 6, protein 9

Special Mint Zucchini

It's a really special Paleo side you should really try soon!

Preparation time: 10 minutes
Cooking time: 7 minutes
Servings: 4

Ingredients:
- 2 tablespoons mint
- 2 zucchinis, cut into halves and then slice into half moons
- 1 tablespoon coconut oil
- ½ tablespoon dill, chopped
- A pinch of cayenne pepper

Directions:
Heat up a pan with the oil over medium high heat, add zucchinis, stir and cook for 6 minutes. Add cayenne, dill and mint, stir, cook for 1 minute more, divide between plates and serve. Enjoy!

Nutritional value: calories 80, fat 0, fiber 1, carbs 1, protein 5

Lovely Kale Dish

It goes perfectly with a tasty pork dish!

Preparation time: 10 minutes
Cooking time: 20 minutes
Servings: 4

Ingredients:
- 2 celery stalks, chopped
- 5 cups kale, torn
- 1 small red bell pepper, chopped
- 3 tablespoons water
- 1 tablespoon coconut oil

Directions:
Heat up a pan with the oil over medium high heat, add celery, stir and cook for 10 minutes. Add kale, water, and bell pepper, stir and cook for 10 minutes more. Divide between plates and serve really soon! Enjoy!

Nutritional value: calories 90, fat 1, fiber 2, carbs 2, protein 6

Kale, Mushrooms and Red Chard Side Dish

This is one of the best and most delicious ways to use kale!

Preparation time: 10 minutes
Cooking time: 15 minutes
Servings: 4

Ingredients:
- ½ pound brown mushrooms, sliced
- 5 cups kale, roughly chopped
- 1 and ½ tablespoons coconut oil
- 3 cups red chard, chopped
- 2 tablespoons water
- Black pepper to the taste

Directions:
Heat up a pan with the oil over medium high heat, add mushrooms, stir and cook for 5 minutes. Add red chard, kale and water, stir and cook for 10 minutes. Add black pepper to the taste, stir and cook for a couple more minutes. Divide between plates and serve. Enjoy!

Nutritional value: calories 100, fat 1, fiber 1, carbs 5, protein 3

Tasty Kale and Beets

The combination is really delicious!

Preparation time: 10 minutes
Cooking time: 30 minutes
Servings: 4

Ingredients:
- 1 tablespoon coconut oil
- 4 cups kale, torn
- 3 beets, cut into quarters and thinly sliced
- 2 tablespoons water
- A pinch of cayenne pepper

Directions:
Put water in a pot, add beets, bring to a boil over medium high heat, cover, reduce temperature, cook for 20 minutes and drain. Heat up a pan with the oil over medium high heat, add kale and the water, stir and cook for 10 minutes. Add beets and cayenne pepper, stir, cook for 2 minutes more, divide between plates and serve as a side dish! Enjoy!

Nutritional value: calories 120, fat 2, fiber 1, carbs 2, protein 4

Amazing Spicy Sweet Potatoes

This sweet potatoes side dish is divine!

Preparation time: 10 minutes
Cooking time: 40 minutes
Servings: 4

Ingredients:
- 4 sweet potatoes, peeled and thinly sliced
- 2 teaspoons nutmeg
- 2 tablespoon coconut oil, melted
- Cayenne pepper to the taste

Directions:
In a bowl, mix sweet potato slices with nutmeg, cayenne, and oil and toss to coat really well. Spread these on a lined baking sheet, place in the oven at 350 degrees F and bake for 25 minutes. Take potatoes out of the oven, flip them, put them back into the oven and bake for 15 minutes more. Serve as a tasty Paleo side dish! Enjoy!

Nutritional value: calories 140, fat 3, fiber 2, carbs 4, protein 10

Delicious Broccoli and Tasty Hazelnuts

You are not going to believe this! It's so tasty!

Preparation time: 10 minutes
Cooking time: 15 minutes
Servings: 4

Ingredients:
- 1 tablespoon olive oil
- 1 garlic clove, minced
- 1 pound broccoli florets
- 1/3 cup hazelnuts
- Black pepper to the taste

Directions:
Heat up a pan with the oil over medium high heat, add hazelnuts, stir and cook for 5 minutes. Transfer hazelnuts to a bowl and leave them aside for now. Heat up the same pan again over medium high heat, add broccoli and garlic, stir, cover and cook for 6 minutes more. Add hazelnuts and black pepper to the taste, stir, divide between plates and serve. Enjoy!

Nutritional value: calories 130, fat 3, fiber 2, carbs 5, protein 6

Tasty Squash and Cranberries

This is so tasty! Just get all the right ingredients and make it as soon as possible!

Preparation time: 10 minutes
Cooking time: 30 minutes
Servings: 2
Ingredients:
- 1 tablespoon coconut oil
- 1 butternut squash, peeled and cubed
- 2 garlic cloves, minced
- 1 small yellow onion, chopped
- 12 ounces canned coconut milk
- 1 teaspoon curry powder
- 1 teaspoon cinnamon powder
- ½ cup cranberries

Directions:
Spread squash pieces on a lined baking sheet, place in the oven at 425 degrees F and bake for 15 minutes. Take squash out of the oven and leave aside for now. Heat up a pan with the oil over medium high heat, add garlic and onion, stir and cook for 5 minutes. Add roasted squash, stir and cook for 3 minutes. Add coconut milk, cranberries, cinnamon and curry powder, stir and cook for 5 minutes more. Divide between plates and serve as a side dish! Enjoy!

Nutritional value: calories 100, fat 2, fiber 4, carbs 8, protein 2

Incredible Chard

This is a perfect side for a seafood based dish!

Preparation time: 10 minutes
Cooking time: 10 minutes
Servings: 2
Ingredients:
- Juice of ½ lemon
- 1 tablespoon coconut oil
- 12 ounces canned coconut milk
- 1 bunch chard
- A pinch of sea salt
- Black pepper to the taste

Directions:
Heat up a pan with the oil over medium high heat, add chard, stir and cook for 5 minutes. Add lemon juice, a pinch of salt, black pepper, and coconut milk, stir and cook for 5 minutes more. Divide between plates and serve as a side. Enjoy!

Nutritional value: calories 150, fat 3, fiber 1, carbs 5, protein 7

Dill Carrots

You must try this Paleo side dish as soon as possible!

Preparation time: 10 minutes
Cooking time: 30 minutes
Servings: 4

Ingredients:
- 1 tablespoon coconut oil, melted
- 2 tablespoons dill, chopped
- 1 pound baby carrots
- 1 tablespoon honey
- A pinch of black pepper

Directions:
Put carrots in a pot, add water to cover, bring to a boil over medium high heat, cover and simmer for 30 minutes. Drain well, put carrots in a bowl, add melted oil, black pepper, dill, and honey, stir very well, divide between plates and serve. Enjoy!

Nutritional value: calories 120, fat 2, fiber 3, carbs 5, protein 6

Paleo Snacks and Appetizers Recipes

Cauliflower Popcorn

If you are on a Paleo diet, you are not allowed to eat corn! So, if you are in the mood for some popcorn, try some cauliflower one!

Preparation time: 5 minutes
Cooking time: 30 minutes
Servings: 1

Ingredients:
- 1 small cauliflower head, chopped
- A pinch of sea salt
- ½ teaspoon chives, dried
- ½ teaspoon onion powder
- A drizzle of avocado oil

Directions:
In a bowl, mix cauliflower popcorn with a pinch of salt and the oil. Toss to coat and spread them on a lined baking sheet. Place in the oven at 450 degrees F and bake for 15 minutes. Take baking sheet out of the oven, flip popcorn and then bake for 15 minutes more. Transfer popcorn to a bowl, add chives and onion powder, stir and serve them. Enjoy!

Nutritional value: calories 80, fat 1, fiber 0, carbs 0, protein 2

Delicious Hummus

Don't worry! This is the Paleo version!

Preparation time: 10 minutes
Cooking time: 0 minutes
Servings: 6

Ingredients:
- ½ cup cashews, soaked for 2 hours and drained
- 1 tablespoon olive oil
- 2 tablespoons lemon juice
- ½ cup pumpkin puree
- 2 tablespoons sesame paste
- 1 garlic clove, minced
- ¼ teaspoon cumin, ground
- A pinch of cayenne pepper
- A pinch of sea salt
- ½ teaspoon pumpkin spice

Directions:
In your food processor, mix soaked cashews with lemon juice, pumpkin puree, sesame paste, garlic, cumin, pepper, sea salt and pumpkin spice and blend really well. Add oil gradually and blend again well. Transfer to a bowl and serve as a Paleo snack. Enjoy!

Nutritional value: calories 60, fat 1, fiber 2, carbs 6, protein 1

Simple Guacamole

This is a popular snack but have you tried the Paleo version?

Preparation time: 10 minutes
Cooking time: 0 minutes
Servings: 4

Ingredients:
- 3 green onions, chopped
- 3 avocados, pitted, peeled and roughly chopped
- A pinch of pink salt
- 1 teaspoon garlic powder
- 4 radishes, chopped
- Juice from 1 lime

Directions:
In your food processor mix onions with avocados, garlic powder, salt and lime juice and pulse a few times. Transfer to a bowl, add radishes, stir and serve cold. Enjoy!

Nutritional value: calories 60, fat 4, fiber 0, carbs 3, protein 1

Delightful and Special Hummus

Did you know you could make different kinds of hummus? Here's another special recipe!

Preparation time: 10 minutes
Cooking time: 40 minutes
Servings: 4

Ingredients:
- 4 tablespoons sesame seeds paste
- 1 cauliflower head, florets separated
- 1 small eggplant, chopped
- 1 small red bell pepper, chopped
- 5 tablespoons olive oil
- 4 tablespoons lemon juice
- 1 teaspoon garlic powder
- Black pepper to the taste
- ½ teaspoon cumin
- A pinch of paprika for serving
- A pinch of sea salt

Directions:
Arrange eggplant, cauliflower and bell pepper pieces on a lined baking sheet. Drizzle 1 tablespoon over them, toss to coat and bake in the oven at 400 degrees F for 40 minutes. Leave veggies to cool down and transfer them to your blender. Add sesame seeds paste, salt, pepper, 4 tablespoons oil, garlic powder, cumin and lemon juice and blend until you obtain a paste. Transfer to a bowl, sprinkle paprika on top and serve as a Paleo snack. Enjoy!

Nutritional value: calories 90, fat 1, fiber 1, carbs 3, protein 6

Sun Dried Tomatoes Spread

This is tasty and very easy to make! Get your ingredients and make it right away!

Preparation time: 10 minutes
Cooking time: 45 minutes
Servings: 6

Ingredients:
- 1 cauliflower head, florets separated
- ½ cup sun-dried tomatoes, chopped
- 10 garlic cloves
- 4 tablespoons tahini
- 4 tablespoons lemon juice
- 5 tablespoons olive oil
- 1 teaspoon basil, dried
- Black pepper to the taste
- 1 teaspoon cumin, ground
- A pinch of sea salt

Directions:
Put cauliflower florets and garlic cloves on a lined baking sheet, drizzle 1 tablespoon oil over them, toss to coat, place in the oven at 400 degrees F and bake for 45 minutes flipping once. Leave cauliflower and garlic to cool down and transfer to your blender. Add sun-dried tomatoes, 4 tablespoons oil, black pepper, ½ teaspoon cumin, tahini paste, a pinch of salt and lemon juice and blend until you obtain a paste. Transfer to a bowl, sprinkle the rest of the cumin and dried basil on top and serve. Enjoy!

Nutritional value: calories 90, fat 2, fiber 2, carbs 3, protein 1

Roasted Eggplant Spread

This is so delicious! It's a Paleo snack you will make over and over again!

Preparation time: 10 minutes
Cooking time: 1 hour
Servings: 4

Ingredients:
- 2 tablespoons lemon juice
- 1 eggplant, cut into halves lengthwise
- 2 tablespoons olive oil
- 1 garlic head, peeled
- Black pepper to the taste
- A pinch of sea salt

Directions:
Place eggplant halves and the garlic head on a lined baking sheet, drizzle some of the oil over them, place in the oven at 350 degrees F and bake for 1 hour. Leave eggplant and garlic to cool down, peel eggplant halves and put everything in your food processor. Add a pinch of salt, black pepper, lemon juice and the rest of the oil and pulse really well. Transfer eggplant spread to a bowl and serve right away. Enjoy!

Nutritional value: calories 100, fat 2, fiber 1, carbs 1, protein 2

Delicious Stuffed Eggs

This is one of the best Paleo appetizers you'll ever try! Your guests will love it!

Preparation time: 10 minutes
Cooking time: 0 minutes
Servings: 8

Ingredients:
- 4 eggs, hard-boiled, peeled and cut in halves
- 1 avocado, pitted, peeled and chopped
- A pinch of sea salt
- Black pepper to the taste
- 1 teaspoon cilantro, chopped
- A pinch of garlic powder

Directions:
Place egg halves on a platter and scoop egg yolks. In a bowl, mix egg yolks with avocado, cilantro, a pinch of sea salt, black pepper to the taste and garlic powder. Mash everything well and then stuff egg whites with this mix. Serve them as a Paleo appetizer. Enjoy!

Nutritional value: calories 60, fat 4, fiber 1, carbs 1, protein 3

Egg Cups

This can be a great snack or even an appetizer! It's up to you!

Preparation time: 10 minutes
Cooking time: 15 minutes
Servings: 12

Ingredients:
- A drizzle of avocado oil
- 12 eggs
- 8 asparagus spears, chopped
- A pinch of sea salt
- Black pepper to the taste
- 12 bacon strips, cooked

Directions:
Divide bacon strips into 12 muffin cups. Crack an egg in each, add asparagus pieces on top, season with a pinch of sea salt and black pepper, place in the oven at 400 degrees F and bake for 15 minutes. Leave egg cups to cool down, transfer them to a platter and serve. Enjoy!

Nutritional value: calories 200, fat 13, fiber 1, carbs 1, protein 10

Avocado Boats

A casual gathering with some of your best friends requires adequate dishes! Well, we give you the perfect Paleo snack for this kind of parties!

Preparation time: 10 minutes
Cooking time: 0 minutes
Servings: 2

Ingredients:
- 5 ounces canned tuna, drained and flaked
- Juice of 1 lemon
- 1 avocado, pitted and cut in halves
- Black pepper to the taste
- 1 tablespoon yellow onion, chopped
- A pinch of sea salt

Directions:
Scoop most of the avocado flesh and put it in a bowl. Add lemon juice, onion, black pepper to the taste, a pinch of salt and tuna and stir everything very well. Fill avocado cups with this mix and serve them. Enjoy!

Nutritional value: calories 100, fat 2, fiber 1, carbs 3, protein 5

Appetizer Salad

Serve this for your guests, and they will really be impressed! It's a wonderful Paleo appetizer!

Preparation time: 10 minutes
Cooking time: 0 minutes
Servings: 4

Ingredients:
- 4 ounces prosciutto, cut into very thin strips
- 1 big romaine lettuce head, chopped
- ½ cup artichoke hearts, chopped
- 4 ounces pepperoni, cubed
- ½ cup pickled hot peppers, chopped
- ½ cup black olives, pitted and chopped
- A drizzle of Italian dressing

For the dressing:
- 1 tablespoon parsley, chopped
- 1 garlic clove, minced
- 1 teaspoon oregano, dried
- Black pepper to the taste
- A pinch of sea salt
- ¾ cup avocado oil
- ¼ cup red wine vinegar

Directions:
In a bowl, mix parsley with garlic, oregano, a pinch of salt, black pepper, oil and vinegar and whisk well. In a salad bowl, mix prosciutto with romaine lettuce, artichoke hearts, pepperoni, hot peppers, and olives. Add salad dressing, toss to coat and serve as a Paleo appetizer. Enjoy!

Nutritional value: calories 100, fat 1, fiber 2, carbs 2, protein 4

Special Mixed Snack

This a very healthy Paleo snack you can make at home for a movie night!

Preparation time: 5 minutes
Cooking time: 1 hour and 30 minutes
Servings: 6

Ingredients:
- 1 cup raw cashews, halved
- 2 and ¼ cup walnuts, chopped
- 1/3 cup stevia
- 5 tablespoons coconut oil
- 1 cup coconut flakes, unsweetened
- 1 teaspoon vanilla extract
- 2 cups banana slices, dried
- ¾ cup dark chocolate chips

Directions:
In your crock pot, mix cashews with walnuts, stevia, oil, vanilla extract and coconut flakes, cover and cook on High for 1 hour. Turn crock pot to Low and cook for 30 minutes. Spread all these on a lined baking sheet and leave them aside to cool down. Mix them with chocolate chips and banana slices, transfer to a bowl and serve as a snack. Enjoy!

Nutritional value: calories 222, fat 12, fiber 3, carbs 10, protein 6

Butternut Squash Bites

This is the best snack you could think of!

Preparation time: 10 minutes
Cooking time: 40 minutes
Servings: 4

Ingredients:
- 15 bacon slices, cut in halves
- 2 pounds butternut squash, cut into medium cubes
- 1 teaspoon chili powder
- 1 teaspoon garlic powder
- 1 teaspoon sweet paprika
- Black pepper to the taste

Directions:
In a bowl, mix butternut squash cubes with chili powder, black pepper, garlic powder and paprika and toss to coat. Wrap squash pieces in bacon slices, place them all on a lined baking sheet, place in the oven at 350 degrees F and bake for 20 minutes. Take baking sheet out of the oven, flip pieces and bake them for 20 minutes more. Arrange squash bites on a platter and serve. Enjoy!

Nutritional value: calories 132, fat 2, fiber 2, carbs 4, protein 6

Baked Zucchini Chips

Make sure you have enough! These are so delicious!

Preparation time: 10 minutes
Cooking time: 12 minutes
Servings: 4

Ingredients:
- 1 zucchini, thinly sliced
- A pinch of sea salt
- Black pepper to the taste
- 1 teaspoon thyme, dried
- 1 egg
- 1 teaspoon garlic powder
- 1 cup almond flour

Directions:
In a bowl, whisk the egg with a pinch of salt. Put flour in another bowl and mix it with thyme, black pepper, and garlic powder. Dredge zucchini slices in the egg mix and then in flour. Arrange chips on a lined baking sheet, place in the oven at 450 degrees F and bake for 6 minutes. Flip chips, cook them for 6 minutes more and transfer to a bowl. Serve your zucchini chips cold. Enjoy!

Nutritional value: calories 110, fat 4, fiber 3, carbs 6, protein 6

Simple and Easy Pepperoni Bites

This is our Paleo suggestion for today: a tasty snack or even appetizer!

Preparation time: 5 minutes
Cooking time: 10 minutes
Servings: 24 pieces

Ingredients:
- 1/3 cup tomatoes, chopped
- ½ cup bell peppers, mixed and chopped
- 24 pepperoni sliced
- ½ cup paleo marinara sauce
- 4 ounces almond cheese, cubed
- 2 tablespoons basil, chopped
- Black pepper to the taste

Directions:
Divide pepperoni slices into a muffin tray. Divide tomato and bell pepper pieces into pepperoni cups. Also divide Paleo marinara sauce, basil and almond cheese cubes. Sprinkle black pepper at the end, introduce cups in the oven at 400 degrees F and bake for 10 minutes. Leave your pepperoni cups to cool down a bit, transfer them to a platter and serve. Enjoy!

Nutritional value: calories 120, fat 2, fiber 1, carbs 3, protein 5

Amazing Party Meatballs

These are easy to make, and they can be a great appetizer!

Preparation time: 10 minutes
Cooking time: 40 minutes
Servings: 20

Ingredients:
- 1 pound turkey meat, ground
- 1 tablespoon coconut oil
- 1 yellow onion, chopped
- 1 egg
- 1 cup almond flour
- 3 tablespoons hot sauce
- 1 teaspoon Italian seasoning
- A pinch of sea salt
- Black pepper to the taste
- 2 tablespoons parsley, chopped
- Paleo marinara sauce for serving

Directions:
In a bowl, mix turkey meat with half of the flour, a pinch of salt, black pepper, Italian seasoning, parsley, onion, egg and hot sauce and stir well. Put the rest of the flour in another bowl. Shape 20 turkey meatballs and dip each one in flour. Heat up a pan with the oil over medium high heat, add meatballs, cook them for 4 minutes on each side, transfer to paper towels, drain grease and place all of them on a platter. Serve them with some Paleo marinara sauce on the side. Enjoy!

Nutritional value: calories 70, fat 3, fiber 0.6, carbs 2, protein 6

Incredible Chicken Strips

These crispy chicken strips are so easy to make! You don't have to be an expert to make this special Paleo appetizer!

Preparation time: 10 minutes
Cooking time: 20 minutes
Servings: 4

Ingredients:
- 1 pound chicken tenders
- 1 egg, whisked
- A pinch of sea salt
- 1/3 cup coconut, unsweetened and shredded
- ¼ cup coconut flour

Directions:
In a bowl, mix coconut with coconut flour and a pinch of sea salt and stir. Put whisked egg in another bowl. Dip chicken pieces in egg, then in coconut mixture and arrange them all on a lined baking sheet. Place in the oven at 350 degrees F and bake for 25 minutes flipping pieces halfway. Transfer chicken strips to a bowl and serve them with a Paleo dip on the side. Enjoy!

Nutritional value: calories 400, fat 23, fiber 5, carbs 8, protein 12

Simple Beef Jerky

Are you looking for a hearty Paleo snack? We think that this one could be what you need!

Preparation time: 6 hours and 10 minutes
Cooking time: 6 hours
Servings: 6

Ingredients:
- ½ cup coconut aminos
- 2 and ½ pounds beef, thinly sliced
- 2 tablespoons gluten free liquid smoke
- ¼ cup coconut sugar
- ¼ cup apple cider vinegar
- A pinch of sea salt
- Small ginger pieces, thinly sliced

Directions:
In a bowl, mix vinegar with coconut sugar, aminos, liquid smoke, ginger and a pinch of salt and stir well. Add meat slices, toss to coat well, cover and keep in the fridge for 6 hours. Transfer meat slices to your preheated dehydrator at 165 degrees F and dehydrate them for 6 hours. Transfer beef jerky to a bowl and serve as a snack. Enjoy!

Nutritional value: calories 140, fat 2, fiber 3, carbs 7, protein 7

Simple Chicken Skewers

This is a Paleo appetizer you can serve on a summer Sunday!

Preparation time: 3 hours
Cooking time: 15 minutes
Servings: 4

Ingredients:
- 2 tablespoons parsley
- 4 chicken breasts, cubed
- ¾ cup lemon garlic powder
- Black pepper to the taste

Directions:
In a bowl, mix chicken with lemon garlic, black pepper, and parsley, stir well, cover and keep in the fridge for 3 hours. Arrange chicken pieces on skewers, place them all on preheated grill and cook for 15 minutes, flipping once. Arrange skewers on a platter and serve. Enjoy!

Nutritional value: calories 150, fat 3, fiber 2, carbs 4, protein 8

Kale Chips and Tasty Dip

This Paleo snack must be served with an aioli dip! This is just perfect!

Preparation time: 10 minutes
Cooking time: 20 minutes
Servings: 6

Ingredients:
- 1 tablespoon avocado oil
- 1 bunch kale, leaves separated
- A pinch of sea salt
- Black pepper to the taste
- *For the aioli dip:*
- ½ teaspoon mustard powder
- 1 egg yolk
- 2 tablespoons lemon juice
- ½ cup olive oil
- ½ cup avocado oil
- 3 rosemary springs, chopped
- 3 garlic cloves, minced

Directions:
Pat dry kale leaves, arrange them on a lined baking sheet, drizzle 1 tablespoon avocado oil, sprinkle a pinch of sea salt and black pepper to the taste, place in the oven at 275 degrees F and bake for 20 minutes. Meanwhile, in your food processor, mix egg yolk with mustard powder, lemon juice, and garlic and blend well. Add olive oil and avocado oil gradually and blend until you obtain a smooth paste. Add rosemary, blend again well and transfer your dip to a bowl. Take kale chips out of the oven, leave them to cool down and arrange them on a platter. Serve with aioli dip on the side. Enjoy!

Nutritional value: calories 100, fat 2, fiber 1, carbs 1, protein 6

Rosemary Crackers

Make this Paleo snack and take it with you at the office!

Preparation time: 10 minutes
Cooking time: 14 minutes
Servings: 40

Ingredients:
- ¼ cup coconut flour
- 1 cup almond flour
- ½ cup sesame seeds, toasted and ground
- 2 tablespoons tapioca flour
- A pinch of sea salt
- Black pepper to the taste
- 1 teaspoon onion powder
- 1 teaspoon rosemary, chopped
- ½ teaspoon thyme, chopped
- 2 eggs
- 3 tablespoons olive oil

Directions:
In a bowl, mix sesame seeds with coconut flour, almond flour, tapioca flour, salt, pepper, rosemary, thyme and onion powder and stir well. In another bowl, whisk eggs with the oil and stir well. Add this to flour mix and knead until you obtain a dough. Shape a disk out of this dough, flatten well and cut 40 crackers out of it. Arrange them all on a lined baking sheet, place in the oven at 375 degrees F and bake for 14 minutes. Leave your crackers to cool down and serve them as a tasty Paleo snack. Enjoy!

Nutritional value: calories 50, fat 3, fiber 1, carbs 2, protein 2

Delicious and Special Crackers

These crackers and simply incredible! They are so tasty and pretty easy to make! It's a great Paleo snack!

Preparation time: 10 minutes
Cooking time: 3 hours
Servings: 40

Ingredients:
- ½ cup chia seeds
- 1 cup flaxseed, ground
- ½ cup pumpkin seeds
- 1/3 cup sesame seeds
- A pinch of sea salt
- 1 and ¼ cups water
- ½ teaspoon garlic powder
- 1 teaspoon thyme, dried
- 1 teaspoon basil, dried

Directions:
Put pumpkin seeds in your food processor, pulse really well and transfer them to a bowl. Add flaxseed, sesame seeds, chia, salt, water, garlic powder, thyme and basil and stir well until they combine. Spread this on a lined baking sheet, press well, cuts into 40 pieces, place in the oven at 200 degrees F and bake for 3 hours. Leave your crackers to cool down before serving them as a snack. Enjoy!

Nutritional value: calories 60, fat 1, fiber 2, carbs 2, protein 3

Simple Coconut Bars

This is a tasty Paleo snack that will give you enough energy to face a hard and stressful day!

Preparation time: 30 minutes
Cooking time: 0 minutes
Servings: 10

Ingredients:
- 1 teaspoon vanilla extract
- 1 cup coconut flakes, unsweetened
- 2 cups cashews
- 1 and ¼ cups figs, dried
- A pinch of sea salt
- 1/3 cup dark chocolate chips
- 1 tablespoon protein powder
- 1 tablespoon cocoa powder

Directions:
In your food processor, mix figs with vanilla, cashews, a pinch of salt, protein powder, cocoa powder and coconut and blend them well. Transfer this into a baking dish and press well. Put chocolate chips in a heatproof bowl, place in your microwave for 1 minute until it melts. Pour this over coconut mix, spread well, place in your freezer for 20 minutes, cut into bars and serve as a Paleo snack. Enjoy!

Nutritional value: calories 234, fat 12, fiber 3, carbs 6, protein 6

Simple Nuts Snack

This can't get any easier! It's such a simple snack idea!

Preparation time: 10 minutes
Cooking time: 16 minutes
Servings: 4

Ingredients:
- 1 egg white
- 16 ounces mixed raw nuts
- Black pepper to the taste
- A pinch of sea salt
- 1 teaspoon sage, dried
- ½ teaspoon smoked paprika
- 1 tablespoon rosemary, chopped
- 1 tablespoon garlic powder

Directions:
In a bowl, whisk egg white with a pinch of sea salt. Put nuts in another bowl and add egg white to them. Add black pepper, sage, paprika, rosemary and garlic powder and stir everything really well. Spread this on a lined baking sheet, place in the oven at 300 degrees F and roast for 8 minutes. Flip nuts and bake them for 8 minutes more. Leave nuts to cool down, divide into bowls and serve as a snack. Enjoy!

Nutritional value: calories 100, fat 3, fiber 1, carbs 5, protein 6

Carrot Balls

This sounds really great, doesn't it? Try this tasty Paleo snack soon!

Preparation time: 10 minutes
Cooking time: 15 minutes
Servings: 14

Ingredients:
- ½ teaspoon cinnamon powder
- 1 cup baby carrots, grated
- ¾ cup pecans
- 1 egg white, whisked well
- 1 tablespoon honey
- 2 tablespoons coconut flour
- 2 tablespoons flaxseed, ground

Directions:
In a bowl, mix baby carrots with egg white, cinnamon, pecans, honey, flaxseed and coconut flour and stir well. Shape 14 balls from this mix, place them on a lined baking sheet, place in the oven at 350 degrees F and bake for 15 minutes. Leave carrot balls to cool down before transferring them to a bowl and serving them. Enjoy!

Nutritional value: calories 120, fat 2, fiber 2, carbs 4, protein 5

Wrapped Olives

Your guests will say you are a genius if you make this appetizer for your next party!

Preparation time: 10 minutes
Cooking time: 35 minutes
Servings: 36

Ingredients:
- 36 almond stuffed green olives
- A pinch of black pepper
- 12 bacon slices, each cut in 3 pieces

Directions:
Wrap each olive with a bacon piece, secure them with a toothpick, sprinkle some black pepper all over, place them on a lined baking sheet, place in the oven at 400 degrees F and bake for 35 minutes. Leave this tasty Paleo appetizer to cool down before arranging on a platter and serving. Enjoy!

Nutritional value: calories 20, fat 2, fiber 0, carbs 0, protein 0.4

Oyster Spread

This is an elegant and very delicious Paleo appetizer you can try for a special and fancy party!

Preparation time: 10 minutes
Cooking time: 0 minutes
Servings: 4

Ingredients:
- 4 ounces canned smoked oysters
- 2 teaspoons coconut cream
- 1 tablespoon red onion, chopped
- 2 pinches cayenne pepper

Directions:
Drain oysters and put them into a bowl. Mash using a fork, add coconut cream, onion, and cayenne, stir well, divide on Paleo crackers and serve as an appetizer! Enjoy!

Nutritional value: calories 120, fat 2, fiber 2, carbs 5, protein 10

Stuffed Mushrooms

Arrange these nicely on a platter, and everyone will be so happy to eat them!

Preparation time: 10 minutes
Cooking time: 20 minutes
Servings: 8

Ingredients:
- 1 pound cremini mushrooms caps
- 3 tablespoons olive oil
- A pinch of cayenne pepper
- A pinch of smoked paprika
- Onion dip

For the dip:
- 1 cup coconut cream
- ½ cup mayonnaise
- 2 tablespoons coconut oil
- 1 yellow onion, finely chopped
- ¼ teaspoon white pepper
- ¼ teaspoon garlic powder
- 2 tablespoons green onions chopped

Directions:
Heat up a pan with 2 tablespoons coconut oil over medium heat, add onion, garlic powder and white pepper, stir, cook for 10 minutes, take off heat and leave aside to cool down. In a bowl, mix mayo with coconut cream, green onions and caramelized onions, stir well and keep in the fridge for now. Season mushroom caps with a pinch of cayenne pepper and paprika and drizzle the olive oil over them. Rub them, place on preheated grill over medium high heat and cook them for 5 minutes on each side. Arrange them on a platter, fill each with some of the onion dip and serve them cold! Enjoy!

Nutritional value: calories 150, fat 3, fiber 2, carbs 4, protein 6

Tasty Apricot Bites

Why should you try the same appetizers over and over again? Here is something really different!

Preparation time: 2 hours
Cooking time: 40 minutes
Servings: 4

Ingredients:
- 10 apricots, dried
- 10 bacon strips, cut in halves
- 10 ounces canned chestnuts
- 2 teaspoons lemongrass, chopped
- 4 tablespoons garlic, minced
- ½ cup coconut aminos

Directions:
Wrap a chestnut and an apricot in bacon and secure with a toothpick. Repeat this with the rest of the chestnuts, apricots and bacon pieces. Heat up a pan over medium heat, add garlic, stir and sauté it for 20 minutes. Transfer garlic to a bowl when it's cold, add lemongrass and coconut aminos. Add apricot bites, cover and leave them aside for 2 hours. Spread apricot bites on a lined baking sheet, place in the oven at 350 degrees F and bake for 20 minutes. Arrange them on a platter and serve as an appetizer. Enjoy!

Nutritional value: calories 130, fat 2, fiber 2, carbs 3, protein 8

Mushroom Boats

These mushroom boats are the best Paleo appetizers!

Preparation time: 10 minutes
Cooking time: 30 minutes
Servings: 4

Ingredients:

- 1 pound Mexican chorizo, chopped
- 1 pound big white mushroom caps, stems separated and chopped
- 3 tablespoons coconut oil
- 1 yellow onion, chopped
- A pinch of black pepper

Directions:
Heat up a pan with 2 tablespoons oil over medium heat, add mushrooms stems, stir and cook them for 3 minutes. Add the rest of the oil, onion and a pinch of black pepper, stir and cook for 7 minutes. Transfer this mix to a bowl, add chorizo and stir well. Stuff mushrooms with this mix, place them on a lined baking sheet and bake in the oven at 400 degrees F for 20 minutes. Arrange mushrooms on a platter and serve them. Enjoy!

Nutritional value: calories 245, fat 23, fiber 2, carbs 4, protein 13

Special Mushroom and Broccoli Appetizer

This is not just a simple and tasty Paleo appetizer! It's a beautiful one as well!

Preparation time: 20 minutes
Cooking time: 10 minutes
Servings: 4

Ingredients:

- 10 mushroom caps
- ½ teaspoon dry mango powder
- ½ teaspoon chili powder
- 1 cup broccoli florets
- 1 teaspoon garam masala
- 1 teaspoon ginger and garlic paste
- ½ teaspoon turmeric powder
- A drizzle of olive oil
- A pinch of sea salt
- Black pepper to the taste

Directions:
In a bowl, mix mango powder with chili powder, garam masala, ginger paste, turmeric, salt, pepper and oil and stir very well. Add mushroom caps and broccoli florets, toss to coat well and keep in the fridge for 20 minutes. Arrange these on skewers, place them on preheated grill over medium high heat, cook for 5 minutes on each side and transfer to a platter. Serve them with a tasty Paleo mayo on the side. Enjoy!

Nutritional value: calories 120, fat 2, fiber 1, carbs 2, protein 5

Zucchini Rolls

Get started! Make this tasty Paleo appetizer now!

Preparation time: 10 minutes
Cooking time: 5 minutes
Servings: 4

Ingredients:
- 3 zucchinis, thinly sliced lengthwise
- 14 bacon slices
- ½ cup sun-dried tomatoes, drained and chopped
- 4 tablespoons raspberry vinegar
- ½ cup basil, chopped
- A pinch of sea salt
- Black pepper to the taste

Directions:
Place zucchini slices in a bowl, sprinkle a pinch of sea salt and vinegar over them and leave aside for 10 minutes. Drain well and season with black pepper to the taste. Divide bacon slices, chopped sun dried tomatoes and basil over zucchini ones, roll each and secure with a toothpick and arrange them on a lined baking sheet. Place in the oven at 400 degrees F for 5 minutes, then arrange them on a platter and serve as an appetizer. Enjoy!

Nutritional value: calories 243, fat 12, fiber 3, carbs 5, protein 14

Special Cauliflower Mini Hot Dogs

This is a great appetizer! It's easy and fun to make! Your kids can help you make this mini dogs!

Preparation time: 10 minutes
Cooking time: 25 minutes
Servings: 6

Ingredients:
- 12 small sausages
- 2 eggs, whisked
- 1 cup cauliflower riced
- 1 and ½ tablespoon coconut oil
- ½ teaspoon baking soda
- 1 teaspoon apple cider vinegar
- ¼ cup coconut flour
- 1 teaspoon red pepper sauce
- A pinch of sea salt
- ¼ teaspoon smoked paprika
- ½ teaspoon mustard powder
- A pinch of chili powder
- 2 teaspoons jalapenos, chopped

Directions:
In a bowl, mix riced cauliflower with coconut flour, eggs, oil, red pepper sauce, mustard, salt, chili powder, paprika and jalapenos. In a bowl, mix baking soda with vinegar and stir well. Add this to cauliflower mix and stir well. Place 12 spoonfuls of this mix on a lined baking sheet, press 1 sausage in the center and top with other 12 spoonfuls of cauliflower mix. Shape place in the oven at 400 degrees F and bake for 25 minutes. Arrange on a platter and serve them. Enjoy!

Nutritional value: calories 140, fat 6, fiber 2, carbs 4, protein 8

Watermelon Wraps

This Paleo appetizer is great for a garden party!

Preparation time: 10 minutes
Cooking time: 0 minutes
Servings: 20

Ingredients:
- 4 watermelon slices
- 1 avocado, peeled, pitted and chopped
- ½ cup cucumber, chopped
- ¼ cup red onion, chopped
- 1 teaspoon coconut aminos
- 1 teaspoon lime juice

Directions:
Cut 20 circles of watermelon using a cookie cutter. In a bowl, mix onion with avocado, aminos, cucumber and lime juice and stir well. Divide this into watermelon circles, place them on a platter and serve right away. Enjoy!

Nutritional value: calories 80, fat 1, fiber 1, carbs 2, protein 2

Cucumber Rolls

These are so convenient and tasty! It's a delicious Paleo snack!

Preparation time: 10 minutes
Cooking time: 0 minutes
Servings: 3

Ingredients:
- 1 cucumber, very thinly sliced
- 6 ham slices
- 1 jalapeno, chopped
- 3 teaspoons Paleo mayonnaise
- 1 teaspoon dill, chopped
- 6 green onions, chopped

Directions:
Arrange ham slices on a working surface. In a bowl, mix mayo with jalapeno, green onions and dill and stir well. Spread some of this mix over 1 ham slice, add a cucumber slice at the end, roll cucumber around ham and secure with a toothpick. Repeat with the remaining ingredients and serve your cucumber rolls right away. Enjoy!

Nutritional value: calories 70, fat 1, fiber 2, carbs 2, protein 5

Crazy Chicken Appetizer

It's such a simple and delicious Paleo appetizer!

Preparation time: 10 minutes
Cooking time: 20 minutes
Servings: 2

Ingredients:
- 3 tablespoons curry powder
- 1 cup coconut flour
- 2 teaspoons turmeric, ground
- 1 tablespoon cumin powder
- 3 chicken breasts, skinless, boneless and cut into small strips
- 1 tablespoon garlic powder
- Black pepper to the taste

Directions:
In a bowl, mix curry powder with flour, turmeric, cumin, garlic powder and black pepper and stir well. Add chicken strips, toss well to coat and arrange them on a lined baking sheet. Place in the oven at 350 degrees F and bake for 20 minutes. Transfer chicken strips to a bowl and serve them cold. Enjoy!

Nutritional value: calories 100, fat 2, fiber 3, carbs 4, protein 2

Fried Peppers

Trust us! This is a Paleo appetizer!

Preparation time: 10 minutes
Cooking time: 13 minutes
Servings: 4

Ingredients:
- 10 shishito peppers
- Juice of ½ lemon
- 2 teaspoons olive oil
- 1 garlic clove, minced
- A pinch of sea salt
- Black pepper to the taste

Directions:
Heat up a pan with the oil over medium high heat, add peppers, lemon juice, garlic, a pinch of salt and black pepper, stir and cook for 10 minutes. Drain excess grease on paper towels, arrange on a small platter and serve. Enjoy!

Nutritional value: calories 60, fat 1, fiber 1, carbs 1, protein 2

Spanish Appetizer Cakes

This Spanish style Paleo appetizer is easy to make and it will help you impress your friends or guests!

Preparation time: 10 minutes
Cooking time: 25 minutes
Servings: 18

Ingredients:
- 2 cups sweet potatoes, peeled, cubed and boiled
- 2 garlic cloves, minced
- 4 tablespoons cilantro, chopped
- 1 teaspoon black pepper
- A pinch of sea salt
- Juice from 2 limes
- A pinch of cayenne pepper
- 2 tablespoons nutritional yeast

Directions:
In a bowl mix sweet potatoes with a pinch of salt and pepper and mash well. Add garlic, cilantro, a black pepper, lime juice, cayenne and nutritional yeast and stir very well. Shape small cakes out of this mix, arrange them on a baking sheet, place in the oven at 350 degrees F and bake for 25 minutes. Arrange cakes on a platter and serve them cold. Enjoy!

Nutritional value: calories 150, fat 2, fiber 2, carbs 4, protein 6

Chicken Bites

These look incredible and they taste even better!

Preparation time: 10 minutes
Cooking time: 45 minutes
Servings: 13

Ingredients:
- 2 pounds chicken breasts, cut into medium pieces
- 1 adobo chili pepper, chopped
- 1/5 cup paleo bbq sauce
- 13 pastrami slices

Directions:
Put bbq sauce in a small pot and heat up over medium high heat. Add chili, stir and bring to a boil. Wrap chicken pieces in pastrami slices, secure them with a toothpick and place them in a baking dish. Spoon the bbq sauce over them, place in the oven at 375 degrees F and bake for 45 minutes. Leave chicken bites to cool down, arrange them on a platter and serve. Enjoy!

Nutritional value: calories 170, fat 3, fiber 2, carbs 4, protein 10

Scallops Bites

Are you looking for something really fancy to offer your guests? Try this recipe!

Preparation time: 10 minutes
Cooking time: 16 minutes
Servings: 4

Ingredients:
- 20 sea scallops
- 4 bacon slices
- ½ cup baby spinach leaves
- ¼ cup red onion, chopped
- ½ teaspoon curry powder
- ½ teaspoon red pepper, ground
- A pinch of sea salt
- 1 tablespoon coconut oil

For the sauce:
- 4 tablespoons balsamic vinegar
- 2 shallots, chopped
- ¼ teaspoon honey
- 1 tablespoon bacon fat

Directions:
Heat up a pan with 1 tablespoon oil over medium high heat, add bacon, stir, cook until it browns, transfer to paper towels, drain grease, cut into medium pieces and leave aside. In a bowl, mix red pepper with curry powder and a pinch of sea salt and stir. Add scallops and rub them well. Heat up the same pan where you cooked the bacon over medium high heat, add scallops and cook them for 3 minutes on each side. Heat up the same pan with 1 tablespoon bacon fat over medium high heat, add shallots, stir and cook them for 2 minutes. Add honey and vinegar, stir, cook until everything thickens and take off heat. Arrange bacon pieces on a platter. Add spinach leaves and onion pieces. Top with scallops, stick a toothpick in the middle of each and drizzle the sauce you've made on top. Enjoy this great Paleo appetizer!

Nutritional value: calories 200, fat 3, fiber 3, carbs 6, protein 10

Delicious Cabbage Chips

You only need a few ingredients to make a healthy and light Paleo snack!

Preparation time: 10 minutes
Cooking time: 2 hours
Servings: 8

Ingredients:
- ½ red cabbage head, leaves separated and halved
- ½ green cabbage head, leaves separated and halved
- A drizzle of olive oil
- Black pepper to the taste
- A pinch of sea salt

Directions:
Spread cabbage leaves on a lined baking sheet, place in the oven at 200 degrees F and bake for 2 hours. Take cabbage chips out of the oven, drizzle oil over them, sprinkle salt and black pepper, rub well, transfer to a bowl and serve as a Paleo snack. Enjoy!

Nutritional value: calories 80, fat 1, fiber 0, carbs 1, protein 2

Paleo Meat Recipes

Chicken Thighs with Tasty Butternut Squash
Try this for dinner tonight and enjoy a marvelous flavor!

Servings: 6
Preparation time: 10 minutes
Cooking time: 30 minutes
Ingredients:

- 6 chicken thighs, boneless and skinless
- ½ pound bacon, chopped
- 2 tablespoons coconut oil
- A pinch of sea salt
- A handful sage, chopped
- Black pepper to the taste
- 3 cups butternut squash, cubed

Directions:

Heat up a pan over medium heat, add bacon, cook until it's crispy, drain on paper towels, transfer to a plate, crumble and leave aside for now. Heat up the same pan over medium heat, add butternut squash, a pinch of salt and black pepper to the taste, stir, cook until it's soft, transfer to a plate and also leave aside. Heat up the pan again with the coconut oil over medium-high heat, add chicken, salt, and pepper and cook for 10 minutes, turning often. Take the pan off the heat, add squash, introduce in the oven at 425 degrees F and bake for 15 minutes. Divide chicken and butternut on plates, top with sage and bacon and serve. Enjoy!

Nutritional value: calories 241, fat 11, carbs 17, fiber 2.5, sugar 3, protein 16

Paleo Turkey Casserole
Make sure you have enough because you will definitely want seconds!

Servings: 6
Preparation time: 10 minutes
Cooking time: 1 hour
Ingredients:

- 1 sweet potato, chopped
- 1 pound turkey meat, ground
- 1 eggplant, thinly sliced
- 1 yellow onion, finely chopped
- 1 tablespoon garlic, finely minced
- A pinch of sea salt
- Black pepper to the taste
- ¼ teaspoon chili powder
- ¼ teaspoon cumin
- 15 ounces canned tomatoes, chopped and drained
- 8 ounces tomato paste
- A drizzle of olive oil
- ½ teaspoon tarragon flakes
- 1/8 teaspoon cardamom, ground
- 1/8 teaspoon oregano

For the sauce:

- 1 tablespoon almond flour
- 1 cup almond milk
- 1 and ½ tablespoons extra virgin olive oil
- 1 tablespoon coconut flour

Directions:

Heat up a pan over medium-high heat, add turkey meat, onion, and garlic, stir and cook until the meat turns brown. Add tomatoes, tomato paste and sweet potatoes, stir and cook for 5 minutes. Add a pinch of sea salt, pepper to the taste, chili powder, cumin, oregano, tarragon flakes and cardamom, stir well and cook for 2 minutes. Grease a baking dish with a drizzle of olive oil, arrange eggplant slices on the bottom and add turkey mix on top. Spread turkey mix evenly, introduce dish in the oven at 350 degrees F and bake for 15 minutes. Meanwhile, heat up a pot over medium-high heat, add the rest of the olive oil, almond flour and coconut one, stir well 1 minute, reduce heat, add almond milk and stir well. Cook this for 10 minutes. Take the baking dish out of the oven and pour this almond milk mix over it. Introduce in the oven again and bake for 45 minutes. Take casserole out of the oven, leave aside a few minutes to cool down, slice and divide between plates and serve. Enjoy!

Nutritional value: calories 278, fat 2.6, carbs 29, fiber 6.7, sugar 13, protein 28.5

Special Paleo Chicken and Veggies Stir Fry

It's a textured dish you can enjoy for dinner today!

Servings: 4
Preparation time: 15 minutes
Cooking time: 20 minutes

Ingredients:
- 1 red bell pepper, chopped
- 1 zucchini, chopped
- 1 yellow onion, finely chopped
- 1 broccoli head, florets separated
- 4 chicken breasts, skinless, boneless and chopped
- A pinch of sea salt
- Black pepper to the taste
- 1 tablespoon coconut oil
- ¼ cup chicken broth
- 2 garlic cloves, finely chopped
- 3 tablespoons coconut amino
- ½ cup orange juice
- 1 tablespoon orange zest
- 1 teaspoon Sriracha sauce
- ¼ teaspoon ginger, grated
- A pinch of red pepper flakes

For the sauce:

Directions:
In a bowl, mix broth with orange juice, zest, amino, ginger, garlic, pepper flakes and Sriracha sauce and stir well. Heat up a pan with the oil over medium heat, add chicken, cook for 8 minutes and transfer to a plate. Heat up the same pan over medium heat, add bell pepper, broccoli florets, onion, and zucchini, stir and cook for 4-5 minutes. Add a pinch of sea salt, pepper, orange sauce you've made, stir, bring to a boil, add chicken, reduce heat and simmer for 8 minutes. Divide between plates and serve hot. Enjoy!

Nutritional value: calories 320, fat 13, carbs 17, protein 45, fiber 3.7, sugar 4

Paleo Stuffed Quail

This is a very elegant recipe you can make for a special occasion!

Servings: 4
Preparation time: 15 minutes
Cooking time: 1 hour

Ingredients:
- 8 bacon slices
- 4 quails
- 1 apple, chopped
- 1 pound grapes
- 1 tablespoon rosemary, chopped
- ½ cup cranberries, chopped
- 2 tablespoons extra virgin olive oil
- 2 garlic cloves, chopped
- 4 rosemary springs
- ½ cup chicken stock
- A pinch of sea salt
- Black pepper to the taste

Directions:
Pat dry quail, season with a pinch of sea salt and pepper and leave aside for now. In a bowl, mix cranberries with chopped rosemary, apple, olive oil, garlic, salt, and pepper to the taste and stir well. Fill quail with this mix, wrap each with 2 bacon slices and tie with cooking twine. Spread half of the grapes in a baking dish, mash gently with a fork, arrange quail on top, spread the rest of the grapes and pour chicken stock at the end. Introduce everything in the oven at 425 degrees F and bake for 1 hour. Divide between plates and serve with baked grapes on the side. Enjoy!

Nutritional value: calories 260, fat 18, carbs 22, fiber 3, protein 29

Paleo Roasted Duck Dish

It's a tasty and very tender dish! Also, it's very nutritious, and of course, it totally respects the paleo diet rules!

Servings: 4
Preparation time: 10 minutes
Cooking time: 2 hours

Ingredients:
- 2 teaspoons allspice, ground
- 4 duck legs
- 4 thyme springs
- 1 lemon, sliced
- 1 orange, sliced
- 1 cup chicken broth
- A pinch of sea salt
- Black pepper to the taste
- ½ cup orange juice

Directions:
Heat up a pan over medium high heat, add duck legs, season with a pinch of salt and pepper to the taste and brown them for 3 minutes on each side. Arrange half of lemon and orange slices on the bottom of a baking dish, place duck legs, top with the rest of the orange and lemon slices and thyme springs. Add chicken stock, orange juice, sprinkle allspice, introduce in the oven at 350 degrees F and bake for 2 hours. Divide between plates and serve hot. Enjoy!

Nutritional value: 255, fat 17, carbs 6, protein 33, fiber 1

Paleo Chicken Meatballs

It's such a versatile dish you will adore sharing with your loved ones!

Servings: 4
Preparation time: 10 minutes
Cooking time: 20 minutes
Ingredients:
- 1 teaspoon sweet paprika
- 1 pineapple, diced
- 1 egg
- 2 pounds chicken meat, ground
- A pinch of sea salt
- Black pepper to the taste
- 1 teaspoon garlic powder
- 1 teaspoon onion powder

For the sauce:
- ¼ cup coconut amino
- 4 tablespoon ketchup
- 1 tablespoon ginger, grated
- ½ cup pineapple juice
- 2 teaspoons raw honey
- ½ teaspoon red pepper flakes
- Salt and black pepper to the taste
- 1 tablespoon garlic, minced

Directions:
In a pot, mix amino with ketchup, ginger, pineapple sauce, garlic, pepper flakes, honey, a pinch of sea salt and pepper to the taste, stir well, bring to a boil over medium heat, simmer for 8 minutes and take off heat. In a bowl, mix chicken meat with paprika, egg, onion powder, garlic powder, salt and black pepper to the taste and stir well. Shape meatballs, arrange them on a lined baking sheet, introduce them in the oven at 475 degrees F and bake for 15 minutes. Heat up a pan over medium heat, add pineapple pieces, stir and cook for 2 minutes. Add baked meatballs, pour sauce you've made at the beginnings, stir gently, cook for 5 minutes, divide between plates and serve. Enjoy!

Nutritional value: calories 264, fat 20, carbs 47, fiber 2, protein 47

Delicious Paleo Beef Casserole

It's a slow cooked meal, full of amazing flavors! It's delicious!

Servings: 4
Preparation time: 10 minutes
Cooking time: 8 hours

Ingredients:

- 2 cups pearl onions
- 3 and ½ pounds grass fed beef meat, cubed
- 4 garlic cloves, minced
- 2 sweet potatoes, chopped
- 2 celery stalks, chopped
- A pinch of sea salt
- Black pepper to the taste
- 2 tablespoons tomato paste
- 2 bay leaves
- 2 cups carrot, chopped
- 2 cups broth
- 1 teaspoon thyme, dried
- 1 tablespoon coconut oil

Directions:
Heat up a pan with the oil over medium-high heat, add beef, stir and brown for 2 minutes on each side and transfer to your slow cooker. Add pearl onions, potatoes, celery, garlic, carrots, tomato paste, stock, bay leaves, thyme, a pinch of salt and pepper to the taste, stir, cover and cook on Low for 8 hours. Uncover cooker, leave stew aside for 10 minutes, divide between plates and serve. Enjoy!

Nutritional value: calories 210, carbs 14, fat 20, fiber 4, protein 38

Paleo Grilled Lamb Chops

We are sure you've never tried this before! It's a very flavored and savory dish!

Servings: 6
Preparation time: 10 minutes
Cooking time: 10 minutes

Ingredients:

- 3 tablespoons coconut amino
- 4 tablespoons extra virgin olive oil
- 8 lamb chops
- A pinch of sea salt
- Black pepper to the taste
- 2 garlic cloves, minced
- 2 tablespoons ginger, minced
- 1 tablespoon parsley leaves, chopped

Directions:
In a bowl, mix olive oil with coconut amino, garlic, ginger and parsley and stir well. Season lamb chops with a pinch of sea salt and pepper to the taste, place them on preheated grill over medium-high heat and cook for 4 minutes on each side, basting all the time with the marinade you've made. Divide lamb chops on plates, leave aside to cool down for 4 minutes and serve. Enjoy!

Nutritional value: calories 214, fat 33, carbs 2, protein 28, fiber 0.2

Paleo Lamb Casserole

It's a very rich Asian style lamb stew! It's perfectly balanced and amazing!

Servings: 4
Preparation time: 2 hours
Cooking time: 1 hour

Ingredients:
- 1 butternut squash, cubed
- 3 pounds lamb shoulder, chopped
- 4 shallots, chopped
- 4 carrots, chopped
- 4 tomatoes, chopped
- 2 Thai chilies, chopped
- 2 tablespoons tomato paste
- 1 cinnamon stick
- 2 and ½ cups warm beef broth
- 2-star anise
- 2 tablespoons tapioca starch
- 1 lemongrass stalk, finely chopped
- 1 teaspoon Chinese five spice powder
- 1 tablespoon ginger, minced
- 2 tablespoon coconut amino
- 1 and ½ tablespoons coconut oil
- 3 garlic cloves, chopped
- Black pepper to the taste

Directions:
In a bowl, mix lamb with coconut amino, tapioca starch, ginger, lemongrass, garlic and pepper, stir well, cover and keep in the fridge for 2 hours. Heat up a pot with the oil over medium-high heat, add marinated lamb, stir and brown for 3 minutes. Add tomato paste and tomatoes, stir and cook for 2 more minutes. Add squash, shallots, Thai chilies, carrots, cinnamon stick, star anise, beef stock and five spices, stir well, introduce in the oven at 325 degrees F and bake for 1 hour. Divide between plates and serve hot. Enjoy!

Nutritional value: calories 456, fat 31, carbs 5, fiber 3, protein 22

Paleo Lamb Chops with Mint Sauce

It's a classic recipe with a special twist! Try it soon!

Servings: 4
Preparation time: 15 minutes
Cooking time: 20 minutes

Ingredients:
- 2 garlic cloves, finely minced
- 8 lamb chops
- 2/3 cup extra virgin olive oil
- 1 tablespoon oregano, finely chopped
- 3 tablespoons Dijon mustard
- 1 tablespoon lemon zest
- 2 tablespoons white wine vinegar
- 1/3 cup mint, chopped
- Black pepper to the taste

Directions:
In a bowl, mix olive oil with oregano, garlic and lemon zest and stir well. Season lamb with black pepper to the taste and brush with the mix you've just made. Heat up your grill over medium high heat, add lamb chops, cook for 5 minutes on each side and transfer to plates. In a bowl, mix mustard with vinegar, pepper and mint and whisk well. Serve lamb chops with vinegar mix drizzled on top. Enjoy!

Nutritional value: calories 160, fat 5.6, carbs 1, fiber 0.2, protein 23.2

Paleo Beef Tenderloin with Special Sauce

We don't want to spoil the surprise! We'll allow you to discover step by step how to make this amazing paleo dish!

Servings: 4
Preparation time: 10 minutes
Cooking time: 40 minutes

Ingredients:
- 3 tablespoons Dijon mustard
- 3 pounds beef tenderloin
- A pinch of sea salt
- Black pepper to the taste
- 1 tablespoon coconut oil
- 3 tablespoons balsamic vinegar

- 3 tablespoons basil leaves, chopped
- ½ cup parsley leaves, chopped
- Zest from 1 lemon
- 2 garlic cloves, finely chopped
- A pinch of sea salt
- Black pepper to the taste
- ¼ cup extra virgin olive oil

For the sauce:

Directions:
In a bowl, mix mustard with vinegar, stir very well and leave aside. Season beef with a pinch of sea salt and pepper to the taste put in a pan heated with the coconut oil over medium-high heat and cook fro 2 minutes on each side. Transfer beef to a baking pan, cover with the mustard mix, introduce in the oven at 475 degrees F and bake for 25 minutes. Meanwhile, in a bowl, mix parsley with basil, lemon zest, garlic, olive oil, a pinch of sea salt, and pepper to the taste and whisk very well. Take beef tenderloin out if the oven, leave aside for a few minutes to cool down, slice and divide between plates. Serve with herbs sauce on the side. Enjoy!

Nutritional value: calories 180, fat 13, carbs 2, fiber 2, protein 7

Paleo Beef Stir Fry

It's an Asian style dish! It's tasty, it's light and very easy to make at home!

Servings: 4
Preparation time: 10 minutes
Cooking time: 20 minutes

Ingredients:
- 10 ounces mushrooms, sliced
- 10 ounces asparagus, sliced
- 1 and ½ pounds beef steak, thinly sliced
- 2 tablespoons honey
- 1/3 cup coconut amino
- 2 teaspoons apple cider vinegar

- ½ teaspoon ginger, minced
- 6 garlic cloves, minced
- 1 chili, sliced
- 1 tablespoon coconut oil
- Black pepper to the taste

Directions:
In a bowl, mix garlic with coconut amino, honey, ginger and vinegar and whisk well. Put some water in a pan, heat up over medium high heat, add asparagus and black pepper, cook for 3 minutes, transfer to a bowl filled with ice water, drain and leave aside. Heat up a pan with the oil over medium-high heat, add mushrooms, cook for 2 minutes on each side, transfer to a bowl and also leave aside. Heat up the same pan over high heat, add meat, brown for a few minutes and mix with chili pepper. Cook for 2 more minutes and mix with asparagus, mushrooms and vinegar sauce you've made at the beginning. Stir well, cook for 3 minutes, take off heat, divide between plates and serve. Enjoy!

Nutritional value: calories 165, fat 7.2, carbs 6.33, fiber 1.3, sugar 3, protein 18.4

Paleo Pork Dish with Delicious Blueberry Sauce

It's such a juicy and delicious dish! You will love it once you try it!

Servings: 4
Preparation time: 10 minutes
Cooking time: 30 minutes

Ingredients:
- 1 cup blueberries
- ½ teaspoon thyme, dried
- 2 pounds pork loin
- 1 tablespoon balsamic vinegar
- ½ teaspoon red chili flakes
- 1 teaspoon ginger powder
- A pinch of sea salt
- Black pepper to the taste
- 2 tablespoon water

Directions:
Put pork loin in a baking dish and season with a pinch of sea salt and pepper to the taste. Heat up a pan over medium heat, add blueberries and mix with vinegar, water, thyme, chili flakes and ginger. Stir well, cook for 5 minutes and pour over pork loin. Introduce in the oven at 375 degrees F and bake for 25 minutes. Take pork out of the oven, leave aside for 5 minutes, slice, divide between plates and serve with blueberries sauce. Enjoy!

Nutritional value: calories 325, fat 23, carbs 6, fiber 1, protein 64

Tasty Paleo Pulled Pork

Are you in the mood for a Mexican dish? Then you should really try this one as soon as possible!

Servings: 4
Preparation time: 12 hours and 10 minutes
Cooking time: 8 hours and 20 minutes

Ingredients:
- ½ cup salsa
- ½ cup beef stock
- ½ cup enchilada sauce
- 3 pounds organic pork shoulder
- 2 green chilies, chopped
- 1 tablespoon garlic powder
- 1 tablespoon chili powder
- 1 teaspoon onion powder
- 1 teaspoon cumin
- 1 teaspoon paprika
- Black pepper to the taste

Directions:
In a bowl, mix chili powder with onion and garlic one. Add cumin, paprika and pepper to the taste and stir everything. Add pork, rub well and keep in the fridge for 12 hours. Transfer pork to your slow cooker, add enchilada sauce, stock, salsa and green chilies, stir, cover and cook on Low for 8 hours. Transfer pork to a plate, leave aside to cool down and shred. Strain sauce from slow cooker into a pan, bring to a boil over medium heat and simmer for 8 minutes stirring all the time. Add shredded pork to the sauce, stir, reduce heat to medium and cook for 20 more minutes. Divide between plates and serve hot. Enjoy!

Nutritional value: calories 250, fat 35, carbs 5, fiber 2, protein 50

Paleo Barbeque Ribs

Take a look at this recipe, get all the ingredients and make it for your loved one's tonight!

Servings: 4
Preparation time: 15 minutes
Cooking time: 2 hours and 47 minutes

Ingredients:

- 1 tablespoon smoked paprika
- ½ tablespoon onion powder
- ½ tablespoon garlic powder
- ½ teaspoon cayenne pepper
- 4 pounds baby ribs
- 1 cup paleo BBQ sauce
- 2 tablespoons raw honey
- 4 teaspoons Sriracha
- ¼ cup cilantro, chopped
- ¼ cup chives, chopped
- ¼ cup parsley, chopped
- Black pepper to the taste

Directions:
In a bowl, mix paprika with onion powder, garlic powder, pepper and cayenne and stir well. Add ribs, toss to coat and arrange them on a lined baking sheet. Introduce in the oven at 325 degrees F and bake them for 2 hours and 30 minutes. In a bowl, mix BBQ sauce with honey and Sriracha and stir well. Take ribs out of the oven, mix them with BBQ sauce, place them on preheated grill over medium-high heat and cook for 7 minutes on each side. Divide ribs on plates, sprinkle chives, cilantro, and parsley on top and serve. Enjoy!

Nutritional value: calories 120, fat 6.4, carbs 2, fiber 03, sugar 0.3, protein 6.2

Special Paleo Pork Chops

It's full of taste and flavors! It's really a special recipe!

Servings: 4
Preparation time: 10 minutes
Cooking time: 30 minutes

Ingredients:

- 8 sage springs
- 4 pork chops, bone-in
- 4 tablespoons ghee
- 4 garlic cloves, crushed
- 1 tablespoon coconut oil
- A pinch of sea salt
- Black pepper to the taste

Directions:
Season pork chops with a pinch of sea salt and pepper to the taste. Heat up a pan with the oil over medium high heat, add pork chops and cook for 10 minutes turning them often. Take pork chops off heat, add ghee, sage, and garlic and toss to coat. Return to heat, cook for 4 minutes often stirring, divide between plates and serve. Enjoy!

Nutritional value: calories 250, fat 41, carbs 1, fiber 1, sugar 0.1, protein 18.3

Paleo Pork with Pear Salsa

It's a great combination of ingredients! It's a well-balanced dish, full of taste and textures!

Servings: 4
Preparation time: 10 minutes
Cooking time: 45 minutes

Ingredients:
- 1 yellow onion, chopped
- 1 organic pork tenderloin
- 2 pears, chopped
- 2 garlic cloves, minced
- 1 tablespoon chives, chopped
- ¼ cup walnuts, chopped
- 3 tablespoons balsamic vinegar
- Black pepper to the taste
- ½ cup chicken stock
- 1 tablespoon coconut oil
- 1 tablespoon lemon juice

Directions:
In a bowl, mix walnuts with pear, chives, pepper and lemon juice and stir well. Heat up a pan with the oil over medium high heat, add tenderloin and brown for 3 minutes on each side. Reduce heat, add onion and garlic, stir and cook for 2 minutes. Add balsamic vinegar, stock, pear mix, stir, introduce in the oven at 400 degrees F and bake for 20 minutes. Take pork out of the oven, leave aside for 4 minutes, slice, divide between plates and serve with pear salsa on top. Enjoy!

Nutritional value: calories 170, fat 3, carbs 19, fiber 4.4, sugar 10, protein 12

Paleo Pork Tenderloin with Carrot Puree

It's a fulfilling dish that will make you want more!

Servings: 4
Preparation time: 10 minutes
Cooking time: 45 minutes

Ingredients:
- 2 sausages, casings removed
- A handful arugula
- Black pepper to the taste
- 1 grass fed pork tenderloin
- 1 tablespoon coconut oil

For the puree:
- 1 sweet potato, chopped
- 3 carrots, chopped
- A pinch of sea salt

- Black pepper to the taste
- 1 tablespoon curry paste

For the sauce:
- 2 tablespoons balsamic vinegar
- 1 teaspoon mustard
- 2 shallots, finely chopped
- Black pepper to the taste
- 4 tablespoons extra virgin olive oil

Directions:
Slice pork tenderloin in half horizontally but not all the way and open it up. Use a meat tenderizer to even it up. Place sausage in the middle, roll pork around it, tie with twine, season pepper to the taste and leave aside. Heat up an oven proof pan with the coconut oil over medium high heat, add pork roll, cook for 3 minutes on each side, introduce in the oven at 350 degrees F and bake for 25 minutes. Meanwhile, put potatoes and carrots in a pot, add water to cover, bring to a boil over medium high heat, cook for 20 minutes, drain and transfer to your food processor. Pulse a few times until you obtain a puree, add a pinch of sea salt and pepper to the taste, blend again, transfer to a bowl and leave aside. Take pork roll out of the oven, slice and divide between plates. Heat up a pan with the olive oil over medium high heat, add shallots, stir and cook for 10 minutes. Add balsamic vinegar, mustard, pepper, stir well and take off heat. Divide carrots puree next to pork slices, drizzle vinegar sauce on to and serve with arugula on the side. Enjoy!

Nutritional value: calories 250, fat 34, carbs 19, fiber 2, protein 53

Paleo Pork with Strawberry Sauce

We are sure you've never tried such a combination before! It's one of the best ones ever!

Servings: 4
Preparation time: 10 minutes
Cooking time: 35 minutes

Ingredients:
- 4 pounds pork tenderloin
- 1 cup strawberries, sliced
- 10 bacon slices
- A pinch of sea salt
- Black pepper to the taste
- 4 garlic cloves, minced
- ½ cup balsamic vinegar
- 2 tablespoons extra virgin olive oil

Directions:
Wrap bacon slices around tenderloin, secure with toothpicks and season with salt and pepper. Heat up your grill over indirect medium high heat, put tenderloin on it and cook for 30 minutes. Heat up a pan with the oil over medium high heat, add garlic, stir and cook for 2 minutes. Add vinegar and half of the strawberries, stir and bring to a boil. Reduce heat to medium and simmer for 10 minutes. Add black pepper to the taste and the rest of the strawberries and stir. Baste pork with some of the sauce and continue cooking over indirect heat until bacon is crispy enough. Transfer pork to a cutting board, leave aside for a few minutes to cool down, slice and divide between plates. Serve with the strawberry sauce right away. Enjoy!

Nutritional value: calories 279, fat 30, carbs 8, fiber 22, protein 125

Paleo Sausage Casserole

It's incredibly easy to make this at home! Why don't you try it tonight?

Servings: 6
Preparation time: 15 minutes
Cooking time: 45 minutes

Ingredients:
- 6 sausage
- 2 green bell peppers, chopped
- 3 sweet potatoes, chopped
- 1-pint grape tomatoes, chopped
- A pinch of sea salt
- Black pepper to the taste
- 2 garlic cloves, minced
- 1 red onion, chopped
- A few thyme springs

Directions:
In a baking dish, mix potatoes with tomatoes, onion, bell pepper, garlic, a pinch of sea salt and pepper and stir gently. Heat up a pan over high heat, add sausages, brown them for 2 minutes on each side and transfer on top of veggies in the baking dish. Add thyme, introduce in the oven at 400 degrees F and bake for 45 minutes. Divide between plates and serve hot. Enjoy!

Nutritional value: calories 355, fat 10, carbs 25, fiber 2, protein 16

Amazing Souvlaki

This is one Greek dish you will adore!

Preparation time: 10 minutes
Cooking time: 20 minutes
Servings: 4

Ingredients:
- 3 sweet potatoes, cubed
- 1 yellow onion, chopped
- 12 mini bell peppers, chopped
- 4 medium round steaks
- ½ cup sun dried tomatoes, chopped
- 1 tablespoon sweet paprika
- 2 tablespoons balsamic vinegar
- Juice of 1 lemon
- 1 tablespoons oregano, dried
- ¼ cup olive oil
- 1 lemon, sliced
- ¼ cup kalamata olives, pitted and chopped
- 4 dill springs
- 2 garlic cloves, minced
- Some bacon fat
- A pinch of sea salt and black pepper

Directions:
Heat up a pan with some bacon fat over medium high heat, add steaks, season them with a pinch of sea salt and some black pepper, brown them for 2 minutes on each side and transfer to a baking dish. Heat up the pan again over medium high heat, add sweet potatoes, cook them for 4 minutes and add them to the baking dish. Also add bell peppers, tomatoes, onion, olives and lemon slices. Meanwhile, in a bowl, mix lemon juice with olive oil, vinegar, garlic, paprika and oregano and whisk well. Pour this over steak and veggies, add dill springs on top, toss to coat, place in the oven at 425 degrees F and bake for 12 minutes. Divide steak and veggies between plates and serve. Enjoy!

Nutritional value: calories 180, fat 11, fiber 0, carbs 0, protein 21

Delicious Mexican Steaks

You should try this tonight! It's so tasty!

Preparation time: 10 minutes
Cooking time: 15 minutes
Servings: 4

Ingredients:
- 2 tablespoons chili powder
- 4 medium sirloin steaks
- 1 teaspoon cumin, ground
- ½ tablespoon sweet paprika
- 1 teaspoon onion powder
- 1 teaspoon garlic powder
- A pinch of sea salt and black pepper to the taste
- 1 small red onion, chopped
- 2 tomatoes, chopped
- 2 garlic cloves, minced
- 2 tablespoons lime juice
- 1 small green bell pepper, chopped
- 1 jalapeno, chopped
- ¼ cup cilantro, chopped
- ¼ teaspoon cumin, ground
- Black pepper to the taste

For the Pico de gallo:

Directions:
In a bowl, mix chili powder with a pinch of salt, black pepper, onion powder, garlic powder, paprika and 1 teaspoon cumin and stir well. Season steaks with this mix, rub well and place them on preheated grill over medium high heat. Cook steaks for 5 minutes on each side and divide them between plates. In a bowl, mix red onion with tomatoes, garlic, lime juice, bell pepper, jalapeno, cilantro, black pepper to the taste and ¼ teaspoon cumin and stir well. Top steaks with this mix and serve. Enjoy!

Nutritional value: calories 200, fat 12, fiber 4, carbs 5, protein 12

Different Grilled Steaks

This is a special Paleo meat recipe you will like for sure!

Preparation time: 10 minutes
Cooking time: 10 minutes
Servings: 4

Ingredients:
- 1 and ½ tablespoons coffee, ground
- 4 rib eye steaks
- ½ tablespoon sweet paprika
- 2 tablespoons chili powder
- 2 teaspoons garlic powder
- 2 teaspoons onion powder
- ¼ teaspoon ginger, ground
- ¼ teaspoon, coriander, ground
- A pinch of cayenne pepper
- Black pepper to the taste

Directions:
In a bowl, mix coffee with paprika, chili powder, garlic powder, onion powder, ginger, coriander, cayenne and black pepper and stir well. Rub steaks with the coffee mix, place them on your preheated grill over medium high heat, cook them for 5 minutes on each side and divide between plates. Leave steaks to cool down for 5 minutes before serving them with a side salad! Enjoy!

Nutritional value: calories 160, fat 10, fiber 1, carbs 4, protein 8

Amazing Beef Lasagna

This is not a regular lasagna! It's so much better!

Preparation time: 10 minutes
Cooking time: 6 hours
Servings: 6

Ingredients:
- 1 red bell pepper, chopped
- 1 eggplant, sliced lengthwise
- 2 zucchinis, sliced lengthwise
- 1 pound beef, ground
- 2 cups tomatoes, chopped
- 2 teaspoons oregano, dried
- 4 cups tomato sauce
- ¼ cup basil, chopped
- 2 garlic cloves, minced
- 1 yellow onion, chopped
- 2 tablespoons tomato paste
- 1 tablespoon parsley, chopped
- 2 tablespoons olive oil
- A pinch of sea salt
- Black pepper to the taste

Directions:
Heat up a pan with the oil over medium high heat, add onion and garlic, stir and cook for 2 minutes. Add beef, stir and brown for 5 minutes more. Add bell pepper, tomatoes, oregano, basil, tomato paste and parsley, stir and cook for 4 minutes more. Add tomato sauce, black pepper to the taste and a pinch of salt and stir well again. Arrange layers of eggplant and zucchini slices with the sauce you've made in your slow cooker. Cover and cook on Low for 4 hours and 45 minutes. Divide your lasagna between plates and serve. Enjoy!

Nutritional value: calories 240, fat 10, fiber 5, carbs 7, protein 12

Steaks and Apricots

The combination is just perfect! Trust us! We know!

Preparation time: 10 minutes
Cooking time: 25 minutes
Servings: 2

Ingredients:
- 2 tablespoons Cajun spice
- ¼ cup coconut oil
- 2 medium skirt steaks
- 1/3 cup lemon juice
- ¼ cup apricot preserves
- ¼ cup coconut aminos

Directions:
In a bowl, mix half of the Cajun spice with lemon juice, aminos, oil and apricot preserves and stir well. Pour this into a pan, bring to a boil over medium high heat and simmer for 8 minutes. Blend this using an immersion blender and leave aside for now. Season steaks with the rest of the Cajun spice, brush them with half of the apricots mix, place them on preheated grill over medium high heat and cook them for 6-minute son each side. Divide steaks on plates and top with the rest of the apricots mix. Enjoy!

Nutritional value: calories 160, fat 6, fiber 0.1, carbs 1, protein 22

Delicious Filet Mignon and Special Sauce

This is such an elegant Paleo dish! You can serve it on a special occasion!

Preparation time: 10 minutes
Cooking time: 25 minutes
Servings: 4

Ingredients:
- 12 mushrooms, sliced
- 1 shallot, chopped
- 4 fillet mignons
- 2 garlic cloves, minced
- 2 tablespoons olive oil
- ¼ cup Dijon mustard
- ¼ cup wine
- 1 and ¼ cup coconut cream
- 2 tablespoons parsley, chopped
- Black pepper to the taste
- A pinch of sea salt

Directions:
Heat up a pan with the oil over medium high heat, add garlic and shallots, stir and cook for 3 minutes. Add mushrooms, stir and cook for 4 minutes more. Add wine, stir and cook until it evaporates. Add coconut cream, mustard, parsley, a pinch of salt and black pepper to the taste, stir and cook for 6 minutes more. Heat up another pan over high heat, add fillets, season them with a pinch of salt and some black pepper and cook them for 4 minutes on each side. Divide fillets between plates and serve with the mushroom sauce on top. Enjoy!

Nutritional value: calories 300, fat 12, fiber 1, carbs 4, protein 23

Amazing Beef Kabobs

It's a succulent Paleo dish you will like! Just try it!

Preparation time: 10 minutes
Cooking time: 12 minutes
Servings: 4

Ingredients:
- 2 red bell peppers, chopped
- 2 pounds sirloin steak, cut into medium pieces
- 1 red onion, chopped
- 1 zucchini, sliced
- Juice from 1 lime
- 2 tablespoons chili powder
- 2 tablespoon hot sauce
- ½ tablespoons cumin powder
- ¼ cup olive oil
- ¼ cup Paleo Salsa
- A pinch of sea salt and black pepper to the taste

Directions:
In a bowl, mix salsa with lime juice, oil, hot sauce, chili powder, cumin, salt and black pepper and whisk well. Layer steaks pieces, bell peppers, zucchini and onion on skewers. Brush kabobs with the salsa mix you made earlier, place them on preheated grill over medium high heat and cook them for 5 minutes on each side. Divide kabobs between plates and serve. Enjoy!

Nutritional value: calories 170, fat 5, fiber 2, carbs 3, protein 8

Delicious Steak

It's a delicious combination between a tasty steak and some wonderful veggies!

Preparation time: 10 minutes
Cooking time: 30 minutes
Servings: 4

Ingredients:
- 2 sweet potatoes, chopped
- 4 sirloin steaks
- 1 red onion, chopped
- 1 broccoli head, florets separated
- 8 cherry tomatoes, halved
- 4 thyme springs
- 4 garlic cloves, minced
- A pinch of sea salt
- Black pepper to the taste
- 4 tablespoons olive oil
- ½ tablespoon sweet paprika

Directions:
In a bowl, mix oil with a pinch of salt, black pepper, garlic and paprika and stir well. Spread broccoli and sweet potatoes on a lined baking sheet, place in the oven at 425 degrees f and bake for 10 minutes. Heat up a pan over medium high heat, add steaks, season them with a pinch of sea salt and black pepper, cook for 2 minutes on each side and add to the baking sheet. Also add onions and tomatoes, drizzle the oil and garlic mix, toss to coat, top with thyme and bake in the oven for 15 minutes more. Divide everything between plates and serve.

Nutritional value: calories 170, fat 2, fiber 2, carbs 4, protein 10

Great Beef Teriyaki

This is so easy to make and it's 100% Paleo!

Preparation time: 10 minutes
Cooking time: 20 minutes
Servings: 4

Ingredients:
- 2 green onions, chopped
- 1 and ½ pounds steaks, sliced
- ¼ cup honey
- ½ cup coconut aminos
- 1 tablespoon ginger, minced
- 1 tablespoon tapioca flour
- 1 tablespoon water
- 2 garlic cloves, minced
- ¼ cup pear juice
- Some bacon fat
- 4 tablespoons white wine

Directions:
Heat up a pan with the bacon fat over medium heat, add ginger and garlic, stir and cook for 2 minutes. Add wine, stir and cook until it evaporates. Add honey, aminos, pear juice, stir, bring to a simmer and cook for 12 minutes. Add tapioca mixed with the water, stir and cook until it thickens. Heat up a pan with some bacon fat over medium high heat, add steak slices and brown them for 2 minutes on each side. Add green onions and half of the sauce you've just made, stir gently and cook for 3 minutes more. Divide steaks between plates and serve with the rest of the sauce on top.

Nutritional value: calories 170, fat 3, fiber 2, carbs 2, protein 8

Delicious Beef and Wonderful Gravy

This is a unique dish you have to try today! It's so amazing!

Preparation time: 10 minutes
Cooking time: 20 minutes
Servings: 4

Ingredients:
- 1 egg, whisked
- 1 tablespoon mustard
- 1 tablespoon tomato paste
- 1 teaspoon garlic powder
- 1 teaspoon onion powder
- Some coconut oil for cooking
- A pinch of sea salt and black pepper to the taste
- 1 and ½ pound beef, ground

For the gravy:
- 2 teaspoons parsley, chopped
- 2 tablespoons ghee
- 1 teaspoon tapioca
- 1 small yellow onion, chopped
- 1 and ¼ cups beef stock
- Black pepper to the taste

Directions:
In a bowl, mix beef with tomato paste, egg, mustard, onion powder, garlic powder, a pinch of salt and black pepper to the taste and stir well. Heat up a pan with the ghee over medium heat, add onion, stir and cook for 2 minutes. Add stock, some black pepper, tapioca mixed with water, stir, cook until it thickens and take off heat. Shape 4 patties from the beef mix. Heat up a pan with the coconut oil over medium high heat, add beef patties and cook for 5 minutes on each side. Pour the gravy over beef patties, sprinkle parsley on top, cook for a couple more minutes, divide between plates and serve. Enjoy!

Nutritional value: calories 200, fat 4, fiber 2, carbs 4, protein 20

Steaks and Scallops

This Paleo dish doesn't need any introductions! Just check it out!

Preparation time: 10 minutes
Cooking time: 20 minutes
Servings: 2

Ingredients:
- 10 sea scallops
- 4 garlic cloves, minced
- 2 beef steaks
- 1 shallot, chopped
- 2 tablespoons lemon juice
- 2 tablespoons parsley, chopped
- 2 tablespoons basil, chopped
- 1 teaspoon lemon zest
- ¼ cup ghee
- ¼ cup veggie stock
- Some bacon fat
- A pinch of sea salt
- Black pepper to the taste

Directions:
Heat up a pan with some bacon fat over medium high heat, add steaks, season them with a pinch of salt and black pepper to the taste and cook for 4 minutes on each side. Add shallot and garlic, stir and cook for 2 minutes more. Add ghee and stir everything. Add stock, basil, lemon juice, parsley and lemon zest and stir. Add scallops, season them with some black pepper as well and cook for a couple more minutes. Divide steaks and scallops between plates and serve with pan juices. Enjoy!

Nutritional value: calories 150, fat 2, fiber 2, carbs 4, protein 14

Sheppard's Pie

You've probably heard about this pie before! Did you know there's a Paleo version as well?

Preparation time: 15 minutes
Cooking time: 45 minutes
Servings: 6

Ingredients:
- 2 pounds sweet potatoes, chopped
- 1 and ½ pounds beef, ground
- 2 cups beef stock
- 1 onion, chopped
- 2 carrots, chopped
- 2 thyme springs
- 2 bay leaves
- 2 garlic cloves, minced
- 2 celery stalks, chopped
- ¼ cup ghee
- Bacon fat
- A handful parsley, chopped
- 2 tablespoons tomato paste
- A pinch of sea salt
- Black pepper to the taste

Directions:
Put sweet potatoes in a pot, add water to cover, bring to a boil over medium high heat, cook for 20 minutes, drain, leave them to cool down and transfer to a bowl. Add ghee, a pinch of salt and pepper and mash potatoes well. Heat up a pan with the bacon fat over medium high heat, add beef, stir and cook for a couple of minutes. Add carrots, garlic, onions, celery, stock, tomato paste, bay leaves, thyme springs, some black pepper and another pinch of salt, stir and cook for 10 minutes. Discard bay leaves and thyme and spread beef mix on the bottom of a baking dish. Top with mashed potatoes, spread well, place in the oven at 375 degrees F and bake for 25 minutes. Leave pie to cool down a bit before slicing and serving it. Enjoy!

Nutritional value: calories 254, fat 7, fiber 4, carbs 7, protein 14

Amazing Lamb Chops

If you like eating lamb chops, then you will definitely like this next recipe!

Preparation time: 10 minutes
Cooking time: 10 minutes
Servings: 6

Ingredients:
- 3 tablespoons coconut aminos
- 4 tablespoons olive oil
- 2 tablespoons ginger, grated
- 8 lamb chops
- 1 tablespoon parsley, chopped
- 2 garlic cloves, minced
- A pinch of sea salt
- Black pepper to the taste

Directions:
In a bowl, mix oil with aminos, parsley, ginger and garlic and stir well. Place lamb chops on a preheated grill over medium high heat, season them with a pinch of salt and black pepper to the taste and grill them for 4 minutes on each side basting them with the oil and ginger mix you've made. Leave lamb chops to cool down for a couple of minutes and then serve. Enjoy!

Nutritional value: calories 160, fat 5, fiber 0, carbs 1, protein 20

Carne Asada

This is one of the best Paleo dishes you'll ever try!

Preparation time: 30 minutes
Cooking time: 25 minutes
Servings: 2

Ingredients:
- ¼ cup olive oil
- ½ teaspoon oregano, dried
- 2 garlic cloves, minced
- Juice from 1 lime
- 2 skirt steaks
- ¼ teaspoon cumin, ground
- 1 Serrano chili pepper, minced
- ¼ cup cilantro, chopped
- A pinch of sea salt
- Black pepper to the taste

For the veggie mix:
- 2 red bell peppers, chopped
- 3 Portobello mushrooms, sliced
- 1 yellow onion, chopped
- 1 tablespoon olive oil
- 1 tablespoon lime juice
- 1 tablespoon taco seasoning

Directions:
In a bowl, mix ¼ cup oil with oregano, garlic, lime juice, cumin, cilantro, chili pepper, a pinch of salt and black pepper and whisk very well. Add steaks, toss to coat and keep in the fridge for 30 minutes. Place steaks on preheated grill over medium high heat, cook them for 4 minutes on each side and transfer to a plate. Heat up a pan with 1 tablespoon oil over medium high heat, add bell pepper and onion, stir and cook for 3 minutes, Add mushrooms, taco seasoning and lime juice, stir and cook for 6 minutes more. Divide steaks between plates and serve with mixed veggies on the side.

Nutritional value: calories 190, fat 2, fiber 1, carbs 4, protein 20

Amazing Slow-Cooked Beef

This is a Paleo dish you can serve during the holidays! Everyone will love it!

Preparation time: 10 minutes
Cooking time: 8 hours and 40 minutes
Servings: 4

Ingredients:
- 2 cups beef stock
- ¼ cup honey
- 1 cup tomato paste
- 1 cup balsamic vinegar
- 4 pounds beef chuck
- 1 tablespoon mustard
- 1 tablespoon sweet paprika
- 1 teaspoon onion powder
- 2 tablespoons chili powder
- 2 garlic cloves, minced
- Black pepper to the taste

Directions:
In a bowl, mix beef chuck with chili powder, paprika, onion powder, garlic and black pepper and rub well. Transfer beef roast to your slow cooker, add stock over it, cover and cook on Low for 8 hours. Meanwhile, heat up a pan over medium heat, add tomato paste, vinegar, mustard, honey and black pepper, stir, bring to a boil and cook for 12 minutes. Transfer beef roast to a cutting board, leave it to cool down a bit, shred with a fork and return to your crock pot. Add the sauce you've made in the pan, cover and cook everything on High for 30 minutes more. Divide this whole mix between plates and serve.

Nutritional value: calories 340, fat 5, fiber 2, carbs 5, protein 24

Beef in Amazing Tomato Marinade

The combination is really good!

Preparation time: 2 hours and 10 minutes
Cooking time: 15 minutes
Servings: 4

Ingredients:
- 2 teaspoons chili powder
- 1 cup tomatoes, crushed
- 4 beef medallions
- 2 teaspoons onion powder
- 2 tablespoons coconut aminos
- 1 jalapeno pepper, chopped
- A pinch of sea salt
- Black pepper to the taste
- 1 tablespoons hot pepper
- 2 tablespoons lime juice

Directions:
In a bowl, mix tomatoes with hot pepper, aminos, chili powder, onion powder, a pinch of salt, black pepper and lime juice and whisk well. Arrange beef medallions in a baking dish, pour the sauce over them and leave them aside for 2 hours. Discard tomato marinade, place beef on preheated grill over medium high heat, cook them for 5 minutes one each side basting them with the marinade. Divide beef medallions on plates, sprinkle jalapeno on top and serve. Enjoy!

Nutritional value: calories 230, fat 4, fiber 1, carbs 3, protein 14

Amazing Lamb Chops and Mint Sauce

How can you resist to such an amazing dish?

Preparation time: 10 minutes
Cooking time: 20 minutes
Servings: 4

Ingredients:
- 2 garlic cloves, minced
- 1 tablespoon lemon zest
- 1 tablespoon oregano, chopped
- 8 lamb chops
- 2/3 cup olive oil
- 1/3 cup mint, chopped
- 2 tablespoons balsamic vinegar
- A pinch of sea salt
- Black pepper to the taste
- 3 tablespoons Dijon mustard

Directions:
In a bowl, mix oil with oregano, garlic and lemon zest and whisk well. Brush lamb chops with this mix, season them with a pinch of salt and black pepper to the taste, place them on preheated grill over medium high heat and cook for 5 minutes on each side. In a bowl, mix mustard with a pinch of salt, mint, vinegar and black pepper and whisk well. Divide lamb chops on plates, drizzle mint sauce over them and serve. Enjoy!

Nutritional value: calories 17, fat 11, fiber 1, carbs 6, protein 14

Amazing Roasted Lamb

It's so rich and intense! You must try this Paleo dish!

Preparation time: 10 minutes
Cooking time: 2 hours and 30 minutes
Servings: 4

Ingredients:
- 15 garlic cloves, peeled
- 2 teaspoons onion powder
- 6 lamb shanks
- 2 teaspoons cumin powder
- 1 cup water
- 3 teaspoons oregano, dried
- ½ cup olive oil
- A pinch of sea salt
- Black pepper to the taste
- ½ cup lemon juice

Directions:
Place garlic cloves in a roasting pan.
Add lamb on top, drizzle half of the oil and season with a pinch of salt and black pepper. Also add onion powder and cumin and rub well. Introduce this in the oven at 450 degrees F and roast for 35 minutes. In a bowl mix the rest of the oil with the water, lemon juice and oregano and whisk very well. Take lamb shanks out of the oven, drizzle this mix, toss to coat well and roast in the oven at 350 degrees F for 2 hours and 30 minutes. Divide lamb pieces between plates and serve. Enjoy!

Nutritional value: calories 170, fat 2, fiber 2, carbs 4, protein 12

Delicious Turkey Casserole

You must try this for dinner sometimes!

Preparation time: 10 minutes
Cooking time: 1 hour
Servings: 6

Ingredients:
- ¼ cup onion, chopped
- 1 pound turkey meat, ground
- 1 sweet potato, cut with a spiralizer
- 1 eggplant, chopped
- 1 tablespoon garlic, minced
- 8 ounces tomato paste
- 15 ounces canned tomatoes, chopped
- A pinch of sea salt
- Black pepper to the taste
- A pinch of oregano, dried
- ¼ teaspoon chili powder
- ¼ teaspoon cumin, ground
- Cooking spray
- A pinch of cardamom, ground
- ½ teaspoon tarragon flakes

For the sauce:
- 1 tablespoon coconut flour
- 1 tablespoon almond flour
- 1 cup almond milk
- 1 and ½ tablespoons olive oil

Directions:
Heat up a pan over medium heat, add onion, turkey and garlic, stir and brown for a few minutes. Add tomatoes, tomato paste and sweet potatoes, stir and cook for a few minutes more. In a bowl, mix eggplant pieces with a pinch of sea salt, black pepper, chili powder, cumin, oregano, cardamom and tarragon flakes and stir well. Spread eggplant into a baking dish after you sprayed it with some cooking spray and top with the turkey mix. Place in the oven at 350 degrees F and bake for 15 minutes. Meanwhile, heat up a pan with the oil over medium heat, add coconut and almond flour and stir for 1 minute. Add almond milk and cook for 10 minutes stirring often. Top turkey casserole with this sauce, place in the oven again and bake for 40 minutes more. Slice and serve hot. Enjoy!

Nutritional value: calories 278, fat 3, fiber 7, carbs 9, protein 18

Indian Beef Patties

This Indian style dish will amaze you!

Preparation time: 10 minutes
Cooking time: 25 minutes
Servings: 4

Ingredients:
- 2 sweet potatoes, boiled and grated
- 1 pound beef, ground
- 1 cup red onion, chopped
- 2 Serrano peppers, chopped
- 1 small ginger piece, grated
- A handful cilantro, chopped
- 4 garlic cloves, minced
- ½ teaspoon meat masala
- A pinch of cayenne pepper
- ¼ teaspoon turmeric powder
- Black pepper to the taste
- 1 egg, whisked
- 4 tablespoons almond meal
- 1 cup water
- 5 tablespoons ghee

Directions:
Heat up a pan over medium high heat, add beef, masala, turmeric, black pepper to the taste and cayenne pepper, stir and brown for a few minutes. Add water, stir, cook for 10 minutes more and take off heat. Heat up a pan with 2 tablespoons ghee over medium heat, add Serrano peppers and onion, stir and cook for 2 minutes. Add garlic and ginger, stir and cook for 1 minute more. Add cilantro and the meat mixture, stir well and take off heat. Add grated sweet potatoes, stir well, cool everything down and shape patties from this mix. Put the egg in a bowl and almond meal in another. Dip patties in egg and then in almond meal. Heat up a pan with the rest of the ghee over medium heat, add beef patties, cook them well on one side, flip, cook on the other as well and transfer them to paper towels. Serve them with a side salad.

Nutritional value: calories 180, fat 3, fiber 3, carbs 6, protein 15

Different Beef Dish

Even your kids will love this Paleo beef dish!

Preparation time: 10 minutes
Cooking time: 35 minutes
Servings: 4

Ingredients:
- 1 pound beef, ground
- 1 teaspoon cumin seeds
- 1 pound sweet potatoes, cubed
- 3 tablespoons ghee
- 2 onions, chopped
- 1 small ginger pieces, grated
- 1 Serrano pepper, chopped
- 2 teaspoons coriander powder
- 2 teaspoons garam masala
- Black pepper to the taste
- 1 cup green peas
- A handful cilantro, chopped

Directions:
Heat up a pan with 2 tablespoons ghee over medium heat, add sweet potato cubes, stir, cook them for 20 minutes and transfer them to a bowl. Heat up the same pan over medium heat, add cumin, stir and brown them for 1 minute. Add Serrano pepper and onion, stir and cook for 4 minutes. Add beef, ginger, coriander, garam masala, cayenne and black pepper, stir and cook for 5 minutes more. Add green peas and sweet potatoes, stir, cook for 5 minutes more, divide between plates and serve with cilantro on top. Enjoy!

Nutritional value: calories 160, fat 3, fiber 1, carbs 5, protein 12

Beef and Cabbage Delight

This is easy to make but we are sure you are going to like it so much!

Preparation time: 10 minutes
Cooking time: 10 minutes
Servings: 4

Ingredients:
- 1 onion, chopped
- 1 pound beef, ground
- 1 napa cabbage head, shredded
- 1 carrot, grated
- A pinch of sea salt
- Black pepper to the taste
- 2 tablespoons coconut oil

Directions:
Heat up a pan with the oil over medium high heat, add onion and beef, stir and brown them for 5 minutes. Add carrots, cabbage, a pinch of salt and black pepper to the taste, stir and cook for 5 minutes more. Divide between plates and serve. Enjoy!

Nutritional value: calories 150, fat 1, fiber 2, carbs 5, protein 9

Simple Beef and Brussels Sprouts

This is such a simple Paleo dish!

Preparation time: 10 minutes
Cooking time: 12 minutes
Servings: 4

Ingredients:
- 1 pound beef, ground
- 1 apple, cored, peeled and chopped
- 1 yellow onion, chopped
- 3 cups Brussels sprouts, shredded
- A pinch of sea salt
- Black pepper to the taste
- 3 tablespoons ghee

Directions:
Heat up a pan with the ghee over medium high heat, add beef, stir and brown for 2 minutes. Add Brussels sprouts, stir and cook for 3 minutes more. Add onion and apple, stir and cook for 5 minutes more. Add a pinch of sea salt and black pepper to the taste, stir, cook for 1 minute more, divide among plates and serve. Enjoy!

Nutritional value: calories 150, fat 1, fiber 2, carbs 3, protein 9

Amazing Beef and Spinach

This is truly impressive and delicious!

Preparation time: 10 minutes
Cooking time: 12 minutes
Servings: 2

Ingredients:
- 1 big oyster mushroom, chopped
- 2 tablespoons almonds, chopped
- 2 tablespoons ghee
- 4 ounces beef, ground
- ½ teaspoon chili flakes
- A pinch of sea salt
- White pepper to the taste
- 1 tablespoon capers
- ¼ cup kalamata olives, pitted
- 1 tablespoon roasted almond butter
- 3 ounces spinach leaves, torn

Directions:
Heat up a pan with the ghee over medium high heat, add mushroom, stir and cook for 3 minutes. Add almonds, stir and cook for 1 minute. Add beef, chili flakes, a pinch of salt and white pepper, stir and cook for 6 minutes. Add almond butter, capers, olives and spinach, stir, cook for a couple more minutes, divide into 2 bowls and serve. Enjoy!

Nutritional value: calories 320, fat 2, fiber 5, carbs 9, protein 23

Incredible Beef and Basil

You will make this so often from now on!

Preparation time: 10 minutes
Cooking time: 16 minutes
Servings: 4

Ingredients:
- 6 garlic cloves, minced
- 2 red chilies, chopped
- 1 tablespoon coconut oil
- 1 yellow onion, chopped
- 1 and ½ pounds beef, ground
- A pinch of sea salt
- Black pepper to the taste
- 3 cups basil, chopped
- ½ cup chicken stock
- 2 cups carrot, grated
- 4 tablespoons lime juice
- 2 tablespoons coconut aminos
- 1 tablespoon olive oil
- ½ tablespoon honey
- Cauliflower rice for serving

Directions:
Heat up a pan with the coconut oil over medium heat, add onions and a pinch of salt, stir and cook for 4 minutes. Add garlic and chili peppers, stir and cook for 1 minute more. Add beef and black pepper, stir and brown everything for 8 minutes. Add stock and half of the basil, stir and cook for 2 minutes more. In a bowl, mix carrots with 1 tablespoon lime juice, the rest of the basil and the olive oil and stir well. In another bowl, mix coconut aminos with the rest of the lime juice and honey and also stir very well. Divide cauliflower rice on plates, add beef and carrot mix on top and drizzle the honey sauce you've made at the end. Enjoy!

Nutritional value: calories 200, fat 3, fiber 5, carbs 7, protein 17

Summer Beef Skillet

This is what you need on a hot summer day!

Preparation time: 10 minutes
Cooking time: 40 minutes
Servings: 4

Ingredients:
- 1 pound beef, ground
- 1 tablespoon parsley flakes
- 2 big tomatoes
- 2 yellow squash, chopped
- 2 green bell peppers, chopped
- 1 yellow onion, chopped
- A pinch of sea salt
- Black pepper to the taste

Directions:
Place tomatoes on a lined baking sheet, place in preheated broiler for 5 minutes, leave them to cool down, peel and roughly chop them. Heat up a pan over medium high heat, add onion and beef, stir and cook for 10 minutes. Add tomatoes, stir and cook for a couple more minutes. Add parsley flakes, black pepper and a pinch of sea salt, stir and cook for 10 minutes more. Add bell pepper pieces and squash ones, stir and cook for 10 minutes. Divide between plates and serve. Enjoy!

Nutritional value: calories 190, fat 3, fiber 4, carbs 6, protein 20

Greek Style Beef Bowls

It's a Mediterranean dish worth trying!

Preparation time: 10 minutes
Cooking time: 25 minutes
Servings: 4

Ingredients:
- 1 pound beef, ground
- 1 tablespoon coconut oil
- 2 garlic cloves, minced
- 1 yellow onion, chopped
- A pinch of sea salt
- Black pepper to the taste
- 1 tablespoon savory, dried
- 1 tablespoon parsley, dried
- 2 tablespoons oregano, dried
- 3 ounces kale, chopped
- 3 ounces endives, chopped
- ¼ cup kalamata olives, pitted and sliced
- ¼ cup green olives, pitted and sliced

Directions:
Heat up a pan with the coconut oil over medium high heat, add garlic, onion, a pinch of salt and black pepper, stir and cook for 3 minutes. Add beef, stir and cook for 10 minutes. Add endives, kale, savory, oregano and parsley, stir and cook for 5 minutes more. Add green and kalamata olives, stir, place in preheated broiler and broil for 4 minutes. Divide into bowls and serve.

Nutritional value: calories 367, fat 7, fiber 4, carbs 9, protein 30

Beef Curry

This Indian style curry is so rich and textured!

Preparation time: 10 minutes
Cooking time: 35 minutes
Servings: 4

Ingredients:
- 1 teaspoon mustard seeds
- 2 tablespoons coconut oil
- 2 curry leaves
- 1 Serrano pepper, chopped
- 1 onion, chopped
- 1 tablespoon garlic, minced
- ¼ cup water
- 2 teaspoons garam masala
- 1 small ginger piece, grated
- ¼ teaspoon chili powder
- ½ teaspoon turmeric powder
- 1 teaspoon coriander powder
- 1 pound beef, ground
- A pinch of sea salt
- Black pepper to the taste
- 3 carrot, chopped
- 10 ounces canned coconut milk

Directions:
Heat up a pan with the oil over medium high heat, add mustard seeds, stir and toast them for 1 minute. Add Serrano pepper, onion and curry leaves, stir and cook for 5 minutes. Add ginger and garlic, stir and cook for 1 minute. Add beef, a pinch of salt, black pepper, coriander powder, turmeric, chili and garam masala, stir and cook for 10 minutes. Add carrot and ¼ cup water, stir and cook for 5 minutes more. Add coconut milk, stir well and cook for 15 minutes. Divide curry into bowls and serve.

Nutritional value: calories 260, fat 4, fiber 5, carbs 9, protein 14

Delicious Thai Curry

You've already tried an Indian curry! Now, it's time you tried a Thai one!

Preparation time: 10 minutes
Cooking time: 30 minutes
Servings: 4

Ingredients:
- 1 yellow onion, chopped
- 3 Thai chilies, chopped
- 2 tablespoons avocado oil
- 1 pound beef, ground
- 1 small ginger pieces, grated
- 3 garlic cloves, minced
- ½ teaspoon cumin
- ½ teaspoon turmeric
- A pinch of sea salt
- Black pepper to the taste
- A pinch of cayenne pepper
- 1 tablespoon red curry paste
- 1 cup tomato sauce
- 1 broccoli head, florets separated
- 1 handful basil, chopped
- 2 teaspoons lime juice
- 2 tablespoons coconut aminos

Directions:
Heat up a pan with the oil over medium heat, add chilies and onion, stir and cook for 5 minutes. Add a pinch of salt, ginger, garlic, cumin, turmeric, black pepper, cayenne and beef, stir and cook for 10 minutes. Add broccoli and curry paste, stir and cook for 1 minute more. Add basil, tomato paste and coconut aminos, stir, bring to a simmer, cover, reduce heat to medium-low and cook for 15 minutes. Add lime juice, stir, divide into bowls and serve. Enjoy!

Nutritional value: calories 200, fat 3, fiber 5, carbs 7, protein 24

Hamburger Salad

Just check this out!

Preparation time: 10 minutes
Cooking time: 8 minutes
Servings: 4

Ingredients:
- 2 garlic cloves, minced
- 1 sweet onion, chopped
- 1 tablespoon coconut oil
- 1 pound beef, ground
- 1 cup cherry tomatoes, chopped
- 1 dill pickle, chopped
- 1 lettuce head, leaves separated and chopped
- A pinch of sea salt
- Black pepper to the taste

For the dressing:
- 2 tablespoons water
- 4 tablespoons mayonnaise
- 2 tablespoons Paleo ketchup
- 1 tablespoon yellow onion, chopped
- 1 teaspoon balsamic vinegar
- 1 tablespoon pickle, minced

Directions:
Heat up a pan with the oil over medium heat, add garlic and onion, stir and cook for 2 minutes. Add beef, a pinch of sea salt and black pepper, stir, cook for 8 minutes more and take off heat. In a salad bowl, combine beef mix and with lettuce leaves, 1 dill pickle and cherry tomatoes. In another bowl, mix water with mayo, ketchup, yellow onion, vinegar and 1 tablespoon pickle and whisk well. Drizzle this over salad, toss to coat and serve. Enjoy!

Nutritional value: calories 170, fat 3, fiber 2, carbs 5, protein 12

Veal Rolls

These are the best rolls you've ever tried!

Preparation time: 10 minutes
Cooking time: 20 minutes
Servings: 4

Ingredients:
- 2 zucchinis, cut in quarters
- 8 veal scallops
- 2 tablespoons olive oil
- 2 teaspoons garlic powder
- ¼ cup balsamic vinegar
- A pinch of sea salt
- Black pepper to the taste

Directions:
Flatten veal scallops with a meat tenderizer, season them with a pinch of sea salt and black pepper to the taste and leave aside. Season zucchini with a pinch of sea salt, black pepper and garlic powder, place on preheated grill over medium high heat, cook for 2 minutes on each side and transfer to a working surface. Roll veal around each zucchini piece. In a bowl, mix oil with balsamic vinegar and whisk well. Brush veal rolls with this mix, place them on your grill and cook for 3 minutes on each side. Serve right away. Enjoy!

Nutritional value: calories 160, fat 3, fiber 2, carbs 5, protein 14

Beef and Tasty Veggies

If you are really hungry and you have no idea what to cook, check out this Paleo recipe!

Preparation time: 10 minutes
Cooking time: 3 hours
Servings: 4

Ingredients:
- 1 yellow onion, sliced
- 3 garlic cloves, minced
- 1 cup beef stock
- 2 tablespoons coconut oil
- 3 pounds beef, cut into cubes
- A pinch of sea salt
- Black pepper to the taste
- 8 ounces carrots, sliced
- 8 ounces mushrooms, sliced
- 1 teaspoon thyme, chopped

Directions:
Heat up a Dutch oven with 1 tablespoon oil over medium high heat, add beef cubes, season with a pinch of sea salt and black pepper, brown for 2 minutes on each side and transfer to a bowl. Heat up the same Dutch oven over medium heat, add garlic, stir and cook for 2 minutes. Add stock, stir well and heat it up. Return meat to the pot, stir, place in the oven at 250 degrees F and roast for 3 hours. In a bowl, mix carrots with mushrooms, 1 tablespoon oil, a pinch of sea salt, black pepper to the taste and thyme and stir well. Spread these into a pan, place in the oven at 250 degrees F and roast them for 15 minutes. Divide beef and juices between plates and serve with roasted veggies on the side. Enjoy!

Nutritional value: calories 200, fat 3, fiber 4, carbs 7, protein 20

Steak and Amazing Blueberry Sauce

This is a really interesting and delicious dish! Try it soon!

Preparation time: 10 minutes
Cooking time: 20 minutes
Servings: 4

Ingredients:
- 1 cup beef stock
- 2 tablespoons shallots, chopped
- 2 garlic cloves, minced
- 1 cup blueberries
- 4 medium flank steaks
- 2 tablespoons ghee
- 1 teaspoon thyme, chopped
- A pinch of sea salt
- Black pepper to the taste

Directions:
Heat up a pan with the ghee over medium heat, add shallot and garlic, stir and cook for 4 minutes. Add thyme, stock, a pinch of salt and black pepper, stir, bring to a simmer and cook for 10 minutes. Add blueberries, stir and cook for 2 minutes more Place steaks on preheated grill over medium high heat, cook for 4 minutes on each side and transfer to plates. Drizzle the blueberry sauce on top and serve them. Enjoy!

Nutritional value: calories 170, fat 4, fiber 3, carbs 7, protein 15

Beef and Bok Choy

Serve this on a casual night! It's so tasty!

Preparation time: 10 minutes
Cooking time: 20 minutes
Servings: 4

Ingredients:
- 1 onion, sliced
- 12 baby bok choy heads, halved
- 2 pound beef sirloin, cut into strips
- 2 garlic cloves, minced
- 3 tablespoons coconut oil
- 5 red chilies, dried and chopped
- A pinch of sea salt
- Black pepper to the taste
- 1 ginger piece, grated

Directions:
Heat up a pan with the oil over high heat, add chilies, garlic and ginger, stir and cook for 1 minute. Add beef, stir, cook for 3 minutes and transfer to a bowl. Heat up the pan again over medium high heat, add onion, stir and cook for 2 minutes. Add bok choy, stir and cook for 4 minutes more. Return beef mix to the pan, stir, cook for 1 minute more, divide between plates and serve hot.
Enjoy!

Nutritional value: calories 140, fat 3, fiber 5, carbs 9, protein 20

Moroccan Lamb

This is just perfect! Find out how to make it!

Preparation time: 10 minutes
Cooking time: 7 minutes
Servings: 4

Ingredients:
- 8 lamb chops
- 2 tablespoons ras el hanout
- 1 teaspoon olive oil

For the sauce:
- ¼ cup parsley, chopped
- 2 tablespoons mint, chopped
- 3 garlic cloves, minced
- 2 tablespoons lemon zest
- ¼ cup olive oil
- ½ teaspoon smoked paprika
- 1 teaspoon red pepper flakes
- 2 tablespoons lemon juice
- A pinch of sea salt
- Black pepper to the taste

Directions:
Rub lamb chops with ras el hanout and 1 teaspoon oil, place them on preheated grill over medium high heat, cook them for 2 minutes on each side and divide them between plates. In your food processor, mix parsley with mint, garlic, lemon zest, ¼ cup oil, paprika, pepper flakes, lemon juice, a pinch of salt and black pepper and pulse really well. Drizzle this over lamb chops and serve. Enjoy!

Nutritional value: calories 400, fat 23, fiber 1, carbs 3, protein 32

Delicious Rosemary Lamb Chops

We can assure you that this is an amazing combination!

Preparation time: 10 minutes
Cooking time: 10 minutes
Servings: 4

Ingredients:
- 4 lamb chops
- 12 rosemary springs
- 4 garlic cloves, halved
- ½ teaspoon black peppercorns
- 3 tablespoons avocado oil
- A pinch of sea salt

Directions:
In a bowl, mix lamb chops with a pinch of salt, black peppercorns and oil and massage well. Spread lamb chops on a lined baking sheet and add garlic next to them. Rub rosemary into your palms and add over lamb chops. Introduce everything in preheated broiler over medium high heat for 10 minutes, divide between plates and serve. Enjoy!

Nutritional value: calories 160, fat 3, fiber 1, carbs 2, protein 20

Lavender Lamb Chops

This is so flavored!

Preparation time: 2 hours
Cooking time: 10 minutes
Servings: 4

Ingredients:
- 4 lamb chops
- 2 garlic cloves, minced
- 1 tablespoon lavender, chopped
- 2 tablespoons rosemary, chopped
- A pinch of sea salt
- Black pepper to the taste
- 1 tablespoon ghee
- 3 small orange peel, grated

Directions:
In a bowl, mix lamb chops with garlic, lavender, rosemary, orange peel, a pinch of salt and black pepper, rub well and keep in the fridge for 2 hours. Heat up your grill over medium high heat, grease it with the ghee, place lamb chops on it, grill for 5 minutes on each side, divide between plates and serve with a side salad on the side. Enjoy!

Nutritional value: calories 160, fat 2, fiber 1, carbs 4, protein 10

Lamb and Eggplant Puree

We are sure you never tried this before!

Preparation time: 15 minutes
Cooking time: 3 hours and 10 minutes
Servings: 4

Ingredients:
- 4 lamb shoulder chops
- 1 tablespoon ghee
- A pinch of sea salt
- Black pepper to the taste
- 1 cup yellow onion, chopped
- 7 ounces tomato paste
- 2 garlic cloves, minced
- 3 cups water
- 8 ounces white mushrooms, halved

For the eggplant puree:
- Juice of 1 lemon
- ¼ teaspoon white pepper
- 2 eggplants
- 4 tablespoons ghee
- A pinch of sea salt

Directions:
Place eggplants on your preheated grill, cook for 30 minutes, flipping them from time to time, leave them to cool down and peel. In your food processor, mix eggplant flesh with a pinch of salt, white pepper, lemon juice and 4 tablespoons ghee and pulse really well. Spoon eggplant puree on plates and leave aside for now. Heat up a pot with 1 tablespoon ghee, add lamb chops, season with a pinch of salt and black pepper to the taste, stir, brown them for a few minutes on each side and transfer to a plate. Heat up the pot again over medium high heat, add onion, stir and cook for a couple of minutes. Add garlic, stir and cook for 1 minute more. Add mushrooms and tomato paste, stir and cook for 3 minutes more. Add water, return lamb chops, stir, bring to a simmer, cover pot, reduce heat to medium-low heat and cook everything for 2 hours and 20 minutes. Divide lamb chops on eggplant puree and serve. Enjoy!

Nutritional value: calories 200, fat 3, fiber 3, carbs 5, protein 10

Thai Lamb Chops

Get all the ingredients and make this Paleo dish tonight!

Preparation time: 1 hour
Cooking time: 15 minutes
Servings: 4

Ingredients:
- 1/3 cup basil, chopped
- 2 garlic cloves, chopped
- 2 tablespoons Thai green curry paste
- 2 tablespoons avocado oil
- 1 tablespoon gluten free tamari sauce
- 1 small ginger piece, grated
- 2 pounds lamb chops
- 1 tablespoon coconut oil
- 1 tablespoon coconut aminos

Directions:
In your food processor, mix basil with garlic, curry paste, avocado oil, tamari sauce, aminos and ginger and blend really well. Put lamb chops in a bowl, add basil mix over them, toss well and keep in the fridge for 1 hour. Heat up a pan with the coconut oil over medium high heat, add lamb chops, cook for 2 minutes on each side, introduce pan in the oven and roast lamb at 400 degrees F for 10 minutes. Serve lamb chops with a side salad. Enjoy!

Nutritional value: calories 170, fat 3, fiber 2, carbs 5, protein 14

Slow Cooked Lamb Shanks

This flavored and rich dish is perfect if you are on a Paleo diet!

Preparation time: 10 minutes
Cooking time: 4 hours
Servings: 4

Ingredients:
- 2 big lamb shanks
- A pinch of sea salt
- 1 garlic head, cloves peeled
- 4 tablespoons olive oil
- Juice of ½ lemon
- Zest from ½ lemon, grated
- ½ teaspoon oregano, dried

Directions:
Put lamb shanks in your slow cooker, sprinkle a pinch of sea salt, add garlic cloves, cover and cook on High for 4 hours. In a bowl, mix olive oil with lemon juice, lemon zest and oregano and whisk well. Transfer lamb shanks to a cutting board, discard bones, shred meat and divide between plates. Drizzle the lemon dressing on top and serve with a Paleo side salad. Enjoy!

Nutritional value: calories 180, fat 2, fiber 2, carbs 4, protein 9

Paleo Seafood and Fish Recipes

Amazing Paleo Shrimp Dish
This dish is just great! You can serve it to your friends for a casual gathering, but you can also make it for a special occasion!

Servings: 4
Preparation time: 10 minutes
Cooking time: 10 minutes

Ingredients:
- 1 small red bell pepper, chopped
- 1 small yellow onion, chopped
- 20 shrimp, peeled and deveined
- 1 garlic clove, finely chopped
- 5 dried red chilies
- 1 inch ginger, minced
- ¼ cup coconut aminos
- A pinch of sea salt
- Black pepper to the taste
- 2 tablespoons coconut oil
- 2 tablespoons water
- 1 tablespoon lime juice
- 1 teaspoon apple cider vinegar
- 1 teaspoon raw honey
- A handful cilantro, finely chopped for serving

Directions:
In a bowl, mix aminos with vinegar, honey, water and lime juice and whisk well. Heat up a pan with the coconut oil over medium heat, add garlic and ginger, stir and cook for 2 minutes. Add red chilies, onion, bell pepper, stir and cook for 4 minutes. Add shrimp, a pinch of salt and pepper to the taste and the vinegar mix you've made, stir and cook for 5 minutes. Divide between plates and serve with cilantro sprinkled on top. Enjoy!

Nutritional value: calories 157, fat 7, carbs 11, fiber 0, protein 5

Special Paleo Fish Dish
It's a light paleo dish that will be ready for you to enjoy in only a few minutes!

Servings: 4
Preparation time: 10 minutes
Cooking time: 10 minutes

Ingredients:
- ¼ cup ghee, melted
- 4 halibut fish fillets
- 4 garlic cloves, minced
- 2 tablespoons parsley, chopped
- Zest and juice from 1 lemon
- 1 lemon, sliced
- A pinch of sea salt
- Black pepper to the taste

Directions:
In a bowl, mix garlic with ghee, lemon zest, juice, parsley, a pinch of sea salt and pepper and stir well. Arrange fish in a baking dish, season with pepper to the taste, drizzle the mix you've made, top with lemon slices, introduce in the oven at 425 degrees F and bake for 15 minutes. Divide between plates and serve warm. Enjoy!

Nutritional value: calories 150, fat 19, carbs 5, fiber 0.4, protein 31

Paleo Glazed Salmon

This dish combines some amazing flavors in a perfect paleo way!

Servings: 4
Preparation time: 10 minutes
Cooking time: 15 minutes

Ingredients:
- 2 tablespoons pure maple syrup
- 4 salmon fillets, skin on
- A pinch of sea salt
- White pepper to the taste
- 2 teaspoons Dijon mustard
- Juice and zest from 1 orange
- 2 garlic cloves, finely chopped

Directions:
In a bowl, mix maple syrup with orange zest, juice, mustard, a pinch of sea salt, pepper and garlic and whisk well. Arrange salmon in a baking dish, brush with the maple syrup and orange mix, introduce in the oven at 400 degrees F and bake for 15 minutes. Divide between plates and serve right away. Enjoy!

Nutritional value: calories 190, fat 10, carbs 12, fiber 0.6, sugar 13, protein 26

Paleo Lobster with Sauce

Who doesn't love a tasty lobster? Try this recipe! This is much better than any other lobster recipes you've tried before!

Servings: 4
Preparation time: 10 minutes
Cooking time: 10 minutes

Ingredients:
- ¼ cup ghee, melted
- 4 lobster tails
- A pinch of sea salt
- Black pepper to the taste
- 2 tablespoons Sriracha sauce
- 1 tablespoon lime juice
- 1 tablespoon chives, chopped
- Some parsley leaves, chopped for serving

Directions:
In a bowl, mix Sriracha sauce with ghee, chives, a pinch of sea salt, pepper and lime juice and whisk well. Cut lobster tails halfway through in the center, open with your fingers, fill them with half of the Sriracha mix, arrange on preheated grill over medium high heat, cook for 4 minutes, flip and cook for 3 minutes more. Divide lobster tails on plates, drizzle the rest of the Sriracha sauce, sprinkle parsley on top and serve. Enjoy!

Nutritional value: calories 240, fat 16, carbs 2, fiber 0.5, protein 19

Paleo Steamed Clams

It's not only very healthy! It's also very easy to make, and it tastes amazing!

Servings: 2
Preparation time: 10 minutes
Cooking time: 10 minutes

Ingredients:
- 3 tablespoons ghee
- 1 and ½ pounds shell clams, scrubbed
- ¼ cup white wine
- 3 garlic cloves, finely chopped
- A pinch of sea salt
- Black pepper to the taste
- ½ cup chicken stock
- 2 tablespoons parsley, chopped
- Lemon wedges

Directions:
Heat up a pot with the ghee over medium heat, add garlic, stir and cook for 1 minute. Add wine, bring to a boil and simmer for a few minutes. Add stock and clams, cover pot and cook for 4-5 minutes. Divide clams on plates, sprinkle parsley on top, a pinch of sea salt and pepper and serve with lemon wedges on the side. Enjoy!

Nutritional value: calories 79, fat 23, carbs 9, fiber 0.4, protein 22

Paleo Salmon Pie

We think you should make this pie tonight for dinner! Everyone will like it!

Servings: 4
Preparation time: 15 minutes
Cooking time: 1 hour

Ingredients:
- 8 sweet potatoes, thinly sliced
- 4 cups salmon, already cooked and shredded
- 1 red onion, chopped
- 2 carrots, chopped
- 1 celery stalk, chopped
- A pinch of sea salt
- Black pepper to the taste
- 2 tablespoons chives, chopped
- 2 cups coconut milk
- 1 tablespoons tapioca starch
- 2 garlic cloves, minced
- 3 tablespoons ghee

Directions:
Heat up a pan with the ghee over medium heat, add garlic and tapioca, stir and cook for 1 minute. Add coconut milk, stir and cook for 3 minutes. Add a pinch of sea salt and pepper and stir again. In a bowl, mix carrots with salmon, celery, chives, onion and pepper to the taste and stir well. Arrange a layer of potatoes in a baking dish, add some of the coconut sauce, add half of the salmon mix, the rest of the potatoes and top with the remaining sauce. Introduce in the oven at 375 degrees F and bake for 1 hour. Divide between plates and serve hot. Enjoy!

Nutritional value: calories 260, fat 11, carbs 20, fiber 12, protein 14

Paleo Grilled Calamari

It's the best dinner idea and it's 100% paleo!

Servings: 4
Preparation time: 10 minutes
Cooking time: 5 minutes

Ingredients:
- 2 pounds calamari, tentacles and tubes sliced into rings
- 1 lime, sliced
- 1 lemon, sliced
- 1 orange, sliced
- 2 tablespoons parsley, chopped
- A pinch of sea salt
- Black pepper to the taste
- 3 tablespoons lemon juice
- ¼ cup extra virgin olive oil
- 2 garlic cloves, minced

Directions:
In a bowl, mix calamari with sliced lemon, lime, orange, lemon juice, a pinch of sea salt, pepper, parsley, garlic and olive oil and toss to coat. Heat up your kitchen grill over medium high heat, add calamari and fruits slices, cook for 5 minutes, divide between plates and serve. Enjoy!

Nutritional value: calories 90, fat 3, carbs 0.2, fiber 0, protein 15

Paleo Shrimp and Zucchini Noodles

It's a simple dish you can make really fast!

Servings: 2
Preparation time: 10 minutes
Cooking time: 15 minutes

Ingredients:
- 2 zucchinis, sliced in thin noodles
- 1 pound shrimp, peeled and deveined
- 4 garlic cloves, minced
- A pinch of sea salt
- Black pepper to the taste
- ¼ cup white wine
- 2 tablespoons chives, chopped
- 2 tablespoons lemon juice
- 2 tablespoons coconut oil

Directions:
Heat up a pan with the coconut oil over medium high heat, add garlic, stir and cook for 3 minutes. Add shrimp, stir and cook for 3 minutes and transfer them to a plate. Pour lemon juice and wine into the pan, bring to a boil over medium heat and simmer for a few minutes. Add zucchini noodles, the shrimp, a pinch of sea salt and pepper to the taste stir gently and divide among plates. Sprinkle chives on top and serve. Enjoy!

Nutritional value: calories 140, fat 12, carbs 6, fiber 3, protein 18

Paleo Scallops with Delicious Puree

It's rather simple to make this recipe, but it's a fancy one, perfect for a special dinner party!

Servings: 4
Preparation time: 10 minutes
Cooking time: 25 minutes

Ingredients:
- 3 garlic cloves, minced
- 2 cups cauliflower florets, chopped
- 2 cups sweet potatoes, chopped
- 2 rosemary springs
- 12 sea scallops
- A pinch of sea salt
- Black pepper to the taste
- ¼ cup pine nuts, toasted
- 2 cups veggie stock
- 2 tablespoons extra virgin olive oil
- A handful chives, chopped

Directions:
Put cauliflower, potatoes, and stock in a pot, bring to a boil over medium high heat, reduce temperature and simmer until veggies are soft. Drain veggies, transfer them to your blender, add a pinch of sea salt and pepper to the taste and pulse until you obtain a puree. Heat up a pan with the oil over medium high heat, add rosemary and garlic, stir and cook for 1 minute. Add scallops, cook them for 2 minutes, often stirring, season them with pepper to the taste and take them off heat. Divide puree on small plates, arrange scallops on top, sprinkle chives and pine nuts at the end and serve. Enjoy!

Nutritional value: calories 170, fat 10, fiber 0, carbs 2, protein 22

Paleo Salmon with Avocado Sauce

These ingredients work perfectly together! The dish tastes amazing!

Servings: 5
Preparation time: 20 minutes
Cooking time: 10 minutes

Ingredients:
- 1 teaspoon cumin
- 1 teaspoon sweet paprika
- 1 teaspoon chili powder
- 1 teaspoon onion powder
- ½ teaspoon garlic powder
- 2 pounds salmon filets, cut into 4 pieces
- A pinch of sea salt
- Black pepper to the taste
- 2 avocados, pitted, peeled and chopped
- 1 garlic clove, minced
- Juice from 1 lime
- 1 red onion, chopped
- 1 tablespoon extra virgin olive oil
- Black pepper to the taste
- 1 tablespoon cilantro, finely chopped

For the avocado sauce:

Directions:
In a bowl, mix paprika with cumin, onion powder, garlic powder, chili powder, a pinch of sea salt and pepper to the taste. Add salmon pieces, toss to coat and keep in the fridge for 20 minutes. Put avocado in a bowl and mash well with a fork. Add red onion, garlic clove, lime juice, olive oil, chopped cilantro, and pepper to the taste and stir very well. Take salmon out of the fridge, place it on preheated grill over medium high heat and cook it for 3 minutes. Flip salmon, cook for 3 more minutes and divide on serving plates. Top each salmon piece with avocado sauce and serve. Enjoy!

Nutritional value: calories 150, fat 12, carbs 9, fiber 6, protein 24

Paleo Fish Tacos

A casual dinner at home requires a simple dinner recipe! Why don't you try this idea?

Servings: 4
Preparation time: 15 minutes
Cooking time: 10 minutes

Ingredients:
- 4 tilapia fillets, cut into medium pieces
- ¼ cup coconut flour
- 2 eggs
- ¾ cup tapioca starch
- ½ cup tapioca starch
- ¼ cup sparkling water
- 2 cups cabbage, shredded
- 2 cups coconut oil
- A pinch of sea salt
- Black pepper to the taste
- Lime wedges for serving
- Cauliflower tortillas

For the Pico de Gallo:
- 2 tomatoes, chopped
- 2 tablespoons jalapeno, finely chopped
- 6 tablespoons yellow onion, finely chopped
- 2 tablespoons lime juice
- 1 tablespoon cilantro, finely chopped

For the mayo:
- 1 tablespoon Sriracha sauce
- ¼ cup homemade mayonnaise
- 2 teaspoons lime juice

Directions:
In a bowl, mix tomatoes with tomatoes with onion, jalapeno, cilantro, 2 tablespoons lime juice and stir well, cover and keep in the fridge for now. In another bowl, mix mayo with Sriracha and 2 teaspoons lime juice, stir well, cover and also keep in the fridge. In a bowl, mix ¾ cup tapioca starch with coconut flour, sparkling water, a pinch of sea salt, pepper and eggs and whisk very well. Put the rest of the tapioca starch in a separate bowl. Pat dry tapioca pieces, coat with tapioca starch and dip each piece in eggs mix. Heat up a pan with the coconut oil over medium high heat, transfer fish fillets to pan, cook for 1 minute, flip them, cook for 1 more minute, transfer to paper towels and drain excess fat. Arrange tortillas on a working surface, divide cabbage on them, add a piece of fish on each, add some of the Pico de Gallo and top with mayo. Serve with lime wedges. Enjoy!

Nutritional value: calories 230, fat 10, carbs 12, fiber 4, protein 13

Smoked Salmon and Fresh Veggies

It might seem like a very simple dish, but it's a delicious and fresh one!

Servings: 2
Preparation time: 10 minutes
Cooking time: 0 minutes

Ingredients:
- 2 cups cherry tomatoes, cut in halves
- 1 red onion, thinly sliced
- 8 ounces smoked salmon, thinly sliced
- 1 cucumber, thinly chopped
- 6 tablespoons extra virgin olive oil
- ½ teaspoon garlic, minced
- 2 tablespoons lemon juice
- Black pepper to the taste
- 1 teaspoon balsamic vinegar
- Some dill, finely chopped
- ½ teaspoon oregano, dried

Directions:
In a bowl, mix oil with garlic, balsamic vinegar, oregano and garlic and whisk well. Add black pepper to the taste and stir well again. In a bowl, mix cucumber with tomatoes and onion. Drizzle the dressing over veggies and toss to coat. Roll salmon pieces and divide them among plates. Add mixed veggies on the side, sprinkle dill all over and serve. Enjoy!

Nutritional value: calories 159, fat 23, carbs 2, fiber 3, protein 14

Paleo Roasted Trout

It's always so refreshing when you find a unique and delicious recipe! This is one of them!

Servings: 4
Preparation time: 10 minutes
Cooking time: 20 minutes

Ingredients:
- 3 trout, cleaned and gutted
- 1 bunch dill
- 2 lemons, sliced
- 1 bunch rosemary
- 2 fennel bulbs, sliced
- A pinch of sea salt
- Black pepper to the taste
- 2 tablespoons extra virgin olive oil

Directions:
Grease a baking dish with some oil, spread fennel slices on the bottom and add trout after you've seasoned them with a pinch of sea salt and pepper. Fill each fish with lemon slices, dill and rosemary springs. Top fish with the rest of the herbs and lemon slices, drizzle the rest of the oil, introduce everything in the oven at 500 degrees F and bake for 10 minutes. Reduce heat to 425 degrees F and bake for 12 more minutes. Leave fish to cool down, divide between plates and serve. Enjoy!

Nutritional value: calories 143, fat 2.3, carbs 1, fiber 0, protein 6

Paleo Roasted Cod

There are a lot of paleo fish recipes, and we are determined to show you the best ones! Here is another delicious paleo fish based dish.

Servings: 4
Preparation time: 10 minutes
Cooking time: 20 minutes

Ingredients:
- ¼ cup ghee
- 4 medium cod fillets, skinless
- 2 garlic cloves, minced
- 1 tablespoon parsley leaves, finely chopped
- 1 teaspoon mustard
- 1 shallot, finely chopped
- 3 tablespoons prosciutto, chopped
- 2 tablespoons lemon juice
- 2 tablespoons coconut oil
- A pinch of sea salt
- Black pepper to the taste
- Lemon wedges for serving

Directions:
In a bowl, mix parsley with ghee, mustard, garlic, shallot, prosciutto, a pinch of sea salt, pepper and lemon juice and whisk very well. Heat up an oven proof pan with the coconut oil over medium high heat, add fish, season with black pepper to the taste and cook for 4 minutes on each side. Spread ghee mix over fish, introduce in the oven at 425 degrees F and bake for 10 minutes. Divide between plates and serve with lemon wedges on the side.
Enjoy!

Nutritional value: calories 138, fat 4, carbs 1, fiber 0, protein 23

Superb Tuna Dish

It's a simple recipe, but it's also a very special and tasty one!

Servings: 4
Preparation time: 15 minutes
Cooking time: 10 minutes

Ingredients:
- 1 teaspoon fennel seeds
- 1 teaspoon mustard seeds
- 4 medium tuna steaks
- ¼ teaspoon black peppercorns
- A pinch of sea salt
- Black pepper to the taste
- 4 tablespoons sesame seeds
- 3 tablespoons coconut oil

Directions:
In your grinder, mix peppercorns with fennel and mustard seeds and grind well. Add sesame seeds, a pinch of sea salt, and pepper to the taste and grind again well. Spread this mix on a plate, add tuna steaks and toss to coat. Heat up a pan with the oil over medium high heat, add tuna steaks and cook for 3 minutes on each side. Divide between plates and serve with a side salad. Enjoy!

Nutritional value: calories 240, fat 2, carbs 0, fiber 0, protein 53

Paleo Salmon Tartar

This is a good idea for a party appetizer! It's really good!

Servings: 4
Preparation time: 15 minutes
Cooking time: 0 minutes

Ingredients:
- 7 ounces smoked salmon, minced
- 14 ounces salmon fillet, cut into very small cubes
- 3 tablespoons red onion, minced
- 2 tablespoons pickled cucumber, minced
- Zest and juice from 1 lemon
- 1 garlic clove, finely minced
- 2 tablespoons basil, minced
- 2 teaspoons oregano, dried
- Black pepper to the taste
- 2 tablespoons mint leaves, minced
- 2 tablespoons Dijon mustard
- 5 tablespoons extra virgin olive oil
- Lime wedges for serving

Directions:
In a bowl, mix onion with cucumber, garlic, lemon zest and juice, basil, mint, oregano, mustard, oil and pepper and stir well. Add smoked and fresh salmon and stir well again. Divide tartar between plates and serve with lime wedges on the side. Enjoy!

Nutritional value: calories 230, fat 16, carbs 2.3, fiber 0.4, protein 17

Grilled Salmon with Peaches

Try this combination as soon as possible! It's really amazing and easy to make!

Servings: 4
Preparation time: 10 minutes
Cooking time: 15 minutes

Ingredients:
- 2 red onions, cut into wedges
- 3 peaches, cut in wedges
- 4 salmon steaks
- 1 teaspoon thyme, chopped
- 1 tablespoon ginger, grated
- A pinch of sea salt
- Black pepper to the taste
- 1 tablespoon white wine vinegar
- 3 tablespoons extra virgin olive oil

Directions:
In a bowl, mix wine with ginger, vinegar, thyme, a pinch of sea salt, pepper and olive oil and whisk very well. In a bowl, mix peaches with onion, salt and pepper and toss to coat. Heat up your kitchen grill over medium high heat, add salmon steaks after you've seasoned them with pepper to the taste, grill for 6 minutes on each side and divide between plates. Add peaches and onions to grill, cook for 4 minutes on each side and transfer next to salmon on plates. Drizzle the vinaigrette you've made all over salmon, onions, and peaches and serve right away. Enjoy!

Nutritional value: calories 448, fat 26, carbs 13, fiber 2, sugar 8, protein 40

Paleo Shrimp Burgers

Combine these delicious and healthy shrimp burgers with the salsa we recommend you and enjoy a divine dish!

Servings: 4
Preparation time: 15 minutes
Cooking time: 15 minutes

Ingredients:
- 2 tablespoons cilantro, chopped
- 1 and ½ pounds shrimp, peeled and deveined
- 2 tablespoons chives, chopped
- Black pepper to the taste
- 1 garlic clove, minced
- ¼ cup radishes, minced
- 1 teaspoon lemon zest
- ¼ cup celery, minced
- 1 egg, whisked
- 1 tablespoon lemon juice
- ¼ cup almond meal

For the salsa:
- 1 avocado, pitted, peeled and chopped
- 1 cup pineapple, chopped
- 2 tablespoons red onion, chopped
- ¼ cup bell peppers, chopped
- 1 tablespoon lime juice
- 1 tablespoon cilantro, finely chopped
- A pinch of sea salt
- Black pepper to the taste

Directions:
In a bowl, mix pineapple with avocado, bell peppers, 2 tablespoons red onion, 1 tablespoon lime juice, pepper to the taste and 1 tablespoon cilantro, stir well and keep in the fridge for now. In your food processor, mix shrimp with 2 tablespoons cilantro, chives, and garlic and blend well. Transfer to a bowl and mix with radishes, celery, lemon zest, lemon juice, egg, almond meal, a pinch of sea salt and pepper to the taste and stir well. Shape 4 burgers, place them on preheated grill over medium high heat and cook for 5 minutes on each side. Divide shrimp burgers between plates and serve with the salsa you've made earlier on the side. Enjoy!

Nutritional value: calories 238, fat 12, carbs 13.2, fiber 3, protein 15.4

Paleo Scallops Tartar

It's a tasty dish with a very sophisticated taste!

Servings: 2
Preparation time: 15 minutes
Cooking time: 0 minutes

Ingredients:
- 6 scallops, diced
- A pinch of sea salt
- Black pepper to the taste
- 3 strawberries, chopped
- 1 tablespoon extra virgin olive oil
- 1 tablespoon green onions, minced
- Juice from ½ lemon
- ½ tablespoon basil leaves, finely chopped

Directions:
In a bowl, mix strawberries with scallops, basil and onions and stir well. Add olive oil, a pinch of salt, pepper to the taste and lemon juice and stir well again. Keep in the fridge until you serve. Enjoy!

Nutritional value: calories 180, fat 27, carbs 3, fiber 0, protein 24

Paleo Shrimp Skewers

A Sunday gathering requires simple and delicious dishes! Here is one idea you can use next time!

Servings: 4
Preparation time: 10 minutes
Cooking time: 10 minutes

Ingredients:
- ½ pound sausages, chopped and already cooked
- ½ pound shrimp, peeled and deveined
- 2 tablespoons extra virgin olive oil
- 2 zucchinis, cubed
- A pinch of sea salt
- Black pepper to the taste
- ½ tablespoon garlic powder
- 2 tablespoons paprika
- ½ tablespoon onion powder
- ¼ tablespoon oregano, dried
- ½ tablespoon chili powder
- ¼ tablespoon thyme, dried

For the Creole seasoning:

Directions:
In a bowl, mix paprika with garlic powder, onion one, chili powder, oregano, and thyme and stir well. In another bowl, mix shrimp with sausage, zucchini, and oil and toss to coat. Pour paprika mix over shrimp mix and stir well. Arrange sausage, shrimp, and zucchini on skewers alternating pieces, season with a pinch of sea salt and black pepper, place them on preheated grill over medium high heat and cook for 8 minutes, flipping skewers from time to time. Arrange on a platter and serve. Enjoy!

Nutritional value: calories 360, fat 32, carbs 4.3, fiber 0.8, sugar 1, protein 18.1

Salmon Skewers

These are so fresh and easy to make!

Preparation time: 10 minutes
Cooking time: 15 minutes
Servings: 4

Ingredients:
- 1 pound wild salmon, skinless, boneless and cubed
- 2 Meyer lemons, sliced
- ¼ cup balsamic vinegar
- ¼ cup orange juice
- 1/3 cup Paleo orange marmalade
- A pinch of pink salt
- Black pepper to the taste

Directions:
Heat up a small pot with the vinegar over medium heat, add marmalade and orange juice, stir, bring to a simmer for 1 minute and take off heat. Skewer salmon cubes and lemon slices, season with a pinch of salt and black pepper, brush them with half of the vinegar mix, place on preheated grill over medium heat, cook for 4 minutes on each side. Brush skewers with the rest of the vinegar mix, grill for 1 minute more, divide between plates and serve. Enjoy!

Nutritional value: calories 150, fat 1, fiber 2, carbs 4, protein 10

Tuna and Chimichurri Sauce

This will be perfect for tonight!

Preparation time: 10 minutes
Cooking time: 5 minutes
Servings: 4

Ingredients:
- 1 small red onion, chopped
- ½ cup cilantro, chopped
- 1/3 cup olive oil
- 2 tablespoons olive oil
- 1 jalapeno pepper, chopped
- 2 tablespoons basil, chopped
- 3 tablespoons vinegar
- 3 garlic cloves, minced
- 1 teaspoon red pepper flakes
- 1 teaspoon thyme, chopped
- A pinch of sea salt
- Black pepper to the taste
- 1 pound sushi grade tuna
- 2 avocados, pitted, peeled and chopped
- 6 ounces arugula

Directions:
In a bowl, mix 1/3 cup oil with onion, jalapeno, cilantro, basil, vinegar, garlic, parsley, pepper flakes, thyme, a pinch of salt and black pepper and whisk well. Heat up a pan with 2 tablespoons oil over medium high heat, add tuna, season with a pinch of sea salt and black pepper, cook for 2 minutes on each side, transfer to a cutting board, leave aside to cool down and slice. In a bowl, mix arugula with half of the chimichurri sauce you've made earlier, toss to coat well and divide between plates. Divide tuna slices, avocado pieces and drizzle the rest of the sauce on top.

Nutritional value: calories 140, fat 1, fiber 1, carbs 2, protein 6

Salmon and Chili Sauce

It's a spicy Paleo dish you can serve for a movie night!

Preparation time: 10 minutes
Cooking time: 15 minutes
Servings: 12

Ingredients:
- 1 and ¼ cups coconut, shredded
- 1 pound salmon, cut into medium cubes
- 1/3 cup coconut flour
- A pinch of sea salt
- Black pepper to the taste
- 1 egg
- 2 tablespoons coconut oil
- ¼ cup water
- ¼ teaspoon agar agar
- 4 red chilies, chopped
- 3 garlic cloves, minced
- ¼ cup balsamic vinegar
- ½ cup honey

Directions:
In a bowl, mix coconut flour with a pinch of salt and stir. In another bowl, whisk the egg with black pepper. Put coconut in a third bowl. Dip salmon cubes in flour, egg and coconut and place them all on a working surface. Heat up a pan with the oil over medium high heat, add salmon cubes, fry them for 3 minutes on each side, transfer them to paper towels, drain grease and divide them between plates. Heat up a pan with the water over medium high heat. Add chilies, cloves, vinegar, honey and agar agar, stir very well, bring to a gentle boil and simmer until all ingredients combine. Drizzle this over salmon cubes and serve.

Nutritional value: calories 140, fat 1, fiber 2, carbs 4, protein 15

Infused Clams

These clams are just so special!

Preparation time: 10 minutes
Cooking time: 12 minutes
Servings: 2

Ingredients:
- 1 tablespoon olive oil
- 3 ounces pancetta
- 3 tablespoons ghee
- 2 pound little clams, scrubbed
- 1 shallot, minced
- 2 garlic cloves, minced
- 1 bottle infused cider
- 1 apple, cored and chopped
- Juice of ½ lemon

Directions:
Heat up a pan with the oil over medium high heat, add pancetta and brown for 3 minutes. Add ghee, shallot and garlic, stir and cook for 3 minutes. Add cider, stir well and cook for 1 minute. Add clams and thyme, cover and simmer for 5 minutes. Add apple and lemon juice, stir, divide everything into bowls and serve. Enjoy!

Nutritional value: calories 120, fat 1, fiber 2, carbs 4, protein 10

Delightful Salmon Dish

This is so tasty and elegant!

Preparation time: 10 minutes
Cooking time: 30 minutes
Servings: 6

Ingredients:
- 2 tablespoons ghee
- A pinch of sea salt
- Black pepper to the taste
- 3 cups apple cider
- ½ teaspoon fennel seeds
- 1 teaspoon mustard seeds
- 1 fennel bulb, chopped
- 1 apple, cored, peeled and chopped
- 4 salmon fillets, skin on and bone in

Directions:
Put cider in a pot and heat up over medium heat. Add mustard seeds, a pinch of salt, black pepper and fennel seeds, stir and boil for 25 minutes. Strain this into a bowl, add half of the ghee, stir well and leave aside for now. Heat up a pan with the rest of the ghee over medium heat, add fennel and apple pieces, stir and cook for 6 minutes. Brush salmon pieces with some of the cider mix, season with a pinch of salt and black pepper, place on a lined baking sheet. Add fennel and apple pieces as well, introduce everything in the oven at 350 degrees F and bake for 25 minutes. Divide salmon between plates and serve with the rest of the cider sauce on top. Enjoy!

Nutritional value: calories 150, fat 3, fiber 2, carbs 4, protein 10

Amazing Shrimp Dish

You must try this as soon as possible if you like shrimp and you are on a Paleo diet!

Preparation time: 10 minutes
Cooking time: 5 minutes
Servings: 4

Ingredients:
- 1 pound big shrimp, peeled and deveined
- 2 teaspoons olive oil
- 1 cup cilantro, chopped
- 1 cup parsley, chopped
- Juice from 2 limes
- ½ cup olive oil
- ¼ cup onion, chopped
- A pinch of sea salt
- ½ teaspoon smoked paprika
- 2 garlic cloves, minced

Directions:
Heat up a pan with 2 teaspoons olive oil over medium heat, add shrimp, cook them for 5 minutes and reduce heat to low. In your food processor, mix ½ cup oil with onion, sea salt, paprika, garlic, lime juice, parsley and cilantro and pulse really well. Divide shrimp on plates, top with the chimichurri and serve. Enjoy!

Nutritional value: calories 120, fat 2, fiber 1, carbs 3, protein 8

Delicious Scallops

This Paleo dish is just fabulous!

Preparation time: 10 minutes
Cooking time: 13 minutes
Servings: 3

Ingredients:

- 1 romanesco head, cut in halves
- 1 shallot, minced
- 3 garlic cloves, minced
- 3 tablespoons olive oil
- 1 and ½ cups chicken stock
- ¼ cup walnuts, toasted and chopped
- 1 and ½ cups grapes, halved
- 2 cups spinach
- 1 tablespoon avocado oil
- 1 pound scallops
- A pinch of sea salt
- Black pepper to the taste

Directions:

Put half of the romanesco in a food processor, blend well and put into a bowl. Put the other half of the romanesco in your food processor, blend well again and add to the bowl. Heat up a pan with 2 tablespoons oil over medium high heat, add garlic and shallot, stir and cook for 1 minute. Add romanesco rice, stir and cook for 3 minutes. Add 1 cup stock, some salt and pepper, spinach and 1 cup grapes, stir and blend using an immersion blender. Add the rest of the stock, blend again, cook for 5 minutes, take off heat and divide between plates. Heat up another pan with the rest of the oil over medium high heat, add scallops, season them with a pinch of sea salt and black pepper, cook for 2 minutes, flip, cook for 1 minute more and add next to romanesco rice. Top with walnuts and the rest of the grapes and serve. Enjoy!

Nutritional value: calories 200, fat 3, fiber 3, carbs 7, protein 15

Amazing Crab Cakes and Red Pepper Sauce

This delightful dish can be served on a special occasion!

Preparation time: 10 minutes
Cooking time: 7 minutes
Servings: 8

Ingredients:

- 1 cup crab meat
- 2 tablespoons parsley, chopped
- 2 tablespoons old bay seasoning
- 2 teaspoons Dijon mustard
- 1 egg, whisked
- 1 tablespoons lemon juice
- 2 tablespoons coconut oil
- 1 and ½ tablespoons coconut flour
- *For the sauce:*
- 1 tablespoons olive oil
- ¼ cup roasted red peppers
- 1 tablespoon lemon juice
- ¼ cup avocado, peeled and chopped

Directions:

In a bowl, mix crabmeat with old bay seasoning, parsley, mustard, egg, 1 tablespoon lemon juice and coconut flour and stir everything very well. Shape 8 patties from this mix and place them on a plate. Heat up a pan with 2 tablespoons coconut oil over medium high heat, add crab patties, cook for 3 minutes on each side and divide between plates. In your food processor, mix olive oil with red peppers, avocado and 1 tablespoon lemon juice and blend really well. Spread this on your crab patties and serve. Enjoy!

Nutritional value: calories 100, fat 4, fiber 3, carbs 5, protein 7

Delicious Grilled Oysters

Make sure you read the whole recipe! It's amazing!

Preparation time: 10 minutes
Cooking time: 7 minutes
Servings: 4

Ingredients:
- ¼ cup red onion, chopped
- 2 tomatoes, chopped
- A handful cilantro, chopped
- 1 jalapeno, chopped
- A pinch of sea salt
- Black pepper to the taste
- Juice from 1 lime
- 2 limes, cut into wedges
- 24 oysters, scrubbed

Directions:
In a bowl, tomatoes with onion, cilantro, jalapeno, a pinch of salt, black pepper and juice from 1 lime, stir well and leave aside. Heat up your grill over medium high heat, add oysters, grill them for 7 minutes. Open them completely and divide oysters between plates. Top with the tomatoes mix and serve with lime wedges on the side. Enjoy!

Nutritional value: calories 140, fat 2, fiber 2, carbs 4, protein 8

Delicious Squid and Guacamole

Did you every try something like this before? It's so impressive!

Preparation time: 10 minutes
Cooking time: 5 minutes
Servings: 2
Ingredients:
- 2 medium squid, cleaned, tentacles and tubes separated
- A pinch of sea salt
- Black pepper to the taste
- 1 tablespoon olive oil
- Juice of ½ lime
- 1 tablespoon coriander, chopped
- 2 red chilies, chopped
- 2 avocados, pitted, peeled and chopped
- 1 tomato, chopped
- 1 red onion, chopped
- Juice from 2 limes

For the guacamole:

Directions:
In a bowl, mix chilies with avocados, coriander, tomato, red onion and juice from 2 limes and stir well. Heat up your grill over medium high heat, add squid pieces after you've rubbed it with 1 tablespoon olive oil, season with salt and pepper to the taste, grill for 3 minutes, flip and cook for 2 minutes on the other side. Transfer squid to a cutting board, slice, drizzle juice from ½ lime toss to coat and divide between plates. Serve with the guacamole on the side.

Nutritional value: calories 360, fat 7, fiber 5, carbs 8, protein 17

Delicious Shrimp and Cauliflower Rice

This sound really tasty, doesn't it?

Preparation time: 10 minutes
Cooking time: 15 minutes
Servings: 4

Ingredients:
- 1 tablespoon ghee
- 1 cauliflower head, florets separated
- ¼ cup coconut milk
- 1 pound shrimp, peeled and deveined
- 2 garlic cloves, minced
- 8 ounces mushrooms, sliced
- 4 bacon slices
- A pinch of red pepper flakes
- A handful mixed parsley and chives, chopped
- ½ cup beef stock
- Black pepper to the taste

Directions:
Heat up a pan over medium high heat, add bacon slices, cook until they are crispy, drain grease on paper towels and leave them aside for now. Put cauliflower florets in your food processor, blend until you obtain your "rice" and transfer to a heated pan over medium high heat. Cook cauliflower rice for 5 minutes stirring often. Add coconut milk and 1 tablespoon ghee, stir and cook for a couple more minutes. Blend everything using an immersion blender, add black pepper to the taste, stir, reduce heat to low and continue cooking for a few minutes more. Heat up the pan where you cooked the bacon over medium high heat, add shrimp, cook for 2 minutes on each side and transfer them to a plate. Heat up the pan again, add mushrooms, stir and cook for a few minutes as well. Add garlic, pepper flakes and some black pepper, stir and cook for 1 minute. Add stock, return shrimp to pan, stir and cook until stock evaporates. Divide cauliflower rice on plates, top with shrimp and mushrooms mix, top with crispy bacon and sprinkle parsley and chives.

Nutritional value: calories 140, fat 2, fiber 2, carbs 4, protein 9

Stuffed Salmon Fillets

You will find this dish really tasty!

Preparation time: 10 minutes
Cooking time: 20 minutes
Servings: 2

Ingredients:
- 2 medium salmon fillets, boneless
- 5 ounces tiger shrimp, peeled, deveined and chopped
- 6 mushrooms, chopped
- 3 green onions, chopped
- 2 cups spinach, chopped
- ¼ cup macadamia nuts, toasted and chopped
- A pinch of sea salt
- Black pepper to the taste
- A pinch of nutmeg, ground
- ¼ cup Paleo mayonnaise
- Bacon fat for cooking

Directions:
Heat up a pan with some bacon fat over medium heat, add onions and mushrooms, a pinch of salt and black pepper, stir and cook for 4 minutes. Add nuts, stir and cook for 2 minutes more. Add spinach, stir and cook for 1 minute. Add shrimp, stir and cook for another minute. Take this mix off heat, leave it aside to cool down a bit, add Paleo mayo and nutmeg and stir everything. Make an incision lengthwise in each salmon fillet, season with some black pepper and stuff with the shrimp mix. Heat up a pan with some bacon fat over high heat, add salmon fillets and cook skin side down for 1 minute. Cover the pan, reduce temperature to medium-low and cook for 8 minutes more. Introduce pan in preheated broiler and broil for 2 minutes. Divide stuffed salmon fillets on plates and serve.

Nutritional value: calories 450, fat 6, fiber 4, carbs 7, protein 40

Glazed Salmon

Serve this Paleo seafood dish with a sweet potato mash on the side and enjoy a marvelous taste!

Preparation time: 10 minutes
Cooking time: 40 minutes
Servings: 2

Ingredients:
- 1 big salmon fillet, cut in halves
- 2 tablespoons mustard
- 1 tablespoon maple syrup
- A pinch of sea salt
- Black pepper to the taste
- 2 sweet potatoes, peeled and chopped
- 2 teaspoons coconut oil
- ¼ cup coconut milk
- 3 garlic cloves, minced

Directions:

In a bowl, mix maple syrup with mustard and whisk well. Season salmon halves with a pinch of sea salt and black pepper to the taste and brush them with half of the maple mix. Heat up a pan with 1 teaspoon coconut oil over medium high heat, add salmon, skin side down and cook for 4 minutes. Transfer salmon to a baking dish, brush with the rest of the maple syrup mix, place in the oven at 425 degrees F and roast for 10 minutes. Put sweet potatoes in a pot, add water to cover, bring to a boil over medium heat, cover and cook for 20 minutes. Heat up a pan with the rest of the oil over medium heat, add garlic, stir and cook for 1 minute. Add sweet potatoes, stir well and then mash everything with a potato masher. Add coconut milk, a pinch of salt and black pepper to the taste and blend using an immersion blender. Divide this mash between plates, add salmon on the side and serve.

Nutritional value: calories 200, fat 3, fiber 3, carbs 6, protein 20

Amazing Salmon and Spicy Slaw

Salmon is a great fish, full of healthy nutrients! So, try this recipe!

Preparation time: 10 minutes
Cooking time: 6 minutes
Servings: 4

Ingredients:
- 3 cups cold water
- 3 scallions, chopped
- 2 teaspoons sriracha sauce
- 4 teaspoons honey
- 3 teaspoons avocado oil
- 4 teaspoons cider vinegar
- 2 teaspoons flax seed oil
- 4 medium salmon fillets, skinless and boneless
- A pinch of sea salt
- 1 and ½ teaspoons jerk seasoning
- 2 cups cabbage, chopped
- 4 cups baby arugula
- 2 cups radish, julienne cut
- ¼ cup pepitas, toasted

Directions:

Put scallions in a bowl, add cold water to them and leave aside. In a bowl, mix Sriracha with honey and stir well. In another bowl, combine 2 teaspoons of the honey mix with 2 teaspoons avocado oil, vinegar, a pinch of sea salt and black pepper and stir well. Sprinkle salmon fillets with a pinch of sea salt, black pepper and jerk seasoning and rub well. Heat up a pan with the rest of the avocado oil over medium high heat, add salmon, cook for 6 minutes, flip, take off heat, cover pan and leave aside for a few more minutes. In a salad bowl, mix cabbage with arugula, radish, pepitas, a pinch of salt, black pepper, the honey and vinegar salad dressing and flax seed oil and toss to coat well. Divide salmon on plates, drizzle the rest of the Sriracha sauce, add cabbage salad next to them and top with drained scallions.

Nutritional value: calories 180, fat 3, fiber 3, carbs 4, protein 8

Spicy Shrimp

This will be done so fast and it tastes amazing!

Preparation time: 10 minutes
Cooking time: 4 minutes
Servings: 2

Ingredients:
- 12 jumbo shrimp, peeled and deveined
- A pinch of sea salt
- Black pepper to the taste
- 2 garlic cloves, minced
- 2 tablespoons olive oil
- ¼ teaspoon red pepper flakes
- 1 teaspoon steak seasoning
- 1 teaspoon lemon zest
- 1 tablespoon parsley, chopped
- 2 teaspoons lemon juice

Directions:
Heat up a pan with the oil over medium high heat, add pepper flakes, garlic and shrimp, stir and cook for 4 minutes. Season with a pinch of sea salt, black pepper, parsley, lemon juice and lemon zest, stir well, divide between plates and serve. Enjoy!

Nutritional value: calories 152, fat 12, fiber 1, carbs 2, protein 6

Salmon and Lemon Relish

You will find this recipe very attractive!

Preparation time: 10 minutes
Cooking time: 1 hour
Servings: 2

Ingredients:
- 1 big salmon fillet, cut in halves
- Black pepper to the taste
- A drizzle of olive oil
- A pinch of sea salt

For the relish:
- 1 tablespoon lemon juice
- 1 shallot, chopped
- 1 Meyer lemon, cut in wedges and then thinly sliced
- 2 tablespoons parsley, chopped
- ¼ cup olive oil
- Black pepper to the taste

Directions:
Put some water in a dish and place it in the oven. Put the salmon on a lined baking dish, drizzle some olive oil, season with a pinch of sea salt and black pepper, rub well, place in the oven at 370 degrees F and bake for 1 hour. Meanwhile, in a bowl, mix shallot with the lemon juice, a pinch of salt and black pepper, stir and leave aside for 10 minutes. In another bowl, mix marinated shallot with lemon slices, some salt, pepper, parsley and ¼ cup oil and whisk well. Cut salmon in chunks, divide on plates and top with lemon relish. Enjoy!

Nutritional value: calories 200, fat 3, fiber 3, carbs 6, protein 20

Delicious Mussels Mix

This will make you taste buds dance!

Preparation time: 10 minutes
Cooking time: 15 minutes
Servings: 6

Ingredients:
- 3 garlic cloves, minced
- 1 yellow onion, chopped
- 1 tablespoon olive oil
- 1 handful parsley, chopped
- ½ cup white wine
- 1 teaspoon red pepper flakes
- 28 ounces canned tomatoes, chopped
- 2 cups chicken stock
- 29 ounces canned crushed tomatoes
- 2 pounds mussels, scrubbed

Directions:
Heat up a pot with the oil over medium heat, add onions, garlic, parsley and pepper flakes, stir and cook for 2 minutes. Add wine, crushed and chopped tomatoes, black pepper and stock, stir, cover and bring to a boil. Add mussels, stir, cover and cook until they open. Ladle this into bowls and serve. Enjoy!

Nutritional value: calories 150, fat 3, fiber 2, carbs 6, protein 12

Amazing Mahi Mahi Dish

This is so delicious and amazing! It's so tasty and you will love it for sure!

Preparation time: 10 minutes
Cooking time: 10 minutes
Servings: 4

Ingredients:
- 4 mahi-mahi fillets
- ½ tablespoon sweet paprika
- ½ teaspoon garlic powder
- ½ teaspoon oregano, dried
- 1 tablespoon chili powder
- 2 tablespoons olive oil
- 2 tablespoons coconut oil
- ½ teaspoon onion powder
- A handful cilantro, chopped
- Lime wedges

For the cilantro butter:
- Juice of 1 lemon
- 1 garlic clove, minced
- ¼ cup ghee, melted
- 2 tablespoons cilantro, chopped

Directions:
In a bowl, mix ¼ cup ghee with 1 garlic clove, juice from 1 lemon and 2 tablespoons cilantro, whisk very well and leave aside for now. In another bowl, mix garlic powder with onion powder, chili powder, oregano and paprika and stir well. Season mahi-mahi with this mix, drizzle the olive oil over them and rub well. Heat up a pan with the coconut oil over medium high heat, add fish fillets, cook for 4 minutes on each side and divide them between plates. Add cilantro butter over fish and serve. Enjoy!

Nutritional value: calories 160, fat 4, fiber 3, carbs 6, protein 15

Delicious Lobster and Sauce

You will make this again for sure!

Preparation time: 10 minutes
Cooking time: 8 minutes
Servings: 4

Ingredients:
- 2 tablespoons sriracha sauce
- 4 lobster tails, cut halfway through the center
- ¼ cup ghee, melted
- 1 tablespoon chives, chopped
- 1 tablespoon parsley, chopped
- 1 tablespoon lime juice
- A pinch of sea salt
- Black pepper to the taste

Directions:
In a bowl, mix ghee with a pinch of salt, black pepper, lime juice, chives and sriracha sauce and whisk well. Fill lobster tails with half of this mix, place them on heated grill over medium high heat, cook for 5 minutes, flip, grill them for 3 minutes more and divide between plates. Top lobster tails with the rest of the Sriracha sauce and parsley. Enjoy!

Nutritional value: calories 223, fat 12, fiber 0, carbs 2, protein 6

Grilled Salmon and Avocado Sauce

You will find this dish really interesting!

Preparation time: 10 minutes
Cooking time: 15 minutes
Servings: 4

Ingredients:
- 1 avocado, pitted, peeled and chopped
- 4 salmon fillets
- ¼ cup cilantro, chopped
- 1/3 cup coconut milk
- 1 tablespoon lime juice
- 1 tablespoon lime zest
- 1 teaspoon onion powder
- 1 teaspoon garlic powder
- A pinch of sea salt
- Black pepper to the taste

Directions:
Season salmon fillets with a pinch of salt, black pepper and lime zest, rub well, place on heated grill over medium heat, cook for 15 minutes flipping once and divide between plates. In your food processor, mix avocado with cilantro, garlic powder, onion powder, lime juice and coconut milk and blend well. Add a pinch of sea salt and some black pepper, blend again and drizzle this over salmon fillets. Serve right away. Enjoy!

Nutritional value: calories 170, fat 7, fiber 2, carbs 3, protein 20

Grilled Calamari

This Paleo dish has such a pleasant and delicate taste!

Preparation time: 10 minutes
Cooking time: 5 minutes
Servings: 4

Ingredients:
- 2 pounds calamari tentacles and tubes cut into rings
- 2 tablespoons parsley, minced
- 1 lemon, sliced
- 1 lime, sliced
- 2 garlic cloves, minced
- 3 tablespoons lemon juice
- ¼ cup olive oil
- A pinch of sea salt
- Black pepper to the taste

Directions:
In a bowl, mix calamari with parsley, lime slices, lemon slices, garlic, lemon juice, a pinch of salt, black pepper and olive oil and stir well. Place calamari rings on preheated grill over medium high heat, cook for 5 minutes and divide between plates. Serve with the lemon and lime slices and some of the marinade drizzled on top. Enjoy!

Nutritional value: calories 130, fat 4, fiber 1, carbs 3, protein 12

Shrimp and Zucchini Noodles

It's a light and delicious option for dinner!

Preparation time: 10 minutes
Cooking time: 15 minutes
Servings: 2

Ingredients:
- 2 zucchinis, cut with a spiralizer
- 1 pound shrimp, peeled and deveined
- 4 garlic cloves, minced
- 2 tablespoons bacon fat
- 2 tablespoons lemon juice
- 2 tablespoons chives, minced
- A pinch of sea salt
- Black pepper to the taste

Directions:
Heat up a pan with the bacon fat over medium heat, add garlic, stir and cook for 3 minutes. Add shrimp, stir, cook for 4 minutes more and transfer to a plate. Heat up the pan again, add lemon juice and zucchini noodles, stir and cook for 4 minutes. Return shrimp to pan, season with a pinch of salt, black pepper and chives, stir, cook for a couple more minutes and divide between plates. Serve right away. Enjoy!

Nutritional value: calories 140, fat 3, fiber 3, carbs 4, protein 8

Wonderful Crusted Salmon

This is so crunchy, tasty and easy to make at home! Try it today!

Preparation time: 10 minutes
Cooking time: 20 minutes
Servings: 4

Ingredients:
- 1 cup pistachios, chopped
- 4 salmon fillets
- ¼ cup lemon juice
- 2 tablespoons honey
- 1 teaspoon dill, chopped
- A pinch of sea salt
- Black pepper to the taste
- 1 tablespoon mustard

Directions:
In a bowl, mix pistachios with mustard, honey, lemon juice, a pinch of salt, black pepper and dill and stir well. Spread this over salmon fillets, press well, place them on a lined baking sheet, place in the oven at 375 degrees F and bake for 20 minutes. Divide salmon between plates and serve with a side salad. Enjoy!

Nutritional value: calories 150, fat 3, fiber 2, carbs 5, protein 12

Stuffed Calamari

This is just so yummy!

Preparation time: 15 minutes
Cooking time: 50 minutes
Servings: 4

Ingredients:
- 4 big calamari, tentacles separated and chopped
- 2 tablespoons parsley, chopped
- 5 ounces kale, chopped
- 2 garlic cloves, minced
- 1 red bell pepper, chopped
- 1 teaspoon oregano, dried
- 14 ounces canned tomato puree
- Some bacon fat
- 1 onion, chopped
- A pinch of sea salt
- Black pepper to the taste

Directions:
Heat up a pan with some bacon fat over medium heat, add onion and garlic, stir and cook for 2 minutes. Add bell pepper, stir and cook for 3 minutes. Add calamari tentacles, stir and cook for 6 minutes more. Add kale, a pinch of sea salt and black pepper, stir, cook for a couple more minutes and take off heat. Stuff calamari tubes with this mix and secure with toothpicks. Heat up a pan with some bacon fat over medium high heat, add calamari, brown them for 2 minutes on each side and then mix with tomato puree. Also add parsley, oregano and some black pepper to the pan, stir gently, cover, reduce heat to medium-low and simmer for 40 minutes. Divide stuffed calamari on plates and serve. Enjoy!

Nutritional value: calories 222, fat 10, fiber 1, carbs 7, protein 15

Amazing Salmon and Chives

This flavored Paleo dish is just what you need today!

Preparation time: 10 minutes
Cooking time: 12 minutes
Servings: 4

Ingredients:
- 2 tablespoons dill, chopped
- 4 salmon fillets
- 2 tablespoons chives, chopped
- 1/3 cup maple syrup
- Bacon fat
- 3 tablespoons balsamic vinegar
- A pinch of sea salt
- Black pepper to the taste
- Lime wedges for serving

Directions:
Heat up a pan with bacon fat over medium high heat, add fish fillets, season them with a pinch of sea salt and black pepper, cook for 3 minutes, cover pan and cook for 6 minutes more. Add balsamic vinegar and maple syrup and cook for 3 minutes basting fish with this mix. Add dill and chives, cook for 1 minute, divide fillets between plates and serve with lime wedges on the side. Enjoy!

Nutritional value: calories 140, fat 3, fiber 2, carbs 5, protein 10

Roasted Cod

This is so flavored and rich!

Preparation time: 10 minutes
Cooking time: 20 minutes
Servings: 4

Ingredients:
- 1 tablespoon parsley, chopped
- 4 medium cod filets
- ¼ cup ghee
- 2 garlic cloves, minced
- 2 tablespoons bacon fat
- 2 tablespoons lemon juice
- 3 tablespoons prosciutto, chopped
- 1 teaspoon Dijon mustard
- 1 shallot, chopped
- A pinch of sea salt
- Black pepper to the taste
- Lemon wedges

Directions:
In a bowl, mix mustard with ghee, garlic, parsley, shallot, lemon juice, prosciutto, salt and pepper and whisk well. Heat up a pan with the bacon fat over medium high heat, add fish fillets, season them with some black pepper and cook for 4 minutes on each side. Spread mustard and ghee mix over fish, transfer everything to a lined baking sheet, place in the oven at 425 degrees F and bake for 10 minutes. Divide fish between plates and serve with lemon wedges on the side. Enjoy!

Nutritional value: calories 150, fat 4, fiber 1, carbs 3, protein 20

Halibut and Tasty Salsa

This brings summer into your kitchen! Just try it!

Preparation time: 15 minutes
Cooking time: 10 minutes
Servings: 4

Ingredients:
- 4 medium halibut fillets
- 2 teaspoons olive oil
- 4 teaspoons lemon juice
- 1 garlic clove, minced
- 1 teaspoon sweet paprika
- A pinch of sea salt
- Black pepper to the taste

For the salsa:
- ¼ cup green onions, chopped
- 1 cup red bell pepper, chopped
- 4 teaspoons oregano, chopped
- 1 small habanero pepper, chopped
- 1 garlic clove, minced
- ¼ cup lemon juice

Directions:
In a bowl, mix red bell pepper with habanero, green onion, ¼ cup lemon juice, 1 garlic clove, oregano, a pinch of sea salt and black pepper, stir well and keep in the fridge for now. In a large bowl, mix paprika, olive oil, 1 garlic clove and 4 teaspoons lemon juice and stir well. Add fish, rub well, cover bowl and leave aside for 10 minutes. Place marinated fish on preheated grill over medium high heat, season with a pinch of sea salt and black pepper, cook for 4 minutes on each side and divide between plates. Top fish with the salsa you've made earlier and serve. Enjoy!

Nutritional value: calories 150, fat 3, fiber 2, carbs 3, protein 12

Special Salmon

Try something new today! Try this cabbage wrapped salmon!

Preparation time: 10 minutes
Cooking time: 20 minutes
Servings: 4

Ingredients:
- 6 cabbage leaves, sliced in half
- 4 medium salmon steaks, skinless
- 2 red bell peppers, chopped
- Some coconut oil
- 1 yellow onion, chopped
- A pinch of sea salt
- Black pepper to the taste

Directions:
Put water in a pot, bring to a boil over medium high heat, add cabbage leaves, blanch them for 2 minutes, transfer to a bowl filled with cold water and pat dry them. Season salmon steaks with a pinch of sea salt and black pepper to the taste and wrap each in 3 cabbage leaf halves. Heat up a pan with some coconut oil over medium high heat, add onion and bell pepper, stir and cook for 4 minutes. Add wrapped salmon, introduce pan in the oven at 350 degrees F and bake for 12 minutes. Divide salmon and veggies between plates and serve. Enjoy!

Nutritional value: calories 140, fat 3, fiber 1, carbs 2, protein 15

Cod and Herb Sauce

You'll get so much flavor from this great Paleo dish!

Preparation time: 10 minutes
Cooking time: 15 minutes
Servings: 4

Ingredients:
- 1 tablespoon chives, chopped
- 4 medium cod fillets
- 1 tablespoon thyme, chopped
- 1 tablespoon parsley, chopped
- Grated zest from ½ lemon
- 1 shallot, chopped
- ¾ cup coconut milk
- 6 tablespoons ghee
- 2 garlic cloves
- A pinch of sea salt
- Black pepper to the taste

Directions:
In a bowl, mix garlic with ghee, shallots, chives, parsley and thyme and stir well. Season cod with a pinch of salt and black pepper to the taste. Heat up a pan over medium heat, add herbed ghee and fish, toss to coat and cook for 2 minutes on each side. Transfer fish to a lined baking sheet, place in the oven at 400 degrees F and bake for 7 minutes. Heat up the pan with the herbed ghee over medium heat, add lemon zest and coconut milk, stir and bring to a simmer over medium heat. Divide fish on plates, drizzle the herbed sauce on top and serve. Enjoy!

Nutritional value: calories 160, fat 3, fiber 2, carbs 3, protein 14

Salmon and Tomato Pesto

We are completely sure that you've never tried making a tomato pesto! Today you will learn how to combine such a pesto with a tasty salmon!

Preparation time: 10 minutes
Cooking time: 15 minutes
Servings: 4

Ingredients:
- 4 salmon fillets, skin on
- 1 tablespoon red bell pepper, chopped
- 1 shallot, chopped
- 2 tablespoon basil, chopped
- ½ cup cherry tomatoes, cut in quarters
- 2 garlic cloves, minced
- ½ cup sun-dried tomatoes, chopped
- 3 tablespoons olive oil
- A pinch of sea salt
- Black pepper to the taste

Directions:
In your food processor, mix sun-dried tomatoes with garlic, oil, basil, shallots, a pinch of sea salt and black pepper and blend really well. Rub salmon with some of this mix, place on preheated grill over medium high heat, cook for 12 minutes flipping once and divide between plates. Add the rest of the tomato pesto on top and serve with cherry tomatoes and bell pepper pieces on the side. Enjoy!

Nutritional value: calories 140, fat 2, fiber 2, carbs 3, protein 9

Salmon Delight

This is an elegant dinner dish, full of intense flavors!

Preparation time: 10 minutes
Cooking time: 27 minutes
Servings: 4

Ingredients:
- 10 ounces spinach, chopped
- 5 sun-dried tomatoes, chopped
- ¼ teaspoon red pepper flakes
- 4 medium salmon fillets
- A pinch of sea salt
- Black pepper to the taste
- 1 tablespoon coconut oil
- ¼ cup shallots, chopped
- 4 garlic cloves

Directions:
Heat up a pan with the oil over medium high heat, add shallots, stir and cook for 3 minutes. Add garlic, stir and cook for 1 minute. Add tomatoes, pepper flakes and spinach, stir and cook for 3 minutes. Season with a pinch of salt and black pepper to the taste, stir, take off heat and leave aside for now. Arrange salmon fillets on a lined baking sheet, season with a pinch of salt and some black pepper, top with the spinach mix, place in the oven at 350 degrees F and bake for 20 minutes. Divide between plates and serve right away. Enjoy!

Nutritional value: calories 140, fat 2, fiber 2, carbs 3, protein 10

Shrimp with Mango and Avocado Mix

This is what you need to eat on a hot summer day!

Preparation time: 10 minutes
Cooking time: 5 minutes
Servings: 2

Ingredients:
- 1 avocado, pitted, peeled and chopped
- 1 pound shrimp, peeled and deveined
- 1 tomato, chopped
- 1 mango, peeled and chopped
- 1 jalapeno, chopped
- 1 tablespoon lime juice
- Bacon fat
- ¼ cup green onions, chopped
- 4 garlic cloves, minced
- A pinch of sea salt
- Black pepper to the taste

Directions:
In a bowl, mix lime juice with jalapeno, mango, tomato, avocado and green onions, stir well and leave aside. Heat up a pan with some bacon fat over medium high heat, add garlic, stir and cook for 2 minutes. Add shrimp, a pinch of sea salt and black pepper, stir and cook for 5 minutes. Divide shrimp on plates, add mango and avocado mix on the side. Enjoy!

Nutritional value: calories 140, fat 2, fiber 3, carbs 3, protein 8

Thai Shrimp Delight

You can serve this if you have friends over for dinner!

Preparation time: 10 minutes
Cooking time: 50 minutes
Servings: 4

Ingredients:
- 1 pound shrimp, peeled and deveined
- 2 shallots, chopped
- 1 spaghetti squash, cut in halves and seedless
- Juice from 1 lime
- 2 tablespoons coconut aminos
- 1 tablespoon chili sauce
- 1 teaspoon ginger, grated
- 3 garlic cloves, minced
- 3 cups mung beans sprouts
- 3 tablespoons coconut oil
- 2 tablespoons almond butter
- 2 eggs, whisked
- 1 cup carrots, chopped
- ¼ cup nuts, roasted and chopped
- ¼ cup cilantro, chopped
- 4 green onions, chopped
- A pinch of sea salt
- Black pepper to the taste

Directions:
Brush squash halves with 1 tablespoon coconut oil, arrange pieces on a lined baking sheet, place in the oven at 400 degrees F and bake for 40 minutes. Leave squash to cool down and make squash noodles using a fork. Heat up a pan over medium heat, add coconut aminos, lime juice, almond butter and chili sauce and stir well until everything combines. Heat up another pan with the rest of the oil over medium high heat, add shrimp, cook for 4 minutes and transfer to a plate. Heat up the pan again over medium high heat, add ginger, shallots and garlic, stir and cook for 2 minutes. Add carrots and sprouts, stir and cook for 1 minute. Add eggs and stir everything. Add almond butter sauce you've made earlier, squash noodles, cilantro, green onions, nuts, shrimp, a pinch of salt and black pepper, stir well, divide between plates and serve right away.

Nutritional value: calories 150, fat 3, fiber 2, carbs 3, protein 14

Scallops Tartar

If you have some special dinner guests, then you might consider making this Paleo dish for them!

Preparation time: 10 minutes
Cooking time: 0 minutes
Servings: 2

Ingredients:
- Juice of ½ lemon
- 1 tablespoon green onions, chopped
- 1 tablespoon olive oil
- 6 scallops, chopped
- 3 strawberries, chopped
- ½ tablespoons basil, chopped
- A pinch of sea salt
- Black pepper to the taste

Directions:
In a bowl, mix green onions with lemon juice, olive oil, scallops, strawberries, basil, a pinch of sea salt and black pepper to the taste, stir well, divide into small bowls and serve cold. Enjoy!

Nutritional value: calories 140, fat 2, fiber 2, carbs 3, protein 9

Shrimp Cocktail

Are you looking for a great Paleo party food? Try this next one!

Preparation time: 30 minutes
Cooking time: 6 minutes
Servings: 4

Ingredients:
- 20 jumbo shrimp, deveined but shelled
- 2 cups ice
- A pinch of sea salt
- A drizzle of olive oil
- 1 cup water
- 1 cup tomato sauce
- ¼ teaspoon Worcestershire sauce
- Juice of 1 lemon
- Zest from 1 lemon
- 1 tablespoons prepared horseradish
- Chili sauce to the taste

For the cocktail sauce:

Directions:
In a bowl, mix water with ice, a pinch of sea salt and shrimp, stir, cover and keep in the fridge for 30 minutes. Discard water from shrimp, rinse them, pat dry them, drizzle olive oil over them and rub well. Arrange shrimp on a lined baking sheet, place in preheated broiler and broil them for 3 minutes. Flip, broil for 2 minutes more and leave aside. In a bowl, mix tomato sauce with Worcestershire sauce, lemon juice, lemon zest, chili sauce to the taste and horseradish and whisk well. Arrange shrimp on a platter and serve with the cocktail sauce on the side.

Nutritional value: calories 160, fat 3, fiber 2, carbs 3, protein 14

Tilapia Surprise

We don't need to tell you more! It's really a surprise!

Preparation time: 10 minutes
Cooking time: 25 minutes
Servings: 4

Ingredients:
- 28 ounces canned coconut milk
- 2 red bell peppers, seedless and cut in halves
- 4 tilapia fillets
- 2 green onions, chopped
- 4 tablespoons Thai red curry paste
- A drizzle of olive oil
- ½ cup water
- 2 tablespoons coconut aminos
- 8 lime wedges
- 1 cup basil, chopped
- A pinch of sea salt
- Black pepper to the taste

Directions:
In your food processor, mix half of the coconut milk with basil, curry paste and blend well. Heat up a pan over medium heat, add curry mix and cook for 3 minutes. Add the rest of the coconut milk, water and coconut aminos, stir and cook for 10 minutes. In a bowl, mix fish with bell pepper, a drizzle of oil, a pinch of salt and black pepper to the taste. Heat up a grill over medium high heat, add peppers, grill them for 5 minutes and transfer to a plate. Place fish on the grill, cook for 6 minutes and divide between plates. Add bell peppers on the side, sprinkle green onions, drizzle curry sauce and serve with lime wedges on the side. Enjoy!

Nutritional value: calories 160, fat 3, fiber 1, carbs 2, protein 12

Tuna and Salsa

It's rich, tasty and nutritious! What more could you ask for?

Preparation time: 2 hours and 10 minutes
Cooking time: 8 minutes
Servings: 4

Ingredients:
- ½ teaspoon coriander
- 4 tuna pieces
- A pinch of sea salt
- Black pepper to the taste
- 3 cherry tomatoes, cut in quarters
- 1 red onion, chopped
- 2 avocados, pitted, peeled and chopped
- 2 tablespoons cilantro, chopped
- 2 tablespoons lime juice
- 1 jalapeno, chopped

Directions:
In a bowl, mix cherry tomatoes with avocados, cilantro, lime juice, jalapeno, a pinch of sea salt and black pepper, stir well and keep in the fridge for 2 hours. Season tuna with a pinch of sea salt, black pepper and coriander and rub well. Place tune on preheated grill over medium high heat, cook for 3 minutes on each side and divide between plates. Serve with the avocado salsa on the side. Enjoy!

Nutritional value: calories 150, fat 2, fiber 1, carbs 2, protein 14

Amazing Salmon Tartar

We know you want the best Paleo recipes! That's why we recommend you to try this next dish!

Preparation time: 30 minutes
Cooking time: 0 minutes
Servings: 4

Ingredients:
- 1 tablespoon chives, minced
- 1 pound salmon fillet, skinless, boneless and cut into small cubes
- 1 small red onion, chopped
- 1 tablespoon basil, chopped
- Juice from lemon
- 2 tablespoons capers
- ¼ cup olive oil
- 1 teaspoon mustard
- 2 green onions, chopped
- A pinch of sea salt
- Black pepper to the taste

Directions:
In a big bowl mix chives with onion, basil, capers, salmon and green onions and stir. In another bowl, mix lemon juice with mustard, oil, a pinch of salt and black pepper the taste and stir well. Add this dressing over salad, toss to coat well, divide between plates and serve. Enjoy!

Nutritional value: calories 130, fat 1, fiber 2, carbs 2, protein 7

Incredible Swordfish

This will be much more than a Paleo dish! It will be a real feast!

Preparation time: 10 minutes
Cooking time: 6 minutes
Servings: 2

Ingredients:
- 2 medium wild swordfish fillets
- 1 tablespoon cilantro, chopped
- 1 avocado, pitted, peeled and chopped
- 1 mango, peeled and chopped
- 2 teaspoons avocado oil
- 1 teaspoon cumin powder
- 1 teaspoon onion powder
- 1 teaspoon garlic powder
- A pinch of sea salt
- Black pepper to the taste
- ½ cup balsamic vinegar
- Juice of ½ lime

Directions:
Season fish fillets with a pinch of sea salt, black pepper, onion powder, garlic powder and cumin powder and rub well. Heat up a pan with half of the oil over medium high heat, add fish and vinegar, cook for 3 minutes on each side and transfer to plates. In a bowl, mix avocado with mango, lime juice, cilantro and the rest of the oil and stir well. Divide this salsa next to fish fillets and serve.

Nutritional value: calories 120, fat 2, fiber 2, carbs 4, protein 16

Crusted Snapper

It's so simple to cook something as delicious as this!

Preparation time: 10 minutes
Cooking time: 8 minutes
Servings: 1

Ingredients:
- 1 red snapper fillet, skinless
- A pinch of sea salt
- Black pepper to the taste
- 1 tablespoon sesame seeds
- 1 teaspoon coconut oil

Directions:
Season red snapper with a pinch of sea salt and black pepper to the taste and spread sesame seeds on one side. Press seeds down, flip fish and spread the remaining sesame seeds on this side. Heat up a pan with the oil over medium high heat, add crusted red snapper, cook for 3 minutes on each side and transfer to a plate.
Serve with a side salad. Enjoy!

Nutritional value: calories 120, fat 1, fiber 1, carbs 2, protein 10

Paleo Vegetables Recipes

Paleo Falafel

Try this Israeli style paleo dish! It's going to be incredible!

Servings: 4
Preparation time: 15 minutes
Cooking time: 40 minutes

Ingredients:

- 2 cups cauliflower florets
- 1 cup yellow onion, chopped
- 1 zucchini, chopped
- ½ cup parsley, chopped
- 4 garlic cloves, minced
- ¼ teaspoon chili powder
- ½ cup cilantro, chopped
- 2 teaspoons cumin
- A pinch of sea salt
- Black pepper to the taste
- ½ cup almond flour
- ½ teaspoon turmeric
- Zest from 1 lemon
- 1 egg, whisked
- Coconut oil

Directions:
In your food processor, mix cilantro, onion, parsley and garlic, blend well and transfer to a bowl. In your food processor, also mix cauliflower with zucchini, blend very well and pour over onion mix. Add chili powder, lemon zest, cumin, turmeric, egg, almond flour, a pinch of salt and pepper to the taste and stir well. Spread some coconut oil on a lined baking sheet, arrange falafels, introduce in the oven at 375 degrees F and bake for 40 minutes, brushing them with some more coconut oil halfway.

Nutritional value: calories 230, fat 14, carbs 15, fiber 2, protein 22

Paleo Daikon Rolls

It's such a fresh dish, and it also looks so good!

Servings: 4
Preparation time: 15 minutes
Cooking time: 0 minutes

Ingredients:

- ½ cup pumpkin seeds
- 2 green onions, chopped
- ½ bunch cilantro, roughly chopped
- 2 tablespoons avocado oil
- 1 tablespoon lime juice
- 2 teaspoons water
- A pinch of sea salt
- Black pepper to the taste
- 2 daikon radishes, sliced lengthwise into long strips
- 1 small cucumber, cut into matchsticks
- ½ avocado, pitted, peeled and sliced
- Handful microgreens

Directions:
In your food processor, mix pumpkin seeds with a pinch of sea salt, pepper, cilantro and green onions and blend very well. Add avocado oil gradually and lime juice and blend very well again. Add water and blend some more. Spread this on each daikon slice, add cucumber matchsticks, avocado slices, and micro greens, roll them, seal edges, divide between plates and serve.

Nutritional value: calories 140, fat 0, carbs 23, fiber 0, protein 0

Paleo Cauliflower Pizza

It's a great snack you can enjoy with your friends!

Servings: 6
Preparation time: 10 minutes
Cooking time: 30 minutes

Ingredients:
- 1 and ½ cups mashed cauliflower
- A pinch of sea salt
- Black pepper to the taste
- ½ cup almond meal
- 1 and ½ tablespoons flax seed, ground
- 2/3 cup water
- ½ teaspoon oregano, dried
- ½ teaspoon garlic powder
- Pizza sauce for serving
- Spinach leaves, chopped and already cooked for serving
- Mushrooms, sliced and cooked for serving

Directions:
In a bowl, mix flax seed with water and stir well. In a bowl, mix cauliflower with almond meal, flax seed mix, a pinch of sea salt, pepper, oregano and garlic powder, stir well, shape small pizza crusts, spread them on a lined baking sheet and bake them in the oven at 420 degrees F and bake for 15 minutes. Take pizzas out of the oven, spread pizza sauce, spinach, and mushrooms on them, introduce in the oven again and bake 10 more minutes. Divide between plates and serve. Enjoy!

Nutritional value: calories 150, fat 8, carbs 20, fiber 1, protein 9

Paleo Endive Bites

You can serve this as an appetizer! It's fresh, delicious and flavored!

Servings: 4
Preparation time: 10 minutes
Cooking time: 15 minutes

Ingredients:
- 4 slices bacon
- 16 endives leaves
- 2 teaspoons white wine vinegar
- 1 cup cherry tomatoes, sliced
- A pinch of sea salt
- 1 tablespoon chives, chopped
- Black pepper to the taste
- 1 tablespoon extra virgin olive oil

Directions:
Arrange bacon slices on a lined baking sheet, introduce in the oven at 400 degrees F and bake for 20 minutes. Drain grease, transfer bacon to a cutting board, leave aside to cool down, crumble and put in a bowl. In another bowl, mix tomatoes with chives, oil, a pinch of salt, pepper and vinegar and stir well. Divide this mix into endive leaves, sprinkle crumbled bacon on top of each, divide between plates and serve. Enjoy!

Nutritional value: calories 120, fat 1, carbs 10, fiber 10, sugar 1, protein 6

Paleo Veggies Dish with Tasty Sauce

It's a paleo dish you should really enjoy sometimes!

Servings: 4
Preparation time: 15 minutes
Cooking time: 20 minutes

Ingredients:

- 2 carrots, chopped
- 8 mushrooms, sliced
- 4 zucchinis, cut in thin noodles
- 2 cups spinach, torn
- 2 yellow squash, halved and sliced
- 1 tablespoon coconut oil
- 1 cup coconut milk
- Juice of 1 lemon
- A pinch of sea salt
- Black pepper to the taste

For the pesto:

- ½ cup extra virgin olive oil
- 2 cups basil
- 1/3 cup pine nuts
- 3 garlic clove, chopped
- A pinch of sea salt
- Black pepper to the taste

Directions:
In your food processor, mix basil with nuts and garlic and pulse well. Add oil, a pinch of salt and pepper, pulse well again, transfer to a bowl and leave aside. Steam carrots, squash, zucchini, and mushrooms in a bamboo steamer for 8 minutes, transfer them to a colander, season with a pinch of sea salt and pepper, leave aside for 10 minutes, pat dry them and put in a bowl. Heat up a pan with the oil over medium high heat, add half of the coconut milk, salt, and pepper and bring to a boil stirring all the time. Add the pesto you've made, lemon juice and the rest of the coconut milk and stir again. Add steamed veggies, stir and cook for 2 minutes., Add spinach, more salt, and pepper if needed, stir, cook for 2 minutes more, transfer to bowls and serve.

Nutritional value: calories 260, fat 12, carbs 17, fiber 13, sugar 5, protein 18

Paleo-Indian Pancakes

This is a veggie based paleo dish you can serve for dinner with tasty green chutney!

Servings: 4
Preparation time: 10 minutes
Cooking time: 15 minutes

Ingredients:

- ½ cup almond flour
- ½ cup tapioca flour
- Coconut oil for frying
- A pinch of sea salt
- Black pepper to the taste
- 1 cup coconut milk
- ½ teaspoon chili powder
- ¼ teaspoon turmeric
- 1 small red onion, chopped
- 1 Serrano chili pepper, minced
- 1 small piece of ginger, grated
- A handful cilantro, chopped

Directions:
In a bowl, mix almond and tapioca flour with milk, chili powder, a pinch of sea salt, pepper and turmeric and stir well. Add onion, Serrano pepper, cilantro and ginger and stir very well. Heat up a pan with the oil over medium high heat, pour ¼ cup pancakes mix, spread, cook for 4 minutes on each side and transfer to a plate. Repeat with the rest of the batter and serve pancakes with green chutney.

Nutritional value: calories 198, fat 6.2, carbs 30, fiber 5.9, sugar 4, protein 8.5

Paleo Stuffed Mushrooms

Eat this tonight, and you won't need anything else!

Servings: 4
Preparation time: 10 minutes
Cooking time: 10 minutes

Ingredients:
- 12 big mushrooms, stems removed
- A pinch of sea salt
- Black pepper to the taste
- 1 small tomato, diced
- ¼ cup homemade paleo pesto
- 2 tablespoons extra virgin olive oil

Directions:
Brush mushrooms with the olive oil and season them with a pinch of sea salt and pepper to the taste. Heat up a pan over medium high heat, add mushrooms and cook them for 5 minutes on each side. Transfer them to a platter, fill each with pesto sauce, top with diced tomatoes and serve. Enjoy!

Nutritional value: calories 80, fat 4, carbs 5, fiber 0, protein 4

Stuffed Zucchinis

It's an impressive recipe you can try for some special guests!

Servings: 4
Preparation time: 10 minutes
Cooking time: 20 minutes

Ingredients:
- 2 tomatoes, chopped
- 1 eggplant, chopped
- 2 zucchinis, cut into halves lengthwise
- 1 yellow onion, chopped
- A pinch of sea salt
- Black pepper to the taste
- ½ bunch parsley, finely chopped
- 3 tablespoons extra virgin olive oil
- 2 garlic cloves, minced

Directions:
Remove flesh from zucchini halves, season them with a pinch of sea salt and pepper, leave aside for 10 minutes and pat dry them, Heat up a pan with 1 tablespoon oil over medium high heat, add onion, stir and cook for 4 minutes. Add garlic, stir and cook 1 minute. Add the rest of the oil, eggplant and chopped zucchini flesh, stir and cook for 10 minutes. Add tomatoes, parsley and pepper to the taste, stir and cook for 5 minutes more. Fill zucchini halves with this mix, place on preheated grill over medium high heat, cook for 3 minutes, divide between plates and serve right away. Enjoy!

Nutritional value: calories 130, fat 6, carbs 9, fiber 2, sugar 0, protein 8

Paleo Stuffed Eggplant

We love eggplants because they are so easy to use in the kitchen! This next recipe proves it!

Servings: 2
Preparation time: 10 minutes
Cooking time: 1 hour

Ingredients:
- 1 eggplant
- 2 tomatoes, finely chopped
- 3 thyme springs
- 1 garlic clove, minced
- 3 tablespoons extra virgin olive oil
- A pinch of sea salt
- Black pepper to the taste
- Lemon juice from ½ lemon

Directions:
Place eggplant on a lined baking sheet, introduce in the oven at 400 degrees F and bake for 30 minutes. Take eggplant out of the oven, leave aside to cool down, cut in half lengthways, drizzle each half with 1 tablespoon olive oil, introduce in the oven again at 350 degrees F and bake for 25 more minutes. Take eggplant halves out of the oven, leave aside for 5 minutes, discard flesh and sprinkle halves with some of the lemon juice, a pinch of sea salt and pepper. In a bowl, mix tomatoes with thyme, garlic, and chopped eggplant flesh and stir. Add lemon juice, pepper and 1 tablespoon olive oil and stir everything well. Scoop this into eggplant halves, divide on a plate and serve. Enjoy!

Nutritional value: calories 180, fat 22, carbs 8.5, fiber 3.4, sugar 2, protein 10

Paleo Tomato and Mushroom Skewers

It's the best paleo dish for summer! The sauce gives this dish some extra flavors!

Servings: 4
Preparation time: 10 minutes
Cooking time: 10 minutes

Ingredients:
- 1 pound mushroom caps
- 4 cups cherry tomatoes
- 1 tablespoon raw honey
- Black pepper to the taste
- 2 tablespoons Dijon mustard
- 4 tablespoons extra virgin olive oil
- 4 garlic cloves, minced
- ½ cup cilantro, minced
- ¼ cup ghee
- ½ cup parsley, minced

Directions:
In a bowl, mix mustard with olive oil, pepper and honey and whisk well. Arrange mushrooms and tomatoes on skewers alternating pieces, brush them with the mustard mix, arrange on preheated grill over medium high heat and cook for 3 minutes on each side. Heat up a pan with the ghee over medium high heat, add garlic, stir and cook for 3 minutes. Add cilantro, parsley, salt and pepper to the taste and cook for 2 minutes more. Divide skewers on plates, drizzle herb sauce on top and serve. Enjoy!

Nutritional value: calories 138, fat 5, carbs 15, fiber 0, protein 4

Amazing Paleo Potato Bites

It's a tasty dish full of colors and tastes!

Servings: 4
Preparation time: 15 minutes
Cooking time: 25 minutes

Ingredients:
- 2 sweet potatoes, thinly sliced
- 1 cup salsa
- 4 ounces bacon, already cooked and crumbled
- 1 teaspoon chili powder
- ½ teaspoon garlic powder
- ½ teaspoon paprika
- 2 tablespoons extra virgin olive oil
- Black pepper to the taste
- Some cilantro, finely chopped

For the guacamole:
- 1 tablespoon lime juice
- 2 avocados, pitted, peeled and chopped
- 1 garlic clove, minced
- ¼ cup red onions, chopped
- ½ cup tomatoes, finely chopped

Directions:
In a bowl, mix avocados with lime juice, garlic, red onions, and tomatoes, stir well, cover and keep in the fridge for now. In a bowl, mix potato slices with the olive oil, chili powder, garlic powder, paprika and pepper and toss to coat. Spread potatoes on a lined baking sheet, introduce in the oven at 450 degrees F and bake for 10 minutes on each side. Take potato slices out of the oven, top each with guacamole, bacon, salsa and chopped cilantro. Divide between plates and serve. Enjoy!

Nutritional value: calories 240, fat 6, carbs 10, fiber 3, sugar 0.4, protein 17

Paleo Cucumber Salsa

Make sure you serve this with some tortilla chips for your next party!

Servings: 12
Preparation time: 1 hour and 10 minutes
Cooking time: 0 minutes

Ingredients:
- 2 cucumbers, chopped
- ½ cup green bell pepper, chopped
- 2 tomatoes, chopped
- 1 jalapeno pepper, chopped
- 1 yellow onion, chopped
- 1 garlic clove, minced
- 2 teaspoons cilantro, chopped
- 1 teaspoon parsley, chopped
- 2 tablespoons lime juice
- ½ teaspoon dill weed
- A pinch of sea salt
- Black pepper to the taste

Directions:
In a bowl, mix cucumbers with jalapeno, tomatoes, green pepper, garlic, onion, a pinch of sea salt and pepper to the taste. Add parsley, cilantro, dill and lime juice and stir well again. Keep in the fridge for 1 hour and serve. Enjoy!

Nutritional value: calories 70, fat 0.2, carbs 1, fiber 2. protein 17

Paleo Sweet Potatoes and Cabbage Bake

This is a versatile dish! You can serve as a breakfast, lunch or even as a light and delicious dinner!

Servings: 4
Preparation time: 10 minutes
Cooking time: 1 hour and 10 minutes

Ingredients:
- 8 sweet potatoes, cut into thin matchsticks
- 1 carrot, sliced
- 2 and ½ cups green cabbage, shredded
- 2 garlic cloves, minced
- A pinch of sea salt
- Black pepper to the taste
- 4 ounces pancetta, chopped
- 3 tomatoes, sliced
- 1 teaspoon thyme, dried

Directions:
In a baking dish, mix cabbage with potatoes, garlic, and carrot. Add thyme, a pinch of sea salt and pepper and pancetta and toss to coat. Spread tomato slices over veggie mix, cover dish with tin foil, introduce in the oven at 350 degrees F and bake for 35 minutes. Discard tin foil and bake veggies for 30 more minutes. Take the dish out of the oven, leave aside to cool down, divide between plates and serve. Enjoy!

Nutritional value: calories 190, fat 0.5, carbs 43, fiber 7, protein 5.9

Paleo Kohlrabi Dish

This is an exotic dish you can try to make when you need to impress some guests!

Servings: 2
Preparation time: 10 minutes
Cooking time: 1 hour

Ingredients:
- 3 kohlrabi, peeled and thinly sliced
- A pinch of sea salt
- Black pepper to the taste
- 4 tablespoons ghee
- 1/3 cup parsley, chopped
- 2 tablespoons lard, melted

Directions:
Arrange kohlrabi slices on the bottom of a baking dish. Drizzle some of the lard over them, season with a pinch of salt and pepper and some of the parsley. Add another layer of kohlrabi, drizzle more lard, season with pepper and parsley again and continue with kohlrabi slices again. Finish with parsley. Cover dish with tin foil, introduce in the oven at 350 degrees F and bake for 30 minutes. Uncover dish, add ghee, introduce in the oven again and bake for 30 more minutes. Take the dish out of the oven, leave aside to cool down, slice, divide between plates and serve. Enjoy!

Nutritional value: calories 207, fat 11, carbs 18, fiber 9.8, sugar 7, protein 11.1

Paleo Onion Rings

Forget about unhealthy snacks! Try this idea today!

Servings: 40 pieces
Preparation time: 10 minutes
Cooking time: 11 minutes

Ingredients:
- 2/3 cup cashew meal
- A pinch of sea salt
- Black pepper to the taste
- 1 big red onion, sliced and rings separated
- 1 teaspoon garlic powder
- ½ teaspoon sweet paprika
- 1 teaspoon onion powder
- 3 eggs

Directions:
In a bowl, mix eggs with a pinch of sea salt and pepper and whisk well. In another bowl, mix cashew meal with pepper, garlic and onion powder and sweet paprika and stir well. Dip each onion ring in eggs and then in cashew meal mix, spread them on a lined baking sheet, introduce in the oven at 425 degrees F and bake for 10 minutes. Transfer onion rings to preheated broiler and broil for 1 minute. Leave onion rings to cool down, divide between bowls and serve as a snack. Enjoy!

Nutritional value: calories 134, fat 3.6, carbs 14, fiber 1.5, protein 4.5

Paleo Baked Yuka with Tomato Sauce

Your party will become a success with this veggie paleo dish!

Servings: 3
Preparation time: 10 minutes
Cooking time: 25 minutes

Ingredients:
- 1 yucca root, cut into strips
- ½ teaspoon garlic powder
- 2 tablespoons coconut oil
- Black pepper to the taste
- ½ teaspoon smoked paprika
- ½ teaspoon onion powder
- 1 tomato, grated and skin discarded
- 1 garlic clove, grated
- 1 tablespoon vinegar
- 2 tablespoons extra virgin olive oil
- A pinch of sea salt

For the sauce:

Directions:
Put yucca strips in a bowl, drizzle with coconut oil, sprinkle pepper, garlic powder, onion powder and paprika, toss to coat, spread on a lined baking sheet, introduce in the oven at 390 degrees F and bake for 25 minutes. Meanwhile, in a bowl, mix tomato with olive oil, a pinch of sea salt, vinegar and garlic and stir very well. Take yucca out of the oven, transfer to plates and serve with tomato sauce drizzled on top. Enjoy!

Nutritional value: calories 230, fat 2.7, carbs 51, fiber 2.5, protein 2

Paleo Surprise Dinner Dish

It's going to be such a surprising dish! You are going to be so appreciated for it!

Servings: 5
Preparation time: 15 minutes
Cooking time: 1 hour and 30 minutes

Ingredients:
- 1 paleo coconut bread, cubed
- 2 tablespoons ghee, melted
- 1 pound sausage, casings removed
- 3 celery stalks, chopped
- 1 fennel, chopped
- 4 garlic cloves, chopped
- 1 yellow onion, chopped
- 8 ounces mushrooms, chopped
- 1 pear, chopped
- 1 red bell pepper, chopped
- 1 tablespoon thyme, chopped
- 2 tablespoons parsley, chopped
- ½ cup white wine
- A pinch of sea salt
- Black pepper to the taste
- 1 teaspoon oregano, dried
- 3 eggs, whisked
- 2 cups chicken stock

Directions:
Spread paleo bread cubes on a lined baking sheet, introduce in the oven at 300 degrees f and bake for 20 minutes. Toss bread cubes, introduce in the oven again, bake for 20 minutes more, take out of the oven and leave aside for now. Heat up a pan over medium high heat, add sausage, break with a fork, brown for a few minutes, transfer to a bowl and leave aside for now as well. Return pan to medium high heat, add 1 tablespoon ghee, melt and add garlic, fennel, onion, and celery, stir and cook for 10 minutes. Transfer veggies to the bowl along with the sausage and stir everything. Return the pan to medium high heat again, melt the rest of the ghee and add red pepper, mushrooms, and wine. Stir, cook until wine evaporates, take off heat and add this to the bowl with the veggies and the sausage. Add thyme, oregano, a pinch of sea salt, pepper, parsley, bread cubes and 1 and ½ cups stock, stir everything and leave aside for 10 minutes. Add the rest of the stock and stir everything again. Pour the veggies mix in a greased baking dish, spread whisked eggs all over, introduce in the oven at 400 degrees F, cover with tin foil and bake for 30 minutes. Remove foil and bake for 15 more minutes. Divide between plates and serve. Enjoy!

Nutritional value: calories 220, fat 12, carbs 5, fiber 0.6, protein 17.5

Paleo Broccoli and Cauliflower Fritters

It doesn't matter how pretentious you are! You will definitely like this dish!

Servings: 8
Preparation time: 10 minutes
Cooking time: 10 minutes

Ingredients:
- 1 cup broccoli, chopped
- 1 and ½ cups cauliflower, chopped
- A pinch of sea salt
- Black pepper to the taste
- 1 tablespoon coconut flour
- 2 eggs
- 1 tablespoon coconut oil for frying
- 2 tablespoons homemade mayonnaise
- 1 tablespoon extra virgin olive oil
- 1 tablespoon coriander, finely chopped
- ½ garlic clove, grated
- 1 teaspoon lime juice

Directions:
In a bowl, mix cauliflower with broccoli, eggs, coconut flour, a pinch of sea salt and pepper to the taste and stir very well. Shape small patties and arrange them on a plate. Heat up a pan with the coconut oil over medium high heat, add veggies fritters, cook for 4 minutes on each side, transfer them to paper towels, drain grease and arrange on a platter. In a bowl, mix mayo with olive oil, coriander, garlic and lime juice and stir well.
Serve you fritters with mayo mix. Enjoy!

Nutritional value: calories 140, fat 3.8, carbs 13, fiber 3.3, sugar 8, protein 7.3

Paleo Spinach and Mushroom Dish

This combination is very healthy! It's a great way to include more spinach in your daily meals!

Servings: 2
Preparation time: 10 minutes
Cooking time: 15 minutes

Ingredients:
- 6 mushrooms, chopped
- A handful cherry tomatoes, cut in halves
- 3 handfuls spinach, torn
- 1 teaspoon ghee
- 2 tablespoons extra virgin olive oil
- 1 small red onion, sliced
- ½ teaspoon lemon rind, diced
- 1 garlic clove, minced
- A pinch of sea salt
- Black pepper to the taste
- A pinch of nutmeg
- A drizzle of lemon juice

Directions:
Heat up a pan with the ghee over medium high heat, add mushrooms, stir, cook for 4 minutes and transfer them to a plate. Heat up the same pan with the olive oil over medium high heat, add onion, stir and cook for 3 minutes. Add tomatoes, a pinch of sea salt, pepper, lemon rind, nutmeg, and garlic, stir and cook for 3 minutes more. Add spinach, stir and cook for 2-3 minutes. Add lemon juice at the end, stir gently, transfer to plates and serve with mushrooms on top. Enjoy!

Nutritional value: calories 120, fat 4.5, carbs 7, fiber 2.5, protein 3.4

Paleo Celery Casserole

It's something you've never tried until now, but you'll love it!

Servings: 8
Preparation time: 10 minutes
Cooking time: 20 minutes

Ingredients:
- 1 white onion, finely chopped
- 1 celery head, chopped
- 2 and ½ tablespoons ghee
- 1 and ½ tablespoons coconut flour
- ½ teaspoon nutmeg
- A pinch of sea salt
- Black pepper to the taste
- 1 and ½ cups coconut milk
- 2 tablespoons extra virgin olive oil
- ½ cup flax meal

Directions:
Heat up a pan with 1 tablespoon olive oil over medium high heat, add celery, stir and cook for a few minutes until it browns a bit. Add a pinch of sea salt and pepper, stir and transfer to a baking dish. Heat up the same pan with the rest of the olive oil over medium heat, add onions, stir and cook for 4 minutes. Add 1 and ½ tablespoons ghee, stir well and cook for 1-2 minutes. Add coconut flour, stir well for a few minutes and take off heat. Add coconut milk, pepper to the taste and nutmeg and stir very well. Return to medium heat and stir for 2 minutes more. Add the rest of the ghee and flax meal, stir and pour everything over celery. Toss to coat, introduce in the oven at 350 degrees F and bake for 15 minutes until it becomes golden. Take casserole out of the oven, leave aside to cool down, cut, divide between plates and serve.

Nutritional value: calories 147, fat 9.2, carbs 11.3, fiber 1.5, sugar 2.1, protein 3.1

Rutabaga Noodles and Cherry Tomatoes

This will be simply amazing!

Preparation time: 10 minutes
Cooking time: 25 minutes
Servings: 4

Ingredients:
For the sauce:
- 1 tablespoon shallot, chopped
- 1 garlic clove, minced
- ¾ cup cashews, soaked for a couple of hours and drained
- 2 tablespoons nutritional yeast
- ½ cup veggie stock
- A pinch of sea salt
- Black pepper to the taste
- 2 teaspoons lemon juice

For the pasta:
- 1 cup cherry tomatoes, halved
- 5 teaspoons olive oil
- ¼ teaspoon garlic powder
- 2 rutabagas, peeled and cut into thin noodles

Directions:
Place tomatoes and rutabaga noodles on a lined baking sheet, drizzle the oil over them, season with a pinch of sea salt, black pepper and garlic powder, toss to coat, place in the oven at 400 degrees F and bake for 20 minutes. Meanwhile, in a food processor, mix garlic with shallots, cashews, veggie stock, nutritional yeast, lemon juice, a pinch of sea salt and black pepper to the taste and blend well. Divide rutabaga pasta between plates, top with tomatoes and drizzle the sauce over them.

Nutritional value: calories 230, fat 2, fiber 5, carbs 10, protein 8

Simple Garlic Tomatoes

This is so great, light and tasty!

Preparation time: 10 minutes
Cooking time: 50 minutes
Servings: 4

Ingredients:
- 4 garlic cloves, crushed
- 1 pound mixed cherry tomatoes
- 3 thyme springs, chopped
- A pinch of sea salt
- Black pepper to the taste
- ¼ cup olive oil

Directions:
In a baking dish, mix tomatoes with a pinch of sea salt, black pepper, olive oil and thyme, toss to coat, place in the oven at 325 degrees F and bake for 50 minutes. Divide tomatoes and pan juices between plates and serve. Enjoy!

Nutritional value: calories 100, fat 0, fiber 1, carbs 1, protein 6

Tomato Quiche

You can serve this for dinner tonight!

Preparation time: 10 minutes
Cooking time: 20 minutes
Servings: 2

Ingredients:
- 1 bunch basil, chopped
- 4 eggs
- 1 garlic clove, minced
- A pinch of sea salt
- Black pepper to the taste
- ½ cup cherry tomatoes, halved
- ¼ cup almond cheese

Directions:
In a bowl, mix eggs with a pinch of sea salt, black pepper, almond cheese and basil and whisk well. Pour this into a baking dish, arrange tomatoes on top, place in the oven at 350 degrees F and bake for 20 minutes. Leave quiche to cool down, slice and serve. Enjoy!

Nutritional value: calories 140, fat 1, fiber 1, carbs 2, protein 10

Amazing Cherry Mix

The name says it all! This is really amazing!

Preparation time: 30 minutes
Cooking time: 4 minutes
Servings: 4

Ingredients:
- 1 teaspoon coconut sugar
- 3 cups cherry tomatoes, halved
- ¼ teaspoon cumin, ground
- 1 tablespoon sherry vinegar
- A pinch of sea salt
- 1 red onion, chopped
- 2 cucumbers, sliced
- ¼ cup olive oil
- Black pepper to the taste

Directions:
Put cherry tomatoes in a bowl, season with coconut sugar, a pinch of salt and black pepper and leave aside for 30 minutes. Drain tomatoes and pour juices into a pan. Heat this up over medium heat, add cumin and vinegar and bring to a simmer. Cook for 4 minutes, take off heat and mix with olive oil. Add tomatoes, onion and cucumber to this mix, toss well, divide between plates and serve. Enjoy!

Nutritional value: calories 120, fat 1, fiber 2, carbs 2, protein 7

Zucchini Noodles with Tomatoes and Spinach
This Paleo dish is very tasty!

Preparation time: 10 minutes
Cooking time: 20 minutes
Servings: 6

Ingredients:
- 2 tablespoons olive oil
- 3 zucchinis, cut with a spiralizer
- 16 ounces mushrooms, sliced
- ¼ cup sun dried tomatoes, chopped
- 1 teaspoon garlic, minced
- ½ cup cherry tomatoes, halved
- 2 cups marinara sauce
- 2 cups spinach, chopped
- A pinch of sea salt
- Black pepper to the taste
- A pinch of cayenne pepper
- A handful basil, chopped

Directions:
Put zucchini noodles in a bowl, season them with a pinch of salt and black pepper and leave them aside for 10 minutes. Heat up a pan with the oil over medium high heat, add garlic, stir and cook for 1 minute. Add mushrooms, stir and cook for 4 minutes. Add sun dried tomatoes, stir and cook for 4 minutes more. Add cherry tomatoes, spinach, cayenne, marinara and zucchini noodles, stir and cook for 6 minutes more. Sprinkle basil on top, toss gently, divide between plates and serve. Enjoy!

Nutritional value: calories 120, fat 1, fiber 1, carbs 2, protein 9

Simple Roasted Tomatoes
These slow roasted tomatoes must be served with the red pepper sauce we suggest you!

Preparation time: 10 minutes
Cooking time: 1 hour
Servings: 4

Ingredients:
- 1 big red onion, cut into wedges
- 2 red bell peppers, chopped
- 2 garlic cloves, minced
- 1 pound cherry tomatoes, halved
- 1 teaspoon thyme, dried
- 1 teaspoon oregano, dried
- 3 bay leaves
- 2 tablespoons olive oil
- 1 tablespoon balsamic vinegar
- A pinch of sea salt
- Black pepper to the taste

Directions:
In a baking dish mix tomatoes with onions, garlic, a pinch of sea salt, black pepper, thyme, oregano, bay leaves, half of the oil and half of the vinegar, toss to coat, place in the oven at 350 degrees F and roast them for 1 hour. Meanwhile, in your food processor, mix bell peppers with a pinch of sea salt, black pepper, the rest of the oil and the rest of the vinegar and blend very well. Discard bay leaves, divide roasted tomatoes, garlic and onions on plates, drizzle the bell peppers sauce over them and serve.

Nutritional value: calories 123, fat 1, fiber 1, carbs 2, protein 10

Grilled Cherry Tomatoes

Serve these with a green salad on the side and enjoy!

Preparation time: 30 minutes
Cooking time: 6 minutes
Servings: 4

Ingredients:
- 1 romaine lettuce head, chopped
- A handful basil, chopped
- 1 cucumber, sliced
- 3 handfuls spinach, chopped
- 2 avocados, pitted, peeled and cubed
- 2 scallions, chopped
- ½ cup almonds, chopped
- 3 handfuls green beans, blanched and chopped

For the tomatoes skewers:
- 3 tablespoons balsamic vinegar
- 24 cherry tomatoes
- 2 tablespoons olive oil
- 3 garlic cloves, minced
- 1 tablespoons thyme, chopped
- A pinch of sea salt
- Black pepper to the taste

For the salad dressing:
- 2 tablespoons balsamic vinegar
- A pinch of sea salt
- Black pepper to the taste
- 4 tablespoons olive oil

Directions:
In a salad bowl, mix lettuce with spinach, cucumber, basil, avocado pieces, scallions, almonds and green beans. In a smaller bowl, mix 4 tablespoons oil with 2 tablespoons balsamic vinegar, a pinch of sea salt and black pepper and whisk well. Add this to salad, toss to coat and leave aside for now. In a bowl, mix 2 tablespoons oil with 3 tablespoons vinegar, 3 garlic cloves, thyme, a pinch of sea salt and black pepper and whisk well. Add tomatoes, toss to coat and leave aside for 30 minutes. Drain marinade, skewer 6 tomatoes on one skewer and repeat with the rest of the tomatoes. Place skewers on preheated grill over medium high heat, grill for 3 minutes on each side and divide between plates.
Serve with the salad you've made earlier on the side.

Nutritional value: calories 140, fat 1, fiber 1, carbs 2, protein 12

Veggies and Fish Mix

This next Paleo dish is so colored and tasty!

Preparation time: 10 minutes
Cooking time: 32 minutes
Servings: 4

Ingredients:
- 1 cup hot water
- 1 tablespoon maple syrup
- 2 tablespoons olive oil
- 1 eggplant, chopped
- 3 cups cherry tomatoes, halved
- 1 teaspoon Paleo Tabasco sauce
- 1 pound tuna, cubed
- 1 teaspoon balsamic vinegar
- ½ cup basil, chopped
- Black pepper to the taste
- A pinch of sea salt

Directions:
In a bowl, mix eggplant pieces with a pinch of salt and black pepper and stir. Heat up a pan with 1 tablespoon oil over medium heat, add eggplant, cook for 6 minutes stirring often and transfer to a bowl. Heat up the pan again with the rest of the oil over medium heat, add tomatoes, cover pan and cook for 6 minutes shaking the pan from time to time. Return eggplant pieces to the pan, add maple syrup, vinegar and hot water, stir, cover and cook for 10 minutes. Add tuna and Tabasco sauce, stir, cover pan again, reduce heat to medium-low and simmer for 10 minutes more. Sprinkle basil on top, divide veggies and tuna mix between plates and serve.

Nutritional value: calories 120, fat 1, fiber 2, carbs 5, protein 12

Spaghetti Squash and Tomatoes

It's fresh, it's flavored and very delicious!

Preparation time: 10 minutes
Cooking time: 50 minutes
Servings: 4

Ingredients:
- ¼ cup pine nuts
- 2 cups basil, chopped
- 1 spaghetti squash, halved lengthwise and seedless
- Black pepper to the taste
- A pinch of sea salt
- 1 teaspoon garlic, minced
- 1 and ½ tablespoons olive oil
- 1 cup mixed cherry tomatoes, halved
- ½ cup olive oil
- 2 garlic cloves, minced

Directions:
Place spaghetti squash halves on a lined baking sheet, place in the oven at 375 degrees F and bake for 40 minutes. Leave squash to cool down and make your spaghetti out of the flesh. In your food processor, mix pine nuts with a pinch of salt, basil and 2 garlic cloves and blend well. Add ½ cup olive oil, blend again well and transfer to a bowl. Heat up a pan with 1 and ½ tablespoons oil over medium high heat, add tomatoes, a pinch of salt, some black pepper and 1 teaspoon garlic, stir and cook for 2 minutes. Divide spaghetti squash on plates, add tomatoes and the basil pesto on top.

Nutritional value: calories 150, fat 1, fiber 2, carbs 4, protein 12

Noodles and Capers Sauce

This is so easy and fresh! It's the best summer Paleo dish!

Preparation time: 10 minutes
Cooking time: 0 minutes
Servings: 4

Ingredients:
- 1 tablespoon capers, drained
- 1 garlic clove
- A pinch of sea salt
- Black pepper to the taste
- A pinch of red pepper flakes
- 15 kalamata olives, pitted
- 2 tablespoons olive oil
- 8 ounces cherry tomatoes, halved
- A handful basil, torn
- Juice of ½ lemon
- 4 zucchinis, cut with a spiralizer

Directions:
In your food processor, mix capers with a pinch of sea salt, black pepper, pepper flakes and olives and blend well. Transfer this to a bowl, add basil, oil and tomatoes, stir well and leave aside for 10 minutes. Divide zucchini noodles on plates, add tomatoes and capers sauce, toss to coat well and serve.

Nutritional value: calories 100, fat 1, fiber 2, carbs 2, protein 6

Zucchini Noodles and Tasty Pesto

Why don't you try this for dinner tonight?

Preparation time: 10 minutes
Cooking time: 10 minutes
Servings: 4

Ingredients:
- 6 zucchinis, trimmed and cut with a spiralizer
- 1 cup basil
- 1 avocado, pitted and peeled
- A pinch of sea salt
- Black pepper to the taste
- 3 garlic cloves, chopped
- ¼ cup olive oil
- 2 tablespoons olive oil
- 1 pound shrimp, peeled and deveined
- ¼ cup pistachios
- 2 tablespoons lemon juice
- 2 teaspoons old bay seasoning

Directions:
In a bowl, mix zucchini noodles with a pinch of sea salt and some black pepper, leave aside for 10 minutes and squeeze well. In your food processor, mix pistachios with black pepper, basil, avocado, lemon juice and a pinch of salt and blend well. Add ¼ cup oil, blend again and leave aside for now. Heat up a pan with 1 tablespoon oil over medium high heat, add garlic, stir and cook for 1 minute. Add shrimp and old bay seasoning, stir, cook for 4 minutes and transfer to a bowl. Heat up the same pan with the rest of the oil over medium high heat, add zucchini noodles, stir and cook for 3 minutes. Divide on plates, add pesto on top and toss to coat well.
top with shrimp and serve.

Nutritional value: calories 140, fat 1, fiber 1, carbs 5, protein 14

Stuffed Portobello Mushrooms

These are more than you can imagine! They look great and they taste divine!

Preparation time: 10 minutes
Cooking time: 20 minutes
Servings: 4

Ingredients:
- 10 basil leaves
- 1 cup baby spinach
- 3 garlic cloves, chopped
- 1 cup almonds, roughly chopped
- 1 tablespoon parsley
- 2 tablespoons nutritional yeast
- ¼ cup olive oil
- 8 cherry tomatoes, halved
- A pinch of sea salt
- Black pepper to the taste
- 4 Portobello mushrooms, stem removed and chopped

Directions:
In your food processor, mix basil with spinach, garlic, almonds, parsley, nutritional yeast, oil, a pinch of salt, black pepper to the taste and mushroom stems and blend well. Stuff each mushroom with this mix, place them on a lined baking sheet, place in the oven at 400 degrees F and bake for 20 minutes. Divide between plates and serve right away. Enjoy!

Nutritional value: calories 145, fat 3, fiber 2, carbs 6, protein 17

Avocado Spread

Serve this right away and get ready to be delighted!

Preparation time: 10 minutes
Cooking time: 0 minutes
Servings: 4

Ingredients:
- 2 avocados, pitted and peeled
- 4 bacon strips, cooked and crumbled
- 2 garlic cloves, minced
- 5 cherry tomatoes, halved
- 1 jalapeno pepper, chopped
- ½ red onion, chopped
- Juice of ½ lime
- A pinch of sea salt
- Black pepper to the taste

Directions:
Put avocados in a bowl and mash them well. Add garlic, jalapeno, onion, a pinch of salt, black pepper, lime juice and bacon and stir well. Top with cherry tomatoes halves and serve. Enjoy!

Nutritional value: calories 140, fat 2, fiber 2, carbs 4, protein 12

Cucumber Noodles and Shrimp

It's a light Thai-style dish you will love!

Preparation time: 20 minutes
Cooking time: 5 minutes
Servings: 4

Ingredients:
- 1 tablespoon Paleo tamari sauce
- 3 tablespoons coconut aminos
- 1 tablespoon sriracha
- 1 tablespoon balsamic vinegar
- ½ cup warm water
- 1 tablespoon honey
- 3 tablespoons lemongrass, chopped
- 1 tablespoon ginger, dried
- 1 pound shrimp, peeled and deveined
- 1 tablespoon olive oil
- 2 cucumbers, cut with a spiralizer
- 1 carrot, cut into thin matchsticks
- ¼ cup balsamic vinegar
- ¼ cup ghee, melted
- ¼ cup peanuts, roasted
- 2 tablespoons sriracha sauce
- 1 tablespoon coconut aminos
- 1 tablespoon ginger, grated
- A handful mint, chopped

For the cucumber noodles:

Directions:
In a bowl, mix 3 tablespoons coconut aminos with 1 tablespoon vinegar, 1 tablespoon tamari, 1 tablespoons sriracha, warm water, honey, lemongrass, 1 tablespoons ginger, 1 tablespoon olive oil and whisk well. Add shrimp, toss to coat and leave aside for 20 minutes. Heat up your grill over medium high heat, add shrimp, cook them for 3 minutes on each side and transfer to a bowl. In a bowl, mix cucumber noodles with carrot, ghee, ¼ cup vinegar, 2 tablespoons Sriracha, 1 tablespoon coconut aminos, 1 tablespoon ginger, peanuts and mint and stir well. Divide cucumber noodles on plates, top with shrimp and serve.

Nutritional value: calories 140, fat 1, fiber 2, carbs 3, protein 8

Veggie Mix and Tasty Scallops

It's a really amazing combination!

Preparation time: 10 minutes
Cooking time: 4 minutes
Servings: 4

Ingredients:
- 1 cup cauliflower rice, already cooked
- 1 tablespoon ginger, grated
- 2 mangos, peeled and chopped
- 1 cucumber, sliced
- 2 teaspoons lime juice
- ½ cup cilantro, chopped
- 2 teaspoons olive oil
- 1 and ½ pounds sea scallops
- Black pepper to the taste

Directions:
In a bowl, mix cucumber slices with mangos, ginger, lime juice, half of the oil, cilantro and black pepper to the taste and stir well. Pat dry scallops and season them with some pepper. Heat up a pan with the rest of the oil over medium high heat, add scallops and cook for 2 minutes on each side. Divide scallops on plates, add cauliflower rice and mango and cucumber salad on the side and serve.

Nutritional value: calories 180, fat 3, fiber 2, carbs 4, protein 14

Cucumber Wraps

These are so yummy and simple to make at home!

Preparation time: 40 minutes
Cooking time: 0 minutes
Servings: 4

Ingredients:
For the mayo:
- 1 tablespoon coconut aminos
- 3 tablespoons lemon juice
- 1 cup macadamia nuts
- 1 tablespoon agave
- 1 teaspoon caraway seeds
- 1/3 cup dill, chopped
- A pinch of sea salt
- Some water

For the filling:
- 1 cup alfalfa sprouts
- 1 red bell pepper, cut into thin strips
- 2 carrots, cut into thin matchsticks
- 1 cucumber, cut into thin matchsticks
- 1 cup pea shoots
- 4 Paleo coconut wrappers

Directions:
Put macadamia nuts in a bowl, add water to cover, leave aside for 30 minutes and drain well. In your food processor, mix nuts with coconut aminos, lemon juice, agave, caraway seeds, a pinch of salt and dill and blend very well. Add some water and blend again until you obtain a smooth mayo. Divide alfalfa sprouts, bell pepper, carrot, cucumber and pea shoots on each coconut wrappers, spread dill mayo over them, wrap, cut each in half and serve. Enjoy!

Nutritional value: calories 140, fat 3, fiber 3, carbs 5, protein 12

Delicious Stuffed Peppers

These are so nutritious!

Preparation time: 10 minutes
Cooking time: 40 minutes
Servings: 4

Ingredients:
- ¼ cup ghee, melted
- 6 colored bell peppers
- 1 garlic head, cloves peeled and chopped
- 10 anchovy fillets
- 15 walnuts

Directions:
Place bell peppers on a lined baking sheet, place in preheated broiler, cook for 20 minutes and leave them to cool down. Heat up a pan with the ghee over low heat, add garlic, stir and cook for 10 minutes. Grind walnuts in a coffee grinder and add this powder to the pan. Also add anchovy and stir well. Peel burnt skin off peppers, discard tops, cut in halves and remove skins. Divide pepper halves on plates, divide anchovy mix on them and serve. Enjoy!

Nutritional value: calories 140, fat 3, fiber 3, carbs 6, protein 14

Mexican-Style Stuffed Peppers

This Mexican dish is just what you need today!

Preparation time: 10 minutes
Cooking time: 6 hours and 20 minutes
Servings: 4

Ingredients:
- 4 bell peppers, tops cut off and seeds removed
- ½ cup tomato juice
- 2 tablespoons jarred jalapenos, chopped
- 4 chicken breasts
- 1 cup tomatoes, chopped
- ¼ cup yellow onion, chopped
- ¼ cup green peppers, chopped
- 2 cups Paleo salsa
- A pinch of sea salt
- 2 teaspoons onion powder
- ½ teaspoon red pepper, crushed
- 1 teaspoon chili powder
- ½ teaspoons garlic powder
- ¼ teaspoon oregano
- 1 teaspoon cumin, ground

Directions:
In your slow cooker, mix chicken breasts with tomato juice, jalapenos, tomatoes, onion, green peppers, a pinch of salt, onion powder, red pepper, chili powder, garlic powder, oregano and cumin, stir well, cover and cook on Low for 6 hours. Shred meat using 2 forks and stir everything well. Stuff bell peppers with this mix, place them into a baking dish, pour salsa over them, place in the oven at 350 degrees F and bake for 20 minutes. Divide stuffed peppers on plates and serve.

Nutritional value: calories 240, fat 4, fiber 3, carbs 7, protein 20

Delicious Peppers Stuffed with Beef

If you don't want to try the bell peppers stuffed with chicken, then try them stuffed with beef!

Preparation time: 10 minutes
Cooking time: 55 minutes
Servings: 4

Ingredients:
- 1 pound beef, ground
- 1 teaspoon coriander, ground
- 1 onion, chopped
- 3 garlic cloves, minced
- 2 tablespoons coconut oil
- 1 tablespoon ginger, grated
- ½ teaspoon cumin
- ½ teaspoon turmeric
- 1 tablespoon hot curry powder
- A pinch of sea salt
- 1 egg
- 4 bell peppers, cut in halves and seeds removed
- 1/3 cup raisins
- 1/3 cup walnuts, chopped

Directions:
Heat up a pan with the oil over medium high heat, add onion, stir and cook for 4 minutes. Add garlic, stir and cook for 1 minute. Add beef, stir and cook for 10 minutes. Add coriander, ginger, cumin, curry powder, a pinch of salt and turmeric and stir well. Add walnuts and raisins, stir take off heat and mix with egg. Divide this mix into pepper halves, place them on a lined baking sheet, place in the oven at 350 degrees F and bake for 40 minutes. Divide between plates and serve.

Nutritional value: calories 240, fat 4, fiber 3, carbs 7, protein 12

Stuffed Poblanos

Discover one of our favorite Paleo recipes!

Preparation time: 10 minutes
Cooking time: 40 minutes
Servings: 4

Ingredients:
- 2 teaspoons garlic, minced
- 1 white onion, chopped
- 10 poblano peppers, one side of them sliced and reserved
- 1 tablespoon olive oil
- Cooking spray
- 8 ounces mushrooms, chopped
- A pinch of sea salt
- Black pepper to the taste
- ½ cup cilantro, chopped

Directions:
Place poblano boats in a baking dish which you've sprayed with some cooking spray. Heat up a pan with the oil over medium high heat, add chopped poblano pieces, onion and mushrooms, stir and cook for 5 minutes. Add garlic, cilantro, salt and black pepper, stir and cook for 2 minutes. Divide this into poblano boats, introduce them in the oven at 375 degrees F and bake for 30 minutes. Divide between plates and serve. Enjoy!

Nutritional value: calories 150, fat 3, fiber 2, carbs 4, protein 10

Delicious Stuffed Baby Peppers

These look so nice and they taste great!

Preparation time: 10 minutes
Cooking time: 0 minutes
Servings: 4

Ingredients:
- 12 baby bell peppers, cut into halves lengthwise and seeds removed
- ¼ teaspoon red pepper flakes, crushed
- 1 pound shrimp, cooked, peeled and deveined
- 6 tablespoons jarred Paleo pesto
- A pinch of sea salt
- Black pepper to the taste
- 1 tablespoon lemon juice
- 1 tablespoon olive oil
- A handful parsley, chopped

Directions:
In a bowl, mix shrimp with pepper flakes, Paleo pesto, a pinch of salt, black pepper, lemon juice, oil and parsley and whisk very well. Divide this into bell pepper halves, arrange on plates and serve. Enjoy!

Nutritional value: calories 130, fat 2, fiber 1, carbs 3, protein 15

Pork Stuffed Bell Peppers

These bell peppers are so tasty! It's one of our favorite foods!

Preparation time: 10 minutes
Cooking time: 26 minutes
Servings: 4

Ingredients:
- 1 teaspoon Cajun spice
- 1 pound pork, ground
- 1 tablespoon olive oil
- 1 tablespoon tomato paste
- 6 garlic cloves, minced
- 1 yellow onion, chopped
- 4 big bell peppers, tops cut off and seeds removed
- A pinch of sea salt
- Black pepper to the taste

Directions:
Heat up a pan with the oil over medium high heat, add garlic and onion, stir and cook for 4 minutes. Add meat, stir and cook for 10 minutes more. Add a pinch of salt, black pepper, tomato paste and Cajun seasoning, stir and cook for 3 minutes more. Stuff bell peppers with this mix, place them on preheated grill over medium high heat, grill for 3 minutes on each side, divide between plates and serve. Enjoy!

Nutritional value: calories 140, fat 3, fiber 2, carbs 3, protein 10

Bell Peppers Stuffed with Tuna

The combination is really great!

Preparation time: 10 minutes
Cooking time: 10 minutes
Servings: 4

Ingredients:
- 2 bell peppers, tops cut off, cut in halves and seeds removed
- 1 tablespoon capers, chopped
- 2 tablespoons tomato puree
- 4 ounces canned tuna, drained and flaked
- 1 scallion, chopped
- 1 tomato, chopped
- Black pepper to the taste

Directions:
Place bell pepper halves on a lined baking sheet, place in preheated broiler over medium high heat, boil for 4 minutes and then leave them aside to cool down. Meanwhile, in a bowl mix capers with tomato puree, tuna, tomato, black pepper and scallion and stir well. Stuff bell peppers with this mix, place in preheated broiler again and cook for 5 minutes. Divide between plates and serve. Enjoy!

Nutritional value: calories 140, fat 2, fiber 4, carbs 6, protein 15

Liver Stuffed Peppers

We can assure you this is a really special dish!

Preparation time: 10 minutes
Cooking time: 15 minutes
Servings: 4

Ingredients:
- 4 bacon slices, chopped
- 1 white onion, chopped
- ½ pound chicken livers, chopped
- 4 garlic cloves, chopped
- 4 bell peppers, tops cut off and seeds removed
- A pinch of sea salt
- Black pepper to the taste
- ½ teaspoon lemon zest, grated
- ¼ teaspoon thyme, chopped
- ¼ teaspoon dill, chopped
- A drizzle of olive oil
- A handful parsley, chopped

Directions:
Heat up a pan over medium heat, add bacon, stir and cook for 2 minutes. Add onion and garlic, stir and cook for 2 minutes. Add livers, a pinch of salt and black pepper, stir, cook for 5 minutes and take off heat. Transfer this to your food processor, blend very well, transfer to a bowl and aside for 10 minutes. Add thyme, oil, parsley, lemon zest and dill, stir well and Stuff each bell pepper with this mix. Serve right away. Enjoy!

Nutritional value: calories 150, fat 3, fiber 2, carbs 5, protein 12

Baked Eggplant

It's a crispy dish you will adore!

Preparation time: 10 minutes
Cooking time: 30 minutes
Servings: 3

Ingredients:
- 2 eggplants, sliced
- A pinch of sea salt
- Black pepper to the taste
- 1 cup almonds, ground
- 1 teaspoon garlic, minced
- 2 teaspoons olive oil

Directions:
Grease a baking dish with some of the oil and arrange eggplant slices on it. Season them with a pinch of salt and some black pepper and leave them aside for 10 minutes. In your food processor, mix almonds with the rest of the oil, garlic, a pinch of salt and black pepper and blend well. Spread this over eggplant slices, place in the oven at 425 degrees F and bake for 30 minutes. Divide between plates and serve. Enjoy!

Nutritional value: calories 140, fat 1, fiber 1, carbs 3, protein 15

Delicious Eggplant Dish

This is so flavored and delicious!

Preparation time: 10 minutes
Cooking time: 40 minutes
Servings: 3

Ingredients:
- 5 medium eggplants, sliced into rounds
- 1 teaspoon thyme, chopped
- 2 tablespoons balsamic vinegar
- 1 teaspoon mustard
- 2 garlic cloves, minced
- ½ cup olive oil
- Black pepper to the taste
- A pinch of sea salt
- 1 teaspoon maple syrup

Directions:
In a bowl, mix vinegar with thyme, mustard, garlic, oil, salt, pepper and maple syrup and whisk very well. Arrange eggplant round on a lined baking sheet, place in the oven at 425 degrees F and roast for 40 minutes. Divide eggplants between plates and serve. Enjoy!

Nutritional value: calories 120, fat 2, fiber 2, carbs 5, protein 15

Delicious Eggplant Casserole

This is really fulfilling!

Preparation time: 10 minutes
Cooking time: 50 minutes
Servings: 4

Ingredients:
- 2 eggplants, sliced
- 3 tablespoons olive oil
- 1 pound beef, ground
- 1 garlic clove, minced
- ¾ cup tomato sauce
- ½ bunch basil, chopped
- A pinch of sea salt
- Black pepper to the taste

Directions:
Heat up a pan with 1 tablespoon oil over medium high heat, add eggplant slices, cook for 5 minutes on each side, transfer them to paper towels, drain grease and leave them aside. Heat up another pan with the rest of the oil over medium high heat, add garlic, stir and cook for 1 minute. Add beef, stir and cook for 5 minutes more. Add tomato sauce, stir and cook for 5 minutes more. Add a pinch of sea salt and black pepper, stir, take off heat and mix with basil. Place one layer of eggplant slices into a baking dish, add one layer of beef mix and repeat with the rest of the eggplant slices and beef. Place in the oven at 350 degrees F and bake for 30 minutes. Leave eggplant casserole to cool down, slice and serve. Enjoy!

Nutritional value: calories 342, fat 23, fiber 7, carbs 10, protein 23

Eggplant and Garlic Sauce

Eggplants go so well with this garlic sauce!

Preparation time: 10 minutes
Cooking time: 10 minutes
Servings: 4

Ingredients:
- 2 tablespoons avocado oil
- 2 garlic cloves, minced
- 3 eggplants, cut into halves and thinly sliced
- 1 red chili pepper, chopped
- 1 green onion stalk, chopped
- 1 tablespoon ginger, grated
- 1 tablespoon coconut aminos
- 1 tablespoon balsamic vinegar

Directions:
Heat up a pan with half of the oil over medium high heat, add eggplant slices, cook for 2 minutes, flip, cook for 3 minutes more and transfer to a plate. Heat up the pan with the rest of the oil over medium heat, add chili pepper, garlic, green onions and ginger, stir and cook for 1 minute. Return eggplant slices to the pan, stir and cook for 1 minute. Add coconut aminos and vinegar, stir, divide between plates and serve. Enjoy!

Nutritional value: calories 130, fat 2, fiber 4, carbs 7, protein 9

Eggplant Hash

This is simple to make at home for you and all your loved ones!

Preparation time: 20 minutes
Cooking time: 20 minutes
Servings: 4

Ingredients:
- 1 eggplant, roughly chopped
- ½ cup olive oil
- ½ pound cherry tomatoes, halved
- 1 teaspoon Tabasco sauce
- ¼ cup basil, chopped
- ¼ cup mint, chopped
- A pinch of sea salt
- Black pepper to the taste

Directions:
Put eggplant pieces in a bowl, add a pinch of salt, toss to coat, leave aside for 20 minutes and drain using paper towels. Heat up a pan with half of the oil over medium high heat, add eggplant, cook for 3 minutes, flip, cook them for 3 minutes more and transfer to a bowl. Heat up the same pan with the rest of the oil over medium high heat, add tomatoes and cook them for 8 minutes stirring from time to time. Return eggplant pieces to the pan and also add a pinch of salt, black pepper, basil, mint and Tabasco sauce. Stir, cook for 2 minutes more, divide between plates and serve. Enjoy!

Nutritional value: calories 120, fat 1, fiber 4, carbs 8, protein 15

Eggplant Jam

We know this sounds impossible but it's really delicious!

Preparation time: 10 minutes
Cooking time: 1 hour
Servings: 6

Ingredients:
- 3 eggplants, sliced lengthwise
- 2 teaspoons sweet paprika
- 2 garlic cloves, minced
- A pinch of sea salt
- A pinch of cinnamon, ground
- 1 teaspoon cumin, ground
- A splash of hot sauce
- ¼ cup water
- 1 tablespoon parsley, chopped
- 2 tablespoons lemon juice

Directions:
Sprinkle some salt on eggplant slices and leave them aside for 10 minutes. Pat dry eggplant slices, brush them with half of the oil, place on a lined baking sheet, place in the oven at 375 degrees F, bake for 25 minutes flipping them halfway and leave them aside to cool down. In a bowl, mix paprika with garlic, cinnamon, cumin, water and hot sauce and stir well. Add baked eggplant pieces and mash them with a fork. Heat up a pan with the rest of the oil over medium-low heat, add eggplant mix, stir and cook for 20 minutes. Add lemon juice and parsley, stir, take off heat, divide into small bowls and serve. Enjoy!

Nutritional value: calories 150, fat 3, fiber 2, carbs 6, protein 15

Warm Watercress Mix

This is so fresh! We just adore this light Paleo dish!

Preparation time: 10 minutes
Cooking time: 10 minutes
Servings: 4

Ingredients:
- 1 pound watercress, chopped
- ¼ cup olive oil
- 1 garlic clove, cut in halves
- 1 bacon slice, cooked and crumbled
- ¼ cup hazelnuts, chopped
- Black pepper to the taste
- ¼ cup pine nuts

Directions:
Heat up a pan with the oil over medium heat, add garlic clove halves, cook for 2 minutes and discard. Heat up the pan with the garlic oil again over medium heat, add hazelnuts and pine nuts, stir and cook for 6 minutes. Add bacon, black pepper to the taste and watercress, stir, cook for 2 minutes, divide between plates and serve right away. Enjoy!

Nutritional value: calories 100, fat 1, fiber 2, carbs 2, protein 6

Watercress Soup

This will warm up your heart!

Preparation time: 10 minutes
Cooking time: 20 minutes
Servings: 4

Ingredients:
- 8 ounces watercress
- 1 tablespoon lemon juice
- A pinch of nutmeg, ground
- 4 ounces canned coconut milk
- A pinch of sea salt
- Black pepper to the taste
- 14 ounces veggie stock
- 1 celery stick, chopped
- 1 onion, chopped
- 1 tablespoon olive oil
- 12 ounces sweet potatoes, peeled and chopped

Directions:
Heat up a pot with the oil over medium heat, add onion and celery, stir and cook for 5 minutes. Add sweet potato pieces and stock, stir, bring to a simmer, cover and cook on a low heat for 10 minutes. Add watercress, stir, cover pot again and cook for 5 minutes. Blend this with an immersion blender, add a pinch of nutmeg, lemon juice, salt, pepper and coconut milk, bring to a simmer again, divide into bowls and serve.

Nutritional value: calories 159, fat 8, fiber 3, carbs 6, protein 16

Delicious Artichokes Dish

You have to try this at home today!

Preparation time: 30 minutes
Cooking time: 30 minutes
Servings: 4

Ingredients:
- 16 mushrooms, sliced
- 1/3 cup tamari sauce
- 1/3 cup olive oil
- 4 tablespoons balsamic vinegar
- 4 garlic cloves, minced
- 1 tablespoon lemon juice
- 1 teaspoon oregano, dried
- 1 teaspoon rosemary, dried
- ½ tablespoon thyme, dried
- A pinch of sea salt
- Black pepper to the taste
- 1 sweet onion, chopped
- 1 jar artichoke hearts
- 4 cups spinach
- 1 tablespoon coconut oil
- 1 teaspoon garlic, minced
- 1 cauliflower head, florets separated
- ½ cup veggie stock
- 1 teaspoon garlic powder
- A pinch of nutmeg, ground

Directions:
In a bowl, mix vinegar with tamari sauce, lemon juice, 4 garlic cloves, olive oil, oregano, rosemary, thyme, a pinch of salt, black pepper and mushrooms, toss to coat well and leave aside for 30 minutes. Transfer these to a lined baking sheet and bake them in the oven at 350 degrees F for 30 minutes. In your food processor, mix cauliflower with a pinch of sea salt and black pepper and pulse until you obtain your rice. Heat up a pan over medium high heat, add cauliflower rice, toast for 2 minutes, add nutmeg, garlic powder, black pepper and stock, stir and cook until stock evaporated. Heat up a pan with the coconut oil over medium heat, add onion, artichokes, 1 teaspoon garlic and spinach, stir and cook for a few minutes. Divide cauliflower rice on plates, top with artichokes and mushrooms and serve.

Nutritional value: calories 200, fat 3, fiber 2, carbs 7, protein 18

Artichokes with Horseradish Sauce

You will soon recommend this simple Paleo dish to others!

Preparation time: 10 minutes
Cooking time: 45 minutes
Servings: 2

Ingredients:
- 1 tablespoon horseradish, prepared
- 2 tablespoons mayonnaise
- A pinch of sea salt
- Black pepper to the taste
- 1 teaspoon lemon juice
- 3 cups artichoke hearts
- 1 tablespoon lemon juice

Directions:
In a bowl, mix horseradish with mayo, a pinch of sea salt, black pepper and 1 teaspoon lemon juice, whisk well and leave aside for now. Arrange artichoke hearts on a lined baking sheet, drizzle 2 tablespoons olive oil over them, 1 tablespoon lemon juice and sprinkle a pinch of salt and some black pepper. Toss to coat well, place in the oven at 425 degrees F and roast them for 45 minutes. Divide artichoke hearts between plates and serve with the horseradish sauce on top. Enjoy!

Nutritional value: calories 300, fat 3, fiber 12, carbs 16, protein 10

Grilled Artichokes

These are to die for!

Preparation time: 10 minutes
Cooking time: 25 minutes
Servings: 4

Ingredients:
- 2 artichokes, trimmed and halved
- Juice of 1 lemon
- 1 tablespoons lemon zest grated
- 1 rosemary spring, chopped
- 2 tablespoons olive oil
- A pinch of sea salt
- Black pepper to the taste

Directions:
Put water in a pot, add a pinch of salt and lemon juice, bring to a boil over medium high heat, add artichokes, boil for 15 minutes, drain and leave them to cool down. Drizzle olive oil over them, season with black pepper to the taste, sprinkle lemon zest and rosemary, stir well and place them on your preheated grill. Grill artichokes over medium high heat for 5 minutes on each side, divide them between plates and serve. Enjoy!

Nutritional value: calories 120, fat 1, fiber 2, carbs 6, protein 7

Artichokes and Tomatoes Dip

It's perfect for the summer!

Preparation time: 10 minutes
Cooking time: 30 minutes
Servings: 4

Ingredients:
- 2 artichokes, cut in halves and trimmed
- Juice from 3 lemons
- 4 sun-dried tomatoes, chopped
- A bunch of parsley, chopped
- A bunch of basil, chopped
- 1 garlic clove, minced
- 4 tablespoons olive oil
- Black pepper to the taste

Directions:
In a bowl, mix artichokes with lemon juice from 1 lemon, some black pepper and toss to coat. Transfer to a pot, add water to cover, bring to a boil over medium high heat, cook for 30 minutes and drain. In your food processor, mix the rest of the lemon juice with tomatoes, parsley, basil, garlic, black pepper and olive oil and blend really well. Divide artichokes between plates and top each with the tomatoes dip. Enjoy!

Nutritional value: calories 140, fat 1, fiber 1, carbs 3, protein 9

Great Carrot Hash

It's so healthy and delicious!

Preparation time: 10 minutes
Cooking time: 45 minutes
Servings: 4

Ingredients:
- 1 tablespoon olive oil
- 6 bacon slices, chopped
- 3 cups carrots, chopped
- ¾ pound beef, ground
- 1 yellow onion, chopped
- A pinch of sea salt
- Black pepper to the taste
- 2 scallions, chopped

Directions:
Place carrots on a lined baking sheet, drizzle the oil, season with a pinch of salt and some black pepper, toss to coat, place in the oven at 425 degrees F and bake for 25 minutes. Meanwhile, heat up a pan over medium high heat, add bacon and fry for a couple of minutes. Add onion and beef and some black pepper, stir and cook for 7-8 minutes more. Take carrots out of the oven, add them to the beef and bacon mix, stir and cook for 10 minutes. Sprinkle scallions on top, divide between plates and serve. Enjoy!

Nutritional value: calories 160, fat 2, fiber 1, carbs 2, protein 12

Carrots and Lime Delight

You've got to learn how to make this incredibly easy dish!

Preparation time: 10 minutes
Cooking time: 30 minutes
Servings: 6

Ingredients:
- 1 and ¼ pounds baby carrots
- 3 tablespoons ghee, melted
- 8 garlic cloves, minced
- A pinch of sea salt
- Black pepper to the taste
- Zest of 2 limes, grated
- ½ teaspoon chili powder

Directions:
In a bowl, mix baby carrots with ghee, garlic, a pinch of salt, black pepper to the taste and chili powder and stir well. Spread carrots on a lined baking sheet, place in the oven at 400 degrees F and roast for 15 minutes. Take carrots out of the oven, shake baking sheet, place in the oven again and roast for 15 minutes more. Divide between plates and serve with lime on top. Enjoy!

Nutritional value: calories 100, fat 1, fiber 1, carbs 1, protein 7

Incredible Glazed Carrots

These glazed carrots are so delicious and surprising!

Preparation time: 10 minutes
Cooking time: 15 minutes
Servings: 4

Ingredients:
- 1 pound carrots, sliced
- 1 tablespoon coconut oil
- 1 tablespoon ghee
- ½ cup pineapple juice
- 1 teaspoon ginger, grated
- ½ tablespoon maple syrup
- ½ teaspoon nutmeg
- 1 tablespoon parsley, chopped

Directions:
Heat up a pan with the ghee and the oil over medium high heat, add ginger, stir and cook for 2 minutes. Add carrots, stir and cook for 5 minutes. Add pineapple juice, maple syrup and nutmeg, stir and cook for 5 minutes more. Add parsley, stir, cook for 3 minutes, divide between plates and serve. Enjoy!

Nutritional value: calories 100, fat 0.5, fiber 1, carbs 3, protein 7

Delicious Purple Carrots

These looks so beautiful and they taste great!

Preparation time: 10 minutes
Cooking time: 1 hour
Servings: 5

Ingredients:
- 6 purple carrots, peeled
- A drizzle of olive oil
- 2 tablespoons sesame seeds paste
- 6 tablespoons water
- 3 tablespoons lemon juice
- 1 garlic clove, minced
- A pinch of sea salt
- Black pepper to the taste
- White and sesame seeds

Directions:
Arrange purple carrots on a lined baking sheet, sprinkle a pinch of salt, black pepper and a drizzle of oil, place in the oven at 350 degrees F and bake for 1 hour. Meanwhile, in your food processor, mix sesame seeds paste with water, lemon juice, garlic, a pinch of sea salt and black pepper and pulse really well. Spread this over carrots, toss gently, divide between plates and sprinkle sesame seeds on top. Enjoy!

Nutritional value: calories 100, fat 1, fiber 1, carbs 5, protein 10

Paleo Salad Recipes

Paleo Egg Salad

You can make this salad for lunch, and you can even bring it with you to the office!

Servings: 4
Preparation time: 10 minutes
Cooking time: 10 minutes

Ingredients:
- 1 avocado, pitted, peeled and chopped
- 1 small red onion, chopped
- 4 eggs
- 1 small red bell pepper, chopped
- ¼ cup homemade mayonnaise
- A pinch of sea salt
- Black pepper to the taste
- 1 tablespoon lemon juice

Directions:
Put eggs in a pot, add water to cover, place on stove over medium high heat, bring to a boil, reduce heat to low and cook for 10 minutes. Drain eggs, leave them in cold water to cool down, peel, chop them and put in a salad bowl. Add a pinch of sea salt and pepper to the taste, onion, bell pepper, avocado, lemon juice and mayo, toss to coat and serve right away. Enjoy!

Nutritional value: calories 109, fat 4.6, carbs 7.5, fiber 3.3, protein 9

Paleo Pear Salad with Tasty Dressing

It's so colored and full of great tastes!

Servings: 4
Preparation time: 10 minutes
Cooking time: 0

Ingredients:
- 1 pear, sliced
- 5 cups lettuce leaves, torn
- 1 small cucumber, chopped
- ½ cup cherry tomatoes, cut in halves
- ½ cup red grapes, cut in halves
- A pinch of sea salt
- Black pepper to the taste
- 3 tablespoons orange juice
- ¼ cup extra virgin olive oil
- 1 tablespoon orange zest
- 2 teaspoons raw honey
- 1 tablespoon parsley, minced

Directions:
In a bowl, mix orange juice with olive oil, orange zest, honey, a pinch of sea salt, pepper to the taste and parsley and whisk very well. In a salad bowl, mix pear with lettuce, cucumber, tomatoes, and grapes. Add salad dressing, toss to coat and serve right away. Enjoy!

Nutritional value: calories 100, fat 14, carbs 15, fiber 1, protein 3

Paleo Shrimp Salad

If you are looking for a great shrimp salad, you must try this one right away!

Servings: 2
Preparation time: 20 minutes
Cooking time: 10 minutes

Ingredients:
- 5 cups mixed greens
- ½ cup cherry tomatoes, cut in halves
- 1 pound shrimp, peeled and deveined
- 1 small red onion, thinly sliced
- 1 avocado, pitted, peeled and chopped
- Black pepper to the taste
- ½ tablespoon sweet paprika
- ½ teaspoon cumin
- 1 tablespoon chili powder
- 1/3 cup cilantro, finely chopped
- ½ cup lime juice
- ¼ cup extra virgin olive oil

Directions:
In a bowl, mix chili powder with cumin, paprika, ¼ cup lime juice and shrimp, toss to coat and leave aside for 20 minutes. Place shrimps on preheated grill over medium high heat, cook for 4 minutes on each side and transfer to a bowl. In a small bowl, mix cilantro with oil, the rest of the lime juice and pepper to the taste and whisk very well. In a large salad bowl, mix greens with tomatoes, onion, avocado and shrimp. Add salad dressing, toss to coat and serve right away. Enjoy!

Nutritional value: calories 190, fat 40, carbs 19, fiber 3, protein 50

Paleo Eggplant and Tomato Salad

It's a great summer dinner, full of healthy ingredients!

Servings: 4
Preparation time: 10 minutes
Cooking time: 8 minutes

Ingredients:
- ½ cup sun-dried tomatoes, sliced
- 1 eggplant, sliced
- 1 green onion, sliced
- Black pepper to the taste
- 4 cups mixed salad greens
- 1 tablespoon mint leaves, finely chopped
- 1 tablespoon oregano, finely chopped
- 1 tablespoon parsley leaves, finely chopped
- 4 tablespoons extra virgin olive oil

For the salad dressing:
- 2 garlic cloves, minced
- ¼ cup extra virgin olive oil
- ½ tablespoon mustard
- 1 tablespoon lemon juice
- ½ teaspoon smoked paprika
- A pinch of sea salt
- Black pepper to the taste

Directions:
Brush eggplant slices with olive oil, season with black pepper, place them on preheated grill over medium high heat, cook for 3 minutes on each side and transfer them to a salad bowl. Add sun-dried tomatoes, onion, greens, mint, parsley, oregano and pepper to the taste and 4 tablespoons olive oil and toss to coat. In a small bowl, mix ¼ cup olive oil with garlic, mustard, paprika, lemon juice, salt, and pepper to the taste and whisk very well. Pour this over salad, toss to coat gently and serve.

Nutritional value: calories 130, fat 27, carbs 14, fiber 2, protein 4

Paleo Potato Salad

This is a different potato salad! It's a mayo-free version, a much healthier one!

Servings: 4
Preparation time: 15 minutes
Cooking time: 30 minutes
Ingredients:

- 8 sweet potatoes, chopped
- 1 tablespoon coriander seeds
- 1 teaspoon cumin seeds
- 1 red onion, sliced
- ½ tablespoon oregano, dried
- A pinch of sea salt
- Black pepper to the taste
- 4 bacon slices, already cooked and crumbled
- ½ teaspoon chili flakes
- ¼ cup extra virgin olive oil
- 3 tablespoons parsley, chopped
- 1 tablespoon coconut oil
- 2 tablespoons red wine vinegar

Directions:

Put potatoes in a pot, add water to cover, bring to a boil over medium high heat, cook for 20 minutes, drain water and put them in a bowl. Heat up a pan with the coconut oil over medium high heat, add onions, stir, reduce temperature to low, cook for 10 minutes and transfer them to a bowl Return pan to medium high heat, add cumin seeds and coriander seeds, stir, toast for 2 minutes and add them to the bowl with the onions. Also add chili flakes, oregano, bacon, parsley, olive oil, vinegar, a pinch of sea salt and pepper to the taste and stir everything well. Add potatoes, toss to coat and serve cold.

Nutritional value: calories 142, fat 24, carbs 47, fiber 2, protein 10

Paleo Chicken Salad

This homemade salad is such a great option for dinner!

Servings: 4
Preparation time: 10 minutes
Cooking time: 50 minutes
Ingredients:

- 2 chicken breasts, skinless and boneless
- 1 pineapple, sliced
- 6 cups mixed salad greens
- 1 red onion, thinly sliced
- ¼ cup pineapple sauce
- ½ cup cherry tomatoes, cut in halves
- A pinch of sea salt
- Black pepper to the taste
- ¼ cup extra virgin olive oil
- 2 tablespoons apple cider vinegar

For the sauce:
- 1 yellow onion, minced
- 1 garlic clove, minced
- 6 ounces tomato paste
- ½ cup apple cider vinegar
- ½ cup water
- ¼ cup ketchup
- 3 tablespoons mustard
- 1 pinch cloves, ground
- A pinch of cinnamon
- A pinch of smoked paprika

Directions:

Heat up a pan over medium high heat, add 1 yellow onion, stir and brown for 3 minutes. Add garlic and cook 1 more minute. Add tomato paste, ½ cup vinegar, water, ketchup, mustard, cloves, cinnamon and a pinch of smoked paprika, stir everything well, bring to a boil, reduce heat to medium-low and simmer for 30 minutes. Take sauce off heat, reserve 1 cup and keep the rest in the fridge for another occasion. Season chicken breast with a pinch of sea salt and pepper to the taste, place them on preheated grill over medium high heat, cook for 8 minutes on each side. Brush chicken with 1 cup of the sauce you've just made and cook for 4 more minutes on each side. Transfer chicken to a cutting board, leave aside to cool down, slice and put in a salad bowl. Grill pineapple on medium high heat, transfer to a cutting board as well, cut into small cubes and add to chicken. Also add greens, red onion, grape tomatoes and pepper to the taste. In a small bowl, mix pineapple juice with 2 tablespoons vinegar, ¼ cup olive oil, a pinch of sea salt and pepper to the taste and stir well. Pour this over chicken salad, toss to coat and serve. Enjoy!

Nutritional value: calories 120, fat 16, carbs 45, fiber 4, protein 16

Special Paleo Chicken Salad

This is another great way to make a chicken salad!

Servings: 2
Preparation time: 10 minutes
Cooking time: 15 minutes

Ingredients:
- 2 teaspoons parsley, dried
- 2 chicken breasts, skinless and boneless
- ½ teaspoon onion powder
- ½ cup lemon juice
- 2 teaspoons paprika
- A pinch of sea salt
- Black pepper to the taste
- 8 strawberries, sliced
- 1 small red onion, sliced
- 6 cups baby spinach
- 1 avocado, peeled and cut into small chunks
- ¼ cup extra virgin olive oil
- 1 tablespoon tarragon, chopped
- 2 tablespoons balsamic vinegar

Directions:
Put chicken in a bowl, add lemon juice, parsley, onion powder and paprika and toss to coat. Place chicken on preheated grill over medium high heat, cook for 10 minutes on each side, transfer to a cutting board and slice. In a bowl, mix oil with vinegar, a pinch of sea salt, pepper and tarragon and whisk well. In a salad bowl, mix spinach with onion, avocado, and strawberry. Add chicken pieces and the vinaigrette, toss to coat and serve. Enjoy!

Nutritional value: calories 230, fat 42, carbs 13, fiber 5, protein 30

Paleo Radish Salad

It's a very crunchy salad! We think you'll really end up loving it!

Servings: 4
Preparation time: 10 minutes
Cooking time: 0 minutes

Ingredients:
- 8 radishes, sliced
- 1 cucumber, sliced
- 1 apple, chopped
- 1 celery stalk, chopped
- Black pepper to the taste
- ¼ cup homemade mayonnaise
- 2 tablespoons chives, chopped
- 2 tablespoons apple cider vinegar
- 2 tablespoons lemon juice

Directions:
In a bowl, mix radishes with apple, celery, and cucumber. In a small bowl, mix mayo with vinegar, pepper, lemon juice and chives and whisk well. Pour this over salad, toss to coat and keep in the fridge until you serve it. Enjoy!

Nutritional value: calories 50, fat 7, carbs 3, fiber 1, protein 1

Brussels Sprouts Salad

You have no idea what to eat tonight? This is a good option for you!

Servings: 4
Preparation time: 20 minutes
Cooking time: 0 minutes

Ingredients:
- 4 cups Brussels sprouts
- 2 cups red cabbage, shredded
- Black pepper to the taste
- 1 red apple, sliced
- 2 celery stalks, chopped
- 2 tablespoons lemon juice
- ¼ cup walnuts, chopped
- ¼ cup homemade mayonnaise
- 4 tablespoons apple cider vinegar

Directions:
In a bowl, mix lemon juice with mayo, vinegar and pepper to the taste and stir very well. In a big bowl, mix Brussels sprouts with cabbage, celery, apple, and walnuts. Add salad dressing you've just made, toss to coat and keep in the fridge for 10 minutes before you serve it. Enjoy!

Nutritional value: calories 80, fat 1, carbs 3, fiber 1, sugar 1, protein 2

Paleo Carrot and Cucumber Salad

Transform 2 simple veggies into a great salad! See how!

Servings: 4
Preparation time: 15 minutes
Cooking time: 0

Ingredients:
- 3 carrots, thinly sliced with a spiralizer
- 2 cucumbers, thinly sliced with a spiralizer
- 1 green onion, sliced
- 1 tablespoon sesame seeds
- 2 tablespoons lime juice
- A pinch of sea salt
- 2 tablespoons white wine vinegar
- Black pepper to the taste
- 2 tablespoons extra virgin olive oil

Directions:
In a salad bowl, mix cucumbers with green onion and carrots. In a small bowl, mix vinegar with olive oil, lime juice, a pinch of sea salt, and pepper to the taste and stir well. Pour this over salad, toss to coat and keep in the fridge until you serve it. Enjoy!

Nutritional value: calories 60, fat 1.7, carbs 12, fiber 2.5, protein 1.3

Paleo Pomegranate Salad

It's a magnificent salad for you to try right now!

Servings: 4
Preparation time: 15 minutes
Cooking time: 0 minutes

Ingredients:
- 1 avocado, pitted, peeled and chopped
- 8 cups mixed salad greens
- 2 tablespoons pine nuts, toasted
- 6 figs, cut into quarters
- ¾ cup pomegranate seeds
- 4 clementines, peeled and chopped
- ¼ cup extra virgin olive oil
- 1 tablespoon lemon juice
- 4 tablespoons orange juice
- 2 tablespoons white wine vinegar
- 1 teaspoon orange zest
- A pinch of sea salt
- Black pepper to the taste

Directions:
In a salad bowl, mix greens with avocado, figs, clementines, pine nuts and pomegranate seeds. In another bowl, mix orange juice with lemon juice, olive oil, orange zest, vinegar, a pinch of sea salt and pepper to the taste and whisk well. Pour this over salad, toss to coat and serve. Enjoy!

Nutritional value: calories 120, fat 6, carbs 12, fiber 2, protein 4.7

Paleo Lobster Salad

This salad is tasty and colored! It's fresh and easy to prepare!

Servings: 2
Preparation time: 10 minutes
Cooking time: 0 minutes

Ingredients:
- 1 grapefruit, peeled and chopped
- 1 pound lobster meat, cooked and chopped
- 1 avocado, pitted, peeled and chopped
- 1 shallot, chopped
- 3 cups mixed greens
- 2 tablespoons grapefruit juice
- 1 tablespoon chives, chopped
- A pinch of sea salt
- Black pepper to the taste
- 4 tablespoons extra virgin olive oil
- 2 tablespoons white wine vinegar
- Some dill, finely chopped for serving

Directions:
In a bowl, mix grapefruit juice with oil, vinegar, chives, shallot, a pinch of sea salt and pepper to the taste and stir very well. Add lobster meat and toss to coat. In a large bowl, mix avocado with greens and grapefruit. Add lobster meat and dressing on top, sprinkle dill all over and serve. Enjoy!

Nutritional value: calories 180, fat 10, carbs 6.5, fiber 1.4, sugar 3.4, protein 11.1

Paleo Steak Salad

This is a true Thai style salad! It's rich, tasty and healthy!

Servings: 4
Preparation time: 1 hour
Cooking time: 15 minutes

Ingredients:
- 4 cups lettuce leaves, torn
- 1 pound steak
- 1 red bell pepper, cut into strips
- 1 cucumber, sliced
- ¼ cup mint leaves, chopped
- ¼ cup cilantro, chopped
- 1 tablespoon ginger, grated
- ¼ cup coconut aminos
- 1 Thai red chili pepper, chopped
- 3 garlic cloves, minced
- Juice from 1 lime
- A pinch of sea salt
- Black pepper to the taste
- Silvered almonds for serving

For the salad dressing:
- 3 tablespoons coconut aminos
- 2 tablespoons melted coconut oil
- 1 teaspoon fish sauce
- Zest from 1 lime
- Juice from 1 lime
- 1 Thai red chili pepper, chopped

Directions:
In a bowl, mix garlic with ginger, 1 red chili, juice from 1 lime and ¼ cup coconut aminos and stir. Add steak, toss to coat, cover bowl and keep in the fridge for 1 hour. In another bowl, mix 2 tablespoons coconut oil with 3 tablespoons coconut aminos, 1 lime chili pepper, fish sauce, zest and juice from 1 lime, stir well and leave aside for now. Place steak on preheated grill over medium high heat, cook for 4 minutes on each side, transfer to a cutting board, leave aside for 4 minutes, slice very thinly and put in a salad bowl. Add lettuce, cucumber, bell pepper, a pinch of sea salt and pepper to the taste. Add salad dressing you've made, toss to coat, sprinkle cilantro, mint, and almonds and serve. Enjoy!

Nutritional value: calories 300, fat 10, carbs 15, fiber 4, sugar 4, protein 38

Paleo Summer Salad

It's not only just a paleo dish! It's a Greek style salad that tastes wonderful!

Servings: 4
Preparation time: 15 minutes
Cooking time: 0 minutes

Ingredients:
- 1 cucumber, chopped
- 4 medium tomatoes, chopped
- 1 red onion, sliced
- 1 green bell pepper, chopped
- ¾ cup kalamata olives, pitted and chopped
- 1 tablespoon lemon juice
- ¼ cup extra virgin olive oil
- ½ teaspoon oregano, dried
- 2 tablespoons red wine vinegar
- Black pepper to the taste

Directions:
In a small bowl, mix lemon juice with oil, oregano, vinegar and pepper to the taste and whisk very well. In a salad bowl, mix tomatoes with bell pepper, onion, and cucumber. Add salad dressing, toss to coat and serve with olives on top. Enjoy!

Nutritional value: calories 140, fat 9, carbs 3, fiber 5, protein 7

Special Paleo Beef Salad

It's a simple salad, but it's full of very exciting textures!

Servings: 4
Preparation time: 10 minutes
Cooking time: 10 minutes

Ingredients:
- 1 pound organic beef steak, cut into strips
- 3 cups broccoli, florets separated
- 8 cups baby salad greens
- 1 red onion, sliced
- 1 red bell pepper, sliced
  For the vinaigrette:
- 1 tablespoon ginger, minced
- A pinch of sea salt
- Black pepper to the taste
- ½ cup extra virgin olive oil
- 2 tablespoons lime juice
- 1 tablespoon rice wine vinegar
- 2 tablespoons shallots, finely chopped

Directions:
In a bowl, mix ginger with oil, lime juice, vinegar, shallots, a pinch of sea salt and pepper to the taste and stir well. Heat up a pan over medium high heat, add 2 tablespoons of vinaigrette, warm up, add broccoli and cook for 3 minutes. Add beef, stir and cook for 4 more minutes and take off heat. In a salad bowl, mix salad greens with onion, bell pepper, broccoli, and beef. Add some black pepper, drizzle the rest of the vinaigrette, toss to coat and serve. Enjoy!

Nutritional value: calories 260, fat 12, carbs 11, fiber 4.3, protein 32

Warm Paleo Salad

When it's cold outside, and you feel like eating something comforting and warm, try this salad!

Servings: 4
Preparation time: 10 minutes
Cooking time: 20 minutes

Ingredients:
- 2 red onions, cut into medium wedges
- 1 butternut squash, cut into medium wedges
- 6 cups spinach
- 4 parsnips, cut into medium wedges
- Black pepper to the taste
- 2 tablespoons white wine vinegar
- 1/3 cup nuts, roasted
- 1 teaspoon Dijon mustard
- ½ tablespoons oregano, dried
- 1 garlic clove, minced
- 6 tablespoons extra virgin olive oil

Directions:
Spread squash, onions, and parsnips in a baking dish. Drizzle half of the oil, sprinkle oregano and pepper to the taste, toss to coat, introduce in the oven at 400 degrees F and bake for 10 minutes. Take veggies out of the oven, turn them and bake for another 10 minutes. In a bowl, mix vinegar with the rest of the oil, garlic, mustard and pepper to the taste and stir very well. Put spinach in a salad bowl, add roasted veggies, pour salad dressing, sprinkle nuts, toss to coat and serve warm. Enjoy!

Nutritional value: calories 131, fat 5.5, carbs 14, fiber 4.7, sugar 5, protein 5.2

Delicious Paleo Salad

You've already discovered some pretty amazing summer and winter salad. Now it's time for a tasty fall one!

Servings: 4
Preparation time: 15 minutes
Cooking time: 35 minutes

Ingredients:
- 2 tablespoons ghee
- 1 tablespoon balsamic vinegar
- 1 zucchini, cubed
- 4 bacon strips
- 4 eggs
- 2 lettuce heads, leaves, torn
- 2 cups chicken meat, already cooked and shredded
- 4 cups arugula
- 1 small red onion, finely chopped
- 1/3 cup cranberries
- A pinch of sea salt
- Black pepper to the taste
- A pinch of garlic powder
- 1/3 cup pecans, chopped
- 2 apples, chopped
- 2 tablespoons maple syrup
- 1 tablespoon apple cider vinegar
- 1 teaspoon shallot, minced
- 1 teaspoon mustard
- 1 teaspoon garlic, minced
- ¼ cup extra virgin olive oil

Directions:
Spread zucchini cubes on a lined baking sheet, sprinkle with a pinch of sea salt, pepper, garlic powder, drizzle balsamic vinegar and add ghee, toss to coat, introduce in the oven at 400 degrees F and bake for 25 minutes. Meanwhile, put eggs in a pot, add water to cover, bring to a boil over medium high heat, boil for 15 minutes, drain, place in a bowl filled with ice water, leave aside to cool down, peel them, chop and put in a salad bowl. Heat up a pan over medium high heat, add bacon, brown for a few minutes, take off heat, leave to cool down and add to the same bowl with the eggs. Add lettuce leaves, arugula, chicken, onion, pecans, apple pieces, roasted squash cubes, and cranberries. In a small bowl, mix maple syrup with apple cider vinegar, mustard, garlic, shallot, olive oil and pepper and whisk very well. Pour this over salad, toss to coat and serve. Enjoy!

Nutritional value: calories 249, fat 10, carbs 35, fiber 6, sugar 2.8, protein 5

Simple Scallops Salad

Get your hands on some delicious scallops and make this salad as soon as possible!

Servings: 4
Preparation time: 10 minutes
Cooking time: 7 minutes

Ingredients:
- 1 pound bay scallops
- 2 teaspoons cayenne pepper
- Black pepper to the taste
- 3 tablespoons lemon juice
- 1 tablespoon homemade mayonnaise
- 1 teaspoon mustard
- A pinch of cayenne pepper
- ½ cup extra virgin olive oil
- 1 garlic clove, minced
- 2 handfuls mixed greens
- 1 avocado, pitted, peeled and cubed
- 1 red bell pepper, cut into thin strips
- 3 tablespoons melted coconut oil

Directions:
In a salad bowl, mix salad greens with avocado and pepper and leave aside for now. In a bowl, mix lemon juice with mustard, garlic, mayo, pepper and a pinch of cayenne, stir well and leave aside. Add olive oil gradually and whisk very well again. Rinse and pat dry scallops, put them in another bowl, add pepper to the taste and 2 teaspoons cayenne and toss to coat. Heat up a pan with the coconut oil over medium high heat, add scallops, cook for 2 minutes on each side and transfer them to the bowl with the veggies. Add mustard dressing you've made, toss to coat and serve. Enjoy!

Nutritional value: calories 235, fat 4.1, carbs 18, fiber 3.3, protein 30.7

Paleo Pork Salad

If you've already tried a paleo chicken or beef salad, then it's definitely time for a pork salad!

Servings: 4
Preparation time: 10 minutes
Cooking time: 5 minutes

Ingredients:
- 2 lettuce heads, torn
- 2 cups pork, already cooked and shredded
- 1 avocado, pitted, peeled and chopped
- 1 cup cherry tomatoes, cut in halves
- 1 green bell pepper, sliced
- 2 green onions, thinly sliced
- A pinch of sea salt
- Black pepper to the taste
- Juice of ½ lime
- 1 tablespoon apple cider vinegar
- ¼ cup BBQ sauce
- 2 tablespoons extra virgin olive oil

Directions:
In a small bowl, mix oil with lime juice, vinegar, black pepper and BBQ sauce and whisk well. Heat up a pan over medium heat, add pork meat and heat it up. Meanwhile, in a salad bowl, mix lettuce leaves with tomatoes, bell pepper, avocado and green onions. Add pork, drizzle the BBQ dressing, toss to coat and serve. Enjoy!

Nutritional value: calories 322, fat 45, carbs 23, fiber 4, protein 36

Paleo Seafood Salad

This salad is for all you seafood lovers! It's the best one!

Servings: 6
Preparation time: 3 hours and 10 minutes
Cooking time: 0 minutes

Ingredients:
- 8 ounces, baby shrimp, already cooked, peeled, deveined and chopped
- 8 ounces crab meat, already cooked
- 2/3 cup homemade mayonnaise
- 2/3 cup yellow onion, chopped
- 2/3 cup celery, chopped
- 2 tablespoons Dijon mustard
- Black pepper to the taste
- ¼ teaspoon onion powder
- ½ teaspoon garlic powder
- 1 tablespoon hot sauce

Directions:
In a salad bowl, mix shrimp with crab meat, onion, and celery. In another bowl, mix mayo with mustard, pepper, onion powder, garlic powder and hot sauce and stir very well. Pour this over seafood salad, toss to coat and keep in the fridge for 3 hours before you serve it.

Nutritional value: calories 240, fat 22, carbs 3.3, fiber 0.6, protein 24

Amazing Taco Salad

It's so full of intense flavors!

Preparation time: 10 minutes
Cooking time: 15 minutes
Servings: 4

Ingredients:
- 1 tablespoon chili powder
- 1 teaspoon onion powder
- ½ teaspoon garlic powder
- 1 teaspoon cumin, ground
- 2 teaspoons paprika
- 3 tablespoons olive oil
- A pinch of cayenne pepper
- 1 pound beef, ground
- 3 cups cilantro, chopped
- Juice from 1 lime
- A pinch of sea salt
- Black pepper to the taste
- 1 romaine lettuce head, chopped
- 1 avocado, pitted, peeled and chopped
- 1 small red onion, chopped
- Some black olives, pitted and chopped
- 1 red bell pepper, chopped
- ½ cup Pico de gallo

Directions:
In a bowl, mix chili powder with paprika, onion and garlic powder, ½ teaspoon cumin, cayenne and some black pepper and stir. Heat up a pan with 1 tablespoon oil over medium heat, add beef, stir and cook for 7 minutes. Add spice mix, stir and cook until meat is done. Meanwhile, in your food processor, blend 1 cup cilantro with lime juice, ½ teaspoon cumin, a pinch of salt, black pepper to the taste and 2 tablespoons oil and pulse really well. In a salad bowl, mix lettuce leaves with avocado, 2 cups cilantro, onion, bell pepper, olives and Pico de gallo and stir. Divide this between plates, top with beef and drizzle the salad dressing on top.

Nutritional value: calories 190, fat 3, fiber 2, carbs 5, protein 12

Delicious Summer Salad

It's so fresh and easy to make! Everyone will love this salad!

Preparation time: 10 minutes
Cooking time: 0 minutes
Servings: 6

Ingredients:
- 1 cup blackberries, halved
- 2 cups honeydew, sliced
- 8 ounces prosciutto
- 3 tablespoons chives, chopped
- Juice of 1 lemon
- Zest from 1 lemon
- 1 shallot, chopped
- 2 cup cantaloupe, sliced
- A pinch of sea salt
- Black pepper to the taste

Directions:
In a large salad bowl, mix blackberries with prosciutto, honeydew, cantaloupe, chives, lemon juice and zest, shallot, a pinch of sea salt and black pepper to the taste, toss to coat and serve cold. Enjoy!

Nutritional value: calories 80, fat 0.5, fiber 1, carbs 1, protein 3

Great Winter Salad

This is a very hearty salad everyone will enjoy for sure!

Preparation time: 10 minutes
Cooking time: 7 minutes
Servings: 2

Ingredients:
- 1 red onion, chopped
- 12 Brussels sprouts, sliced
- A pinch of sea salt
- Black pepper to the taste
- 1 tablespoon olive oil
- 1/3 cup pecans, chopped
- ¼ cup raisins
- 2/3 cup hemp seeds
- ½ red apple, cored and chopped

Directions:
Heat up a pan with the oil over medium heat, add onion, stir and cook for a few minutes. Add Brussels sprouts, cook for 4 minutes, take off heat and leave aside to cool down. Add apple pieces, hemp seeds, raisins, a pinch of sea salt, black pepper and pecans, stir salad and serve. Enjoy!

Nutritional value: calories 100, fat 0.7, fiber 1, carbs 3, protein 9

Kale and Carrots Salad

This is an energy boost not just a salad!

Preparation time: 10 minutes
Cooking time: 0 minutes
Servings: 1

Ingredients:
- 1 carrot, grated
- A handful kale, chopped
- 1 small lettuce head, chopped
- 1 tablespoon tahini paste
- 1 tablespoon olive oil
- A pinch of sea salt
- Black pepper to the taste
- Juice of ½ lime
- A pinch of garlic powder

Directions:
In a salad bowl, mix carrots with kale and lettuce leaves. In your blender, mix tahini with a pinch of salt, black pepper, garlic powder, lime juice and oil and pulse well. Pour this over salad, toss to coat well and serve. Enjoy!

Nutritional value: calories 100, fat 1, fiber 0, carbs 0, protein 7

Simple Chicken Salad

It's the best chicken salad you'll ever try!

Preparation time: 10 minutes
Cooking time: 0 minutes
Servings: 2

Ingredients:
- 1 smoked chicken breast, sliced
- 2 handfuls lettuce leaves, torn
- 1 avocado, pitted, peeled and cubed
- 2 eggs, hard-boiled and halved
- A handful walnuts, chopped
- 2 tablespoons flaxseed oil

Directions:
In a salad bowl, mix lettuce with avocado, walnuts and chicken slices and toss. Add eggs and oil, toss gently and serve. Enjoy!

Nutritional value: calories 110, fat 0.9, fiber 1, carbs 4, protein 12

Sweet Potato Salad

It's a flavored and savory salad you will adore!

Preparation time: 10 minutes
Cooking time: 30 minutes
Servings: 4

Ingredients:
- 3 sweet potatoes, cubed
- 2 tablespoons coconut oil
- 4 garlic cloves, minced
- ½ pound bacon, chopped
- Juice from 1 lime
- A pinch of sea salt
- Black pepper to the taste
- 2 tablespoons balsamic vinegar
- 2 tablespoons olive oil
- A handful dill, chopped
- 2 green onions, chopped
- A pinch of cinnamon, ground
- A pinch of red pepper flakes

Directions:
Arrange bacon and sweet potatoes on a lined bacon sheet, add garlic and coconut oil, toss well, place in the oven at 375 degrees F and bake for 30 minutes. Meanwhile, in a bowl, mix vinegar with lime juice, olive oil, green onions, pepper flakes, dill, a pinch of sea salt, black pepper and cinnamon and stir well. Transfer bacon and sweet potatoes to a salad bowl, add salad dressing, toss well and serve. Enjoy!

Nutritional value: calories 170, fat 3, fiber 2, carbs 5, protein 12

Rich Salad

The best Paleo salad you can think of is now here!

Preparation time: 10 minutes
Cooking time: 0 minutes
Servings: 1

Ingredients:
- 1 chicken breast, cooked and sliced
- 1 medium lettuce head, chopped
- 1 sweet potato, boiled and cubed
- 1 tablespoon pumpkin seeds
- 6 black olives, pitted and chopped
- 1 tablespoon olive oil
- 1 tablespoon balsamic vinegar

Directions:
In a salad bowl, mix chicken breast slices with lettuce, sweet potato, pumpkin seeds, olives, olive oil and balsamic vinegar, stir well and serve right away. Enjoy!

Nutritional value: calories 130, fat 2, fiber 1, carbs 4, protein 8

Salmon Salad

Have you ever tried a salmon salad? Try this one!

Preparation time: 10 minutes
Cooking time: 5 minutes
Servings: 2

Ingredients:
- 1 lettuce head, chopped
- 2 salmon fillets
- 1 tablespoon olive oil
- 1 tablespoon coconut aminos
- 1 avocado, pitted, peeled and sliced
- 1 cucumber, sliced
- A pinch of sea salt
- Black pepper to the taste

Directions:
Heat up a pan with the oil over medium high heat, add salmon fillets skin side down, cook for 3 minutes, flip and cook for 2 minutes more. In a salad bowl, mix lettuce with cucumber, avocado, a pinch of salt, black pepper and coconut aminos and stir. Flake salmon using a fork, add to salad, drizzle some of the oil from the pan, toss to coat and serve. Enjoy!

Nutritional value: calories 140, fat 3, fiber 2, carbs 6, protein 15

Summer Salad

This is a wonderful veggie mix you will like!

Preparation time: 10 minutes
Cooking time: 0 minutes
Servings: 3

Ingredients:
- 1 lettuce head, chopped
- A handful kale, chopped
- A handful green beans
- A handful walnuts, chopped
- 8 cherry tomatoes, halved
- A handful radishes, chopped
- 1 tablespoon lemon juice
- 8 dates, chopped
- A drizzle of olive oil

Directions:
In a salad bowl, mix lettuce with kale, green beans, walnuts, tomatoes, radishes and dates. In smaller bowl, mix lemon juice with olive oil and whisk well. Add this to salad, toss to coat and serve. Enjoy!

Nutritional value: calories 100, fat 0, fiber 1, carbs 1, protein 6

Tomato Salad

This delicious salad combines perfectly with its creamy dressing!

Preparation time: 10 minutes
Cooking time: 0 minutes
Servings: 4

Ingredients:
- 1 bunch kale, chopped
- 12 cherry tomatoes, halved
- 2 handful green beans
- 3 tablespoons Paleo mayonnaise
- 1 teaspoon mustard

Directions:
In a salad bowl, mix tomatoes with green beans and kale. In a small bowl, mix mayo with mustard and whisk well. Add this to salad, toss to coat and serve. Enjoy!

Nutritional value: calories 110, fat 2, fiber 1, carbs 3, protein 5

Broccoli Salad

Your new favorite Paleo salad is here!

Preparation time: 10 minutes
Cooking time: 2 minutes
Servings: 4

Ingredients:
- ¼ cup walnuts, chopped
- ¼ cup cranberries
- 2 bacon slices
- 4 cups broccoli florets, roughly chopped
- 1 teaspoon lemon juice
- ¼ cup olive oil

Directions:
Heat up a pan over medium high heat, add bacon, cook for 2 minutes, leave aside to cool down and chop. In a salad bowl, mix broccoli with bacon, cranberries, walnuts, lemon juice and olive oil, toss to coat and serve. Enjoy!

Nutritional value: calories 120, fat 2, fiber 1, carbs 5, protein 8

Cabbage and Salmon Slaw

This salmon salad is more that you could expect!

Preparation time: 10 minutes
Cooking time: 8 minutes
Servings: 4

Ingredients:
- 2 salmon fillets, skin on
- 1 and ½ teaspoons coconut aminos
- ½ cup mayonnaise
- 1 teaspoon lime juice
- 1 teaspoon honey
- 1 fennel bulb, sliced
- 1 small red cabbage head, sliced
- A bunch of coriander, chopped
- A pinch of sea salt
- Black pepper to the taste

Directions:
Put water in a pot and bring to a simmer over medium high heat. Place salmon fillets in a vacuum bag, place in water, cook for 8 minutes, leave aside to cool down and cut into medium pieces. Put salmon cubes in a salad bowl, add fennel, cabbage and coriander and toss gently. In another bowl, mix coconut aminos with mayo, lime, honey, salt and pepper and whisk well. Add this to salad, toss to coat well and serve. Enjoy!

Nutritional value: calories 160, fat 3, fiber 2, carbs 5, protein 17

Watermelon Salad

This is refreshing, colored and flavored!

Preparation time: 1 hour and 10 minutes
Cooking time: 0 minutes
Servings: 4

Ingredients:
- 8 cups mixed salad greens
- 4 cups watermelon, cubed
- ¼ cup mayonnaise
- 1 and ½ tablespoons honey
- 2 teaspoons balsamic vinegar
- 1 teaspoon poppy seeds
- A pinch of sea salt
- Black pepper to the taste

Directions:
In a salad bowl, mix salad greens with watermelon cubes. In another bowl, mix mayo with honey, vinegar and poppy seeds, whisk well and keep in the fridge for 1 hour. Drizzle this over salad, season with a pinch of salt and black pepper to the taste, toss to coat well and serve. Enjoy!

Nutritional value: calories 120, fat 0.5, fiber 1, carbs 0, protein 6

Red Cabbage Salad

It has such and intense color! It's wonderful!

Preparation time: 10 minutes
Cooking time: 15 minutes
Servings: 4

Ingredients:
- 1 purple cabbage head, cut into thin strips
- 4 prosciutto slices
- 1 red onion, thinly sliced
- 1 green apple, cored and chopped
- ½ cup pecans, toasted
- A handful watercress
- ½ cup olive oil
- 1 garlic clove, minced
- ¼ cup balsamic vinegar
- 1 teaspoon honey
- ½ teaspoon mustard
- A pinch of sea salt
- Black pepper to the taste

Directions:
Place prosciutto slices on a lined baking sheet, place in the oven at 350 degrees F and cook for 15 minutes. Leave prosciutto to cool down and chop it. In a salad bowl mix cabbage with prosciutto, onion, apple pieces, watercress and pecans and toss. In another bowl, mix olive oil with honey, vinegar, garlic, mustard, a pinch of salt and black pepper and whisk well. Drizzle this over your salad and serve. Enjoy!

Nutritional value: calories 110, fat 0.8, fiber 1, carbs 2, protein 7

Avocado Salad

Combine avocados with some tasty tuna and you will obtain a delicious lunch or dinner salad!

Preparation time: 10 minutes
Cooking time: 0 minutes
Servings: 2

Ingredients:
- Juice of 1 lemon
- 1 avocado, pitted, peeled and chopped
- 1 tablespoon onion, chopped
- 5 ounces canned wild tuna, flaked
- Black pepper to the taste

Directions:
In a salad bowl, mix avocado with onion, tuna, black pepper and lemon juice, toss well and serve. Enjoy!

Nutritional value: calories 90, fat 0, fiber 1, carbs 0, protein 12

Quick and Tasty Salad

It's easy to make something tasty for dinner!

Preparation time: 10 minutes
Cooking time: 0 minutes
Servings: 4

Ingredients:
For the salad dressing:
- 1 tablespoon basil, chopped
- 1 teaspoon rosemary , chopped
- ½ cup avocado mayonnaise
- 1 garlic clove, minced
- A pinch of sea salt
- Black pepper to the taste
- 1 teaspoon lemon juice

For the salad:
- 6 baby lettuce heads, chopped
- 1 cup cherry tomatoes, halved
- ½ pound bacon, cooked and chopped
- 2 green onions, chopped

Directions:
In a bowl, mix basil with rosemary, mayo, garlic, lemon juice, a pinch of salt and black pepper and whisk well. In a salad bowl, mix lettuce with tomatoes, green onions and bacon. Add salad dressing, toss to coat and serve.

Nutritional value: calories 140, fat 3, fiber 2, carbs 4, protein 15

Tasty Sashimi Salad

If you are in the mood for something tasty and exotic tonight, then try this salad!

Preparation time: 10 minutes
Cooking time: 0 minutes
Servings: 2

Ingredients:
- 1 teaspoon balsamic vinegar
- ½ tablespoon honey
- 1 mango, peeled and roughly chopped
- 2 handfuls kale, chopped
- ½ pound salmon sashimi, sliced
- 3 tablespoons tamari sauce
- 2 tablespoons olive oil

Directions:
In a bowl, mix tamari with oil, honey and vinegar and whisk well. In a salad bowl, mix kale with mango and sashimi. Add salad dressing, toss to coat and serve. Enjoy!

Nutritional value: calories 140, fat 1, fiber 2, carbs 2, protein 16

Fresh Salad

It's all about eating healthy and delicious!

Preparation time: 10 minutes
Cooking time: 0 minutes
Servings: 4

Ingredients:
- 2 cup red cabbage, chopped
- 4 cups Brussels sprouts, shredded
- 2 tablespoons lemon juice
- 4 tablespoons balsamic vinegar
- ¼ cup Paleo mayonnaise
- 1 red apple, cored and chopped
- 2 celery sticks, chopped
- ¼ cup walnuts, chopped
- A pinch of sea salt
- Black pepper to the taste

Directions:
In a salad bowl, mix cabbage with Brussels sprouts, apple, celery and walnuts. In another bowl, mix lemon juice with vinegar, a pinch of salt, black pepper and mayo and whisk well. Add this to salad, toss to coat and serve. Enjoy!

Nutritional value: calories 90, fat 0, fiber 1, carbs 1, protein 7

Hearty Chicken Salad

This rich dinner salad is exactly what you need today!

Preparation time: 1 hour and 10 minutes
Cooking time: 0 minutes
Servings: 6

Ingredients:
- 1 rotisserie chicken, chopped
- 1 apple, cored and chopped
- ¼ cup cranberries, dried
- ¼ cup chives, chopped
- ¼ cup red onion, chopped
- 1 celery stalk, chopped
- A pinch of sea salt
- Black pepper to the taste
- 2 cups mayonnaise
- 8 handfuls arugula
- 7 avocados, pitted, peeled and chopped

For the vinaigrette:
- 1 garlic clove, minced
- ½ cup olive oil
- 1 teaspoon mustard
- 3 tablespoons lemon juice
- Black pepper to the taste

Directions:
In a salad bowl, mix chicken meat with apple, cranberries, chives, onion, celery, arugula, avocados, mayo, a pinch of salt and black pepper to the taste and toss well. In a small bowl, mix oil with garlic, mustard, black pepper and lemon juice and whisk well. Add this to salad, toss again well and leave aside at room temperature for 1 hour before serving. Enjoy!

Nutritional value: calories 180, fat 3, fiber 3, carbs 6, protein 20

Tomato and Chicken Salad

Serve as much as you like! It's delicious!

Preparation time: 10 minutes
Cooking time: 0 minutes
Servings: 6

Ingredients:
- 3 tablespoons oil
- 4 tablespoons balsamic vinegar
- A pinch of sea salt
- Black pepper to the taste
- 3 cups chicken, cooked and shredded
- 2 pounds cherry tomatoes, halved
- ½ cup red onion, chopped
- 2 tablespoons basil, chopped
- 2 tablespoons chives, chopped
- 2 tablespoons parsley, chopped
- 1 tablespoon thyme, chopped

Directions:
In a salad bowl, mix chicken with tomatoes, onion, basil, chives, parsley and thyme and stir. In a small bowl, mix oil with vinegar, a pinch of salt and black pepper and whisk well. Add this to salad, toss to coat and serve. Enjoy!

Nutritional value: calories 140, fat 3, fiber 1, carbs 2, protein 16

Kale and Avocado Salad

It's green, healthy and Paleo! It's perfect!

Preparation time: 10 minutes
Cooking time: 0 minutes
Servings: 4

Ingredients:
- 2 tablespoons olive oil
- 1 teaspoon maple syrup
- 3 tablespoons lemon juice
- 2 basil leaves, chopped
- 1 garlic clove, minced
- 1 avocado, pitted, peeled and chopped
- 1 bunch kale, chopped
- 1 cup grapes, seedless and halved
- ¼ cup pumpkin seeds
- 1/3 cup red onion, chopped

Directions:
In a salad bowl, mix kale with avocado, grapes, pumpkin seeds and onion and stir, In another bowl, mix oil with maple syrup, lemon juice, basil and garlic and whisk well. Add this to salad, toss to coat and serve. Enjoy!

Nutritional value: calories 120, fat 1, fiber 1, carbs 2, protein 11

Chicken Salad and Raspberry Dressing

The combination is perfect! The tastes are perfectly balanced!

Preparation time: 10 minutes
Cooking time: 10 minutes
Servings: 4

Ingredients:

For the salad dressing:
- 1 tablespoon raspberry vinegar
- 1 shallot, chopped
- 6 ounces raspberries
- 2/3 cup walnuts, chopped
- A pinch of sea salt
- Black pepper to the taste
- ¼ cup olive oil

For the salad:
- ½ teaspoon garlic powder
- 1 tablespoon olive oil
- ¼ teaspoon smoked paprika
- ¼ teaspoon turmeric
- Black pepper to the taste
- 2 chicken breast halves
- 1 tablespoon ghee
- 5 ounces baby arugula
- 1 yellow bell pepper, chopped
- 8 ounces strawberries, halved
- 1 avocado, pitted, peeled and chopped
- ¼ red cabbage, shredded
- 1 cup blueberries

Directions:
Put walnuts in your food processor, blend well and transfer to a bowl. Add vinegar, raspberries, shallots, oil, a pinch of salt and black pepper, whisk well and leave aside for now. Meanwhile, in a bowl, mix 1 tablespoon oil with garlic powder, black pepper, paprika and turmeric and whisk well. Brush chicken breast halves with this mix, place them on your grill after you've greased it with the ghee and cook them over medium high heat for 4 minutes on each side. Transfer chicken to a cutting board, leave them to cool down a bit, slice and transfer them to a salad bowl. Add strawberries, avocado, cabbage, blueberries, bell pepper and arugula. Add salad dressing you've made at the beginning, toss to coat and serve.

Nutritional value: calories 150, fat 3, fiber 2, carbs 5, protein 18

Delicious Dinner Salad

This is such an amazing option!

Preparation time: 10 minutes
Cooking time: 0 minutes
Servings: 2

Ingredients:
- 1 and ½ tablespoons vinegar
- 3 tablespoons olive oil
- 1 teaspoon thyme, dried
- 2 tablespoons macadamia nuts, chopped
- A pinch of sea salt
- Black pepper to the taste
- ¾ cup chicken, cooked and shredded
- 3 tablespoons onion, chopped
- ¼ cup carrot, grated
- 4 radishes, chopped
- ½ cup red cabbage, shredded
- ½ cup green cabbage, shredded

Directions:
In a salad bowl, mix chicken with macadamia nuts, carrot, onion, radishes, green and red cabbage. In a bowl, mix vinegar with oil, a pinch of salt, black pepper and thyme and whisk well. Add this to salad, toss to coat and serve. Enjoy!

Nutritional value: calories 120, fat 2, fiber 3, carbs 4, protein 12

Broccoli and Carrots Salad

Everyone will ask for more!

Preparation time: 10 minutes
Cooking time: 0 minutes
Servings: 2

Ingredients:
- 3 carrots, sliced
- 1 cup broccoli, chopped
- 1/3 cup mushrooms, sliced
- 2 tablespoons walnuts, chopped
- 3 tablespoons red onion, chopped
- 3 tablespoons black olives, pitted and chopped
- A pinch of sea salt
- Black pepper to the taste
- 1 teaspoon mustard
- 3 tablespoons olive oil
- 1 and ½ tablespoons red vinegar

Directions:
In a salad bowl, mix carrots with olives, onion, walnuts, mushrooms and broccoli. In a small bowl, mix oil with vinegar, mustard, salt and pepper and whisk well. Add this to salad, toss to coat and serve.

Nutritional value: calories 140, fat 1, fiber 3, carbs 4, protein 15

Salmon and Strawberry Salad

We want you to make this Paleo salad right away!

Preparation time: 10 minutes
Cooking time: 8 minutes
Servings: 4

Ingredients:
- 1 pound salmon fillet
- 2 tablespoons olive oil
- ¼ teaspoon coriander, ground
- ½ teaspoon cumin, ground
- 1 teaspoon chili powder
- ¼ teaspoon paprika
- A pinch of sea salt
- Black pepper to the taste
- 6 strawberries, chopped
- ¼ cup red onion, chopped
- 1 jalapeno, chopped
- Juice from 1 lime
- 1 garlic clove, minced
- 5 ounces baby arugula
- ½ avocado, pitted, peeled and chopped
- 3 radishes, chopped

For the vinaigrette:
- ¼ cup balsamic vinegar
- 1/3 cup olive oil
- ½ teaspoon lemon zest
- 3 strawberries, chopped
- 1 tablespoon lemon juice
- 1 and ½ tablespoons maple syrup
- 1 and ½ tablespoons mustard

Directions:
In a bowl, mix 2 tablespoons oil with coriander, cumin, chili powder, paprika, a pinch of salt and black pepper to the taste and whisk well. Brush salmon with this mix, place on preheated grill over medium high heat, cook for 6 minutes skin side down, flip, cook for 2 minutes more, transfer to a cutting board, leave aside to cool down, cut into medium pieces and transfer to a bowl. Add radishes, avocado, 6 strawberries, garlic, arugula, red onion, jalapeno and lime juice and toss gently. In another bowl, mix 1/3 cup oil with 3 strawberries, vinegar, lemon zest, 1 tablespoon lemon juice, maple syrup and mustard and whisk very well. Add this to salad, toss to coat and serve.

Nutritional value: calories 120, fat 2, fiber 2, carbs 4, protein 10

Incredible Autumn Salad

Enjoy a delicious and special Paleo salad today!

Preparation time: 10 minutes
Cooking time: 4 minutes
Servings: 4

Ingredients:
For the salad dressing:
- 1 tablespoon parsley, chopped
- 1/3 cup cashew butter
- 1 tablespoon sesame seeds
- ½ cup green onion, chopped
- 2 tablespoons tamari sauce
- 2 tablespoons lemon juice
- 2 tablespoons vinegar
- A pinch of sea salt
- Black pepper to the taste
- 2 garlic cloves, minced
- 1/3 cup coconut milk
- ¼ cup avocado oil

For the salad:
- 2 tablespoons water
- 3 sweet potatoes, cut with a spiralizer
- 1 tablespoon parsley, chopped

Directions:
In your blender, mix cashew butter with 1 tablespoon parsley, green onion, sesame seeds, vinegar, tamari sauce, lemon juice, garlic, coconut milk, a pinch of salt and black pepper and pulse really well. Add the oil gradually and blend again well. Put sweet potato noodles in a bowl, add the water, place in your microwave and steam at High for 4 minutes. Drain potato noodles, transfer to a bowl and add 1 tablespoon parsley. Add dressing, toss to coat and serve.

Nutritional value: calories 300, fat 4, fiber 4, carbs 10, protein 6

Beetroot Salad

This is so great and delicious!

Preparation time: 10 minutes
Cooking time: 25 minutes
Servings: 2

Ingredients:

- 2 teaspoons oregano, dried
- 2 garlic cloves, minced
- 4 chicken thighs, skin on
- Juice of ½ lemon
- A pinch of sea salt
- Black pepper to the taste
- 2 tablespoons coconut oil
- 2 tablespoons olive oil

For the pumpkin:
- ½ butternut squash, chopped
- 1 and ½ teaspoons fennel seeds
- 1 tablespoons olive oil

For the beetroot:
- 1 tablespoon vinegar
- 2 beetroots, cooked, peeled and cut into medium pieces
- 1/3 cup walnuts, chopped
- ¼ teaspoon cinnamon powder
- 1 tablespoon maple syrup

For the salad dressing:
- ½ teaspoon maple syrup
- 2 tablespoons olive oil
- 1 tablespoon vinegar
- ½ teaspoon mustard
- 3 cups salad leaves, torn
- A pinch of sea salt
- Black pepper to the taste

Directions:

In a bowl, mix chicken thighs with 2 garlic cloves, oregano juice from ½ lemon, 2 tablespoons oil, a pinch of salt and black pepper, stir, leave aside for 10 minutes and discard marinade. Heat up a pan with the coconut oil over medium high heat, add chicken pieces, cook for 5 minutes on each side, transfer to a cutting board, leave aside to cool down, shred and put in a bowl. In a bowl, mix butternut squash with fennel seeds, a pinch of salt, some black pepper and 1 tablespoon oil, toss well, spread on a lined baking sheet, place in the oven at 360 degrees F for 20 minutes. Leave butternut squash pieces to cool down and add them to the bowl with the chicken. In a bowl, mix beetroots with 1 tablespoon vinegar and black pepper to the taste, stir well and add to chicken salad as well. Heat up a pan over medium high heat, add walnuts, maple syrup and cinnamon, stir, toast for a few minutes, take off heat, cool down and add to salad bowl. In a small bowl, mix 2 tablespoon oil with1 tablespoon vinegar, ½ teaspoon maple syrup, mustard, a pinch of salt and some black pepper and whisk well. Add salad leaves to the salad bowl, add salad dressing, toss to coat well and serve. Enjoy!

Nutritional value: calories 160, fat 3, fiber 4, carbs 5, protein 20

Chorizo Salad

It's delicious and very rich! It's great for a cold day!

Preparation time: 10 minutes
Cooking time: 20 minutes
Servings: 4

Ingredients:
- 4 cups arugula
- 1 tablespoon rosemary, chopped
- 2 green onions, chopped
- 2 chorizo sausages, sliced
- 1 tablespoon bacon fat
- 2 garlic cloves, minced
- 4 sweet potatoes, peeled and cubed
- A pinch of sea salt
- Black pepper to the taste
- *For the salad dressing:*
- 2 teaspoons mustard
- 2 tablespoons apple vinegar
- 4 tablespoons olive oil
- ½ teaspoon lemon juice

Directions:
Heat up a pan with the bacon fat over medium heat, add sweet potatoes, stir and cook for 7 minutes. Add a pinch of salt, black pepper, rosemary and garlic, stir and cook for 6 minutes more. Add chorizo slices, stir, cook for 3 minutes, take off heat, cool down and transfer everything to a salad bowl. Add green onions and arugula and stir. In a small bowl, mix olive oil with lemon juice, vinegar, mustard and some black pepper and whisk well. Add this to salad, toss to coat and serve.

Nutritional value: calories 190, fat 3, fiber 2, carbs 5, protein 9

Shrimp and Radish Salad

If you are in the mood for some tasty shrimp today, try this dish!

Preparation time: 10 minutes
Cooking time: 4 minutes
Servings: 4

Ingredients:
- 2 pounds shrimp, deveined
- A pinch of sea salt
- Black pepper to the taste
- 2 tablespoons olive oil
- 4 ounces watermelon radish, thinly sliced
- 4 ounces radishes, sliced
- ½ cup fennel bulb, chopped
- 4 green onions, chopped
- 1 teaspoon maple syrup
- 2 tablespoons lemon juice
- ¼ cup mint, chopped
- 2 tablespoons mayonnaise

Directions:
Heat up a pan with the oil over medium high heat, add shrimp, season with a pinch of salt and some black pepper, cook for 2 minutes on each side and transfer them to a salad bowl. Add watermelon radish, radishes, fennel and onions and stir gently. In a small bowl, mix maple syrup with lemon juice, mint and mayo and whisk well. Add this to salad, toss to coat well and serve. Enjoy!

Nutritional value: calories 170, fat 3, fiber 3, carbs 6, protein 10

Great Steak Salad

It's rich and vibrant!

Preparation time: 10 minutes
Cooking time: 0 minutes
Servings: 4

Ingredients:
- 6 cups romaine lettuce, chopped
- 1 red onion, chopped
- 1 yellow bell pepper, chopped
- 1 red bell pepper, chopped
- A pinch of sea salt
- Black pepper to the taste
- 1 cucumber, sliced
- ½ cup kalamata olives, pitted and sliced
- ¼ cup parsley, chopped
- ¾ pound flank steak, cooked and sliced
- 1 tablespoon olive oil

Directions:
In a salad bowl, mix lettuce with onion, yellow bell pepper, red bell pepper, cucumber, olives, parsley and steak slices and toss well. Add a pinch of salt, black pepper and the oil, toss to coat well and serve. Enjoy!

Nutritional value: calories 150, fat 3, fiber 2, carbs 3, protein 10

Russian Salad

It's the best winter salad!

Preparation time: 10 minutes
Cooking time: 0 minutes
Servings: 4

Ingredients:
- ½ cup walnuts, chopped
- ¼ cup Paleo mayo anise
- 1 and ½ pounds beets, roasted, peeled and grated
- ½ cup raisins
- 2 garlic cloves, minced
- ¼ cup parsley, chopped
- A pinch of sea salt
- Black pepper to the taste

Directions:
In a salad bowl, mix grated beets with walnuts, raisins, garlic, parsley, salt and pepper and stir. Add mayo, stir well and serve cold. Enjoy!

Nutritional value: calories 150, fat 4, fiber 3, carbs 3, protein 8

Cucumber And Tomato Salad

This is probably the most popular combination ever!

Preparation time: 10 minutes
Cooking time: 0 minutes
Servings: 4

Ingredients:
- 2 tablespoons red vinegar
- 3 tablespoons olive oil
- 1 teaspoon oregano, chopped
- 1 and ½ pounds cucumber, sliced
- 1 cup mixed colored tomatoes, halved
- 2 tablespoons mint, chopped
- ½ cup red onion, chopped
- 2 tablespoons parsley, chopped
- 2 tablespoons dill, chopped
- A pinch of sea salt
- Black pepper to the taste

Directions:
In a bowl, mix cucumber with tomatoes, onion, mint, parsley, oregano, dill, salt and pepper and stir. Add vinegar and oil, toss to coat and serve. Enjoy!

Nutritional value: calories 90, fat 0, fiber 1, carbs 0, protein 7

Swiss Chard Salad

We are very excited to introduce to you this great Paleo salad!

Preparation time: 10 minutes
Cooking time: 3 minutes
Servings: 4

Ingredients:
- 1 garlic clove, minced
- 1 shallot, chopped
- 1 tablespoon rosemary, chopped
- A pinch of sea salt
- Black pepper to the taste
- 2 tablespoons avocado oil
- 1 bunch Swiss chard, sliced
- 1 and ½ cup walnuts, halved
- 1 tablespoon vinegar
- 1 tablespoon lemon juice

Directions:
Heat up a pan with the oil over medium high heat, add garlic, rosemary, shallot, a pinch of salt and black pepper, stir and cook for 3 minutes. Add walnuts, stir, reduce heat and cook for a few seconds more. In a salad bowl, mix Swiss chard with vinegar, lemon juice and shallots mix and toss to coat. Enjoy!

Nutritional value: calories 195, fat 2, fiber 2, carbs 4, protein 10

Figs and Cabbage Salad

Are you looking for a Paleo salad you can serve your loved ones tonight? Why don't you try this great salad?

Preparation time: 10 minutes
Cooking time: 6 minutes
Servings: 4

Ingredients:
- 1 red cabbage head, shredded
- 2 tablespoons olive oil
- A pinch of sea salt
- Black pepper to the taste
- ¼ cup balsamic vinegar
- ½ teaspoon oregano, dried
- 1 yellow onion, chopped
- 1 tablespoon maple syrup
- 2 figs, cut into quarters
- A handful oregano, chopped

Directions:
In a bowl mix cabbage with a pinch of salt and some black pepper, stir well and leave aside. Heat up a pan with half of the oil over medium heat, add onion, stir and cook for 4 minutes. Add dried oregano and vinegar, stir, cook for 5 minutes and take off heat. Add maple syrup, some black pepper and stir well. In a salad bowl, mix squeezed cabbage with onions mix, figs and the rest of the oil, toss to coat and serve with fresh oregano on top. Enjoy!

Nutritional value: calories 140, fat 2, fiber 2, carbs 4, protein 9

Tasty Shrimp Cobb Salad

We are sure you've heard about the famous cobb salad but have you tried the Paleo version?

Preparation time: 10 minutes
Cooking time: 4 minutes
Servings: 4

Ingredients:
- 4 bacon strips, cooked and chopped
- 1 tablespoon bacon fat
- 1 pound shrimp, peeled and deveined
- 1 teaspoon garlic powder
- A pinch of sea salt
- Black pepper to the taste
- 6 cups romaine lettuce leaves, chopped
- 4 eggs, hard-boiled, peeled and chopped
- 1-pint cherry tomatoes, halved
- 1 avocado, pitted, peeled and chopped

For the vinaigrette:
- 1 garlic clove, minced
- 2 tablespoons Paleo mayonnaise
- 2 tablespoon vinegar
- 3 tablespoons avocado oil

Directions:
In a bowl mix garlic with mayo, vinegar and avocado oil, whisk well and leave aside for now. Heat up a pan with the bacon fat over medium high heat, add shrimp, season with a pinch of salt, some black pepper and garlic powder, cook for 2 minutes, flip, cook for 2 minutes more and transfer them to a salad bowl. Add tomatoes, avocado pieces, lettuce leaves, bacon and egg pieces and stir. Add the vinaigrette you've made earlier, toss to coat and serve. Enjoy!

Nutritional value: calories 150, fat 1, fiber 2, carbs 6, protein 10

Grilled Shrimp Salad

You need some time and the right ingredients to make this amazing salad!

Preparation time: 1 hour
Cooking time: 8 minutes
Servings: 4

Ingredients:

- ¼ cup ghee, melted
- ½ teaspoon dill, dried
- ¼ teaspoon smoked paprika
- A pinch of sea salt
- Black pepper to the taste
- 4 bacon slices, cooked and crumbled
- 12 ounces shrimp, peeled and deveined
- 4 cups mixed salad greens
- 1 avocado, pitted, peeled and chopped
- A handful cherry tomatoes, halved
- 2 tablespoons scallions, chopped

Directions:

In a bowl, mix ghee with a pinch of salt, black pepper, dill and paprika and stir well. Put shrimp in a bowl, add half of the ghee mix over them toss well and leave aside in the fridge for 1 hour. Heat up a pan over medium high heat, add shrimp, cook for 3 minutes on each side and transfer to a bowl. Add the rest of the ghee mix, bacon, mixed greens, avocado, tomatoes and scallions, toss everything well and serve. Enjoy!

Nutritional value: calories 200, fat 3, fiber 5, carbs 7, protein 15

Green Apple and Shrimp Salad

The combination is just right for a summer dinner!

Preparation time: 10 minutes
Cooking time: 0 minutes
Servings: 3

Ingredients:

- 1 green apple, cored and chopped
- 2 cups shrimp, peeled, deveined, cooked and chopped
- 3 eggs, hard-boiled, peeled and chopped
- 1 small red onion, chopped
- ¼ cup Dijon mustard
- 4 celery stalks, chopped
- 1 tablespoon olive oil
- 2 tablespoons vinegar
- ½ teaspoon thyme, chopped
- ½ teaspoon parsley, chopped
- ½ teaspoon basil, chopped
- A pinch of sea salt
- Black pepper to the taste

Directions:

In a big salad bowl, mix apple pieces with shrimp, eggs, onion and celery and stir. In another bowl, mix mustard with oil, vinegar, thyme, parsley, basil, a pinch of salt and black pepper and whisk well. Add this to your salad, toss well and serve. Enjoy!

Nutritional value: calories 110, fat 2, fiber 4, carbs 7, protein 15

Simple Cucumber Salad

This really special summer salad will be ready in no time!

Preparation time: 10 minutes
Cooking time: 0 minutes
Servings: 4

Ingredients:
- 1 zucchini, cut with a spiralizer
- 3 big cucumbers, cut with a spiralizer
- 2 garlic cloves, minced
- 1 and ½ tablespoons balsamic vinegar
- ¼ teaspoon ginger, grated
- A pinch of sea salt
- Black pepper to the taste
- 2 teaspoons sesame oil
- 1 small red jalapeno pepper, chopped
- 5 mint leaves, chopped

Directions:
In a salad bowl, mix zucchini noodles with cucumber ones, garlic, ginger, salt and pepper and stir. Add vinegar, oil, jalapeno and mint, toss to coat and serve right away. Enjoy!

Nutritional value: calories 90, fat 0, fiber 1, carbs 1, protein 5

Cuban Radish Salad

This is just great!

Preparation time: 10 minutes
Cooking time: 0 minutes
Servings: 4

Ingredients:
- 6 radishes, sliced
- 1 romaine lettuce head, chopped
- 1 avocado, pitted, peeled and chopped
- 2 tomatoes, roughly chopped
- 1 red onion, chopped
- ¼ cup apple cider vinegar
- ½ cup olive oil
- ¼ cup lime juice
- 3 garlic cloves, minced
- A pinch of sea salt
- Black pepper to the taste

For the salad dressing:

Directions:
In a salad bowl, mix radishes with lettuce leaves, avocado, onion and tomatoes and stir. In another bowl, mix vinegar with oil, lime juice, garlic, a pinch of salt and black pepper and whisk well. Add this to salad, toss to coat and serve. Enjoy!

Nutritional value: calories 100, fat 0.6, fiber 1, carbs 2, protein 4

Radish and Eggs Salad

It's a creamy and very healthy Paleo salad!

Preparation time: 10 minutes
Cooking time: 10 minutes
Servings: 2

Ingredients:

- 8 radishes, sliced
- 2 eggs
- ½ cup green onions, chopped
- 1 tablespoon mayonnaise
- ½ teaspoon mustard
- 1 tablespoon lemon juice
- A pinch of sea salt
- Black pepper to the taste
- A few lettuce leaves, chopped

Directions:
Put water in a pot, add eggs, bring to a boil over medium high heat, cook for 10 minutes, transfer eggs to a bowl filled with ice water, leave them to cool down, peel and chop them. In a salad bowl, mix lettuce leaves with chopped eggs, green onions and radishes. Add mustard, mayo, lemon juice, a pinch of salt and black pepper, toss to coat well and serve. Enjoy!

Nutritional value: calories 110, fat 1, fiber 2, carbs 4, protein 10

Paleo Dessert Recipes

Paleo Hazelnut Balls

After a delicious paleo meal, you must enjoy a delicious paleo dessert! Try this one!

Servings: 4
Preparation time: 30 minutes
Cooking time: 0 minute

Ingredients:
- 10 hazelnuts, roasted
- 1 cup hazelnuts, roasted and chopped
- 1 teaspoon vanilla extract
- 2 tablespoons raw cocoa powder
- ¼ cup maple syrup

Directions:
Put ½ cup chopped hazelnuts in your food processor and blend well. Add vanilla extract, cocoa powder, and maple syrup and blend again well. Roll the 10 hazelnuts in cocoa powder mix, dip them in the rest of the chopped hazelnuts and arrange balls on a lined baking sheet. Introduce in the freezer for 20 minutes and then serve them. Enjoy!

Nutritional value: calories 47, fat 2, carbs 11, fiber 0.1, sugar 7, protein 2

Paleo Pumpkin Cookies

These cookies are a real treat! We recommend you to try them soon!

Servings: 4
Preparation time: 10 minutes
Cooking time: 20 minutes

Ingredients:
- ¼ cup apple sauce
- 1 and ½ cup pumpkin puree
- 1 teaspoon vanilla extract
- ¼ cup coconut milk
- 1 cup almond milk
- ½ teaspoon pumpkin pie spice
- ½ cup coconut flour

Directions:
In a bowl, mix applesauce with pumpkin puree, vanilla extract, and coconut milk and stir very well. Add almond meal, pumpkin pie spice, and coconut flour and stir well again. Drop spoonfuls of batter on a lined baking sheet, flatten with a fork, introduce in the oven at 350 degrees F and bake for 25 minutes. Take cookies out of the oven, leave aside to cool down, transfer to a platter and serve. Enjoy!

Nutritional value: calories 140, fat 18, carbs 22, fiber 1.1, protein 10

Paleo Almond Bars

It's so easy to make a delicious paleo dessert! This recipe is the perfect example!

Servings: 9
Preparation time: 30 minutes
Cooking time: 7 minutes

Ingredients:
- ½ cup coconut butter
- ¾ cup melted coconut oil
- ½ cup cocoa powder
- ½ cup maple syrup
- ¼ cup dark chocolate, chopped
- ½ cup raspberries
- ¼ cup almonds, roasted and chopped

Directions:
Heat up a pan over medium heat, add coconut oil, coconut butter, maple syrup and cocoa powder and stir well until everything blends. Add chocolate pieces, almonds, and raspberries and stir again. Pour this mix into a lined baking tray, introduce in the freezer for 20 minutes, slice, arrange on plates and serve. Enjoy!

Nutritional value: calories 120, fat 3.5, carbs 5, fiber 0, protein 1

Paleo Muffins

Make these today, and you can even enjoy them tomorrow for breakfast!

Servings: 8
Preparation time: 10 minutes
Cooking time: 30 minutes

Ingredients:
- 1 cup almond butter
- 1 egg, whisked
- 3 bananas, chopped
- ½ cup cocoa powder
- 2 tablespoons raw honey
- 2 teaspoons vanilla extract

Directions:
In a bowl, mix almond butter with bananas, cocoa powder, egg, vanilla extract and honey and stir very well. Pour this into a muffin tray, introduce in the oven at 375 degrees F and bake for 30 minutes. Leave muffins to cool down for 5 minutes, removed from muffin tray and serve. Enjoy!

Nutritional value: calories 171, fat 19, carbs 24, fiber 1, protein 10

Paleo Stuffed Apples

It may seem like a classic fall dessert, but it's actually more than that!

Servings: 4
Preparation time: 10 minutes
Cooking time: 40 minutes

Ingredients:
- 4 apples, peeled
- 1 cup fresh blueberries
- 2 teaspoons lemon juice
- ½ cup apple juice
- ½ teaspoon cinnamon, ground
- 4 tablespoons almond meal
- 4 tablespoons coconut flakes

Directions:
Scoop the inside of each apple, brush them with lemon juice and place in a baking dish. Fill apples with blueberries and sprinkle cinnamon on top. Spread the rest of the blueberries in the baking dish, pour apple juice, sprinkle almond meal and coconut flakes on each apple, introduce everything in the oven at 375 degrees F and bake for 40 minutes. Take apples out of the oven, leave them to cool down, divide between plates and serve. Enjoy!

Nutritional value: calories 169, fat 1.4, carbs 38, fiber 4.7, sugar 31, protein 3.8

Paleo Raspberry Popsicles

Are you looking for something refreshing to eat on a hot summer day? Try this amazing paleo dessert.

Servings: 4
Preparation time: 2 hours
Cooking time: 15 minutes

Ingredients:
- 1 and ½ cups raspberries
- 2 cups water

Directions:
Put raspberries and water in a pan, heat up over medium heat, bring to a boil and simmer for 15 minutes. Take off heat, pour the mix into an ice cube tray, add a popsicle stick in each, introduce in the freezer and chill for 2 hours. Enjoy!

Nutritional value: calories 58, fat 0.4, carbs 0, fiber 2. protein 1.4

Paleo Pumpkin Pudding

It's so creamy and perfect! It's one of our favorite paleo desserts!

Servings: 4
Preparation time: 10 minutes
Cooking time: 8 minutes

Ingredients:
- 1 and ¾ cup almond milk
- ½ cup pumpkin puree
- 2 tablespoons tapioca starch
- ¼ cup raw honey
- 1 tablespoon water
- 1 egg
- 1 teaspoon vanilla extract
- ¼ teaspoon nutmeg, ground
- ½ teaspoon cinnamon, ground
- 1/8 teaspoon allspice, ground
- ¼ teaspoon ginger, ground

Directions:
In a bowl, mix tapioca starch with water and stir well. Put almond milk in a pot and mix with honey and egg. Stir, bring to a boil and stir in the tapioca starch mix. Cook for 2 minutes and take off heat. In a bowl, mix pumpkin puree with vanilla extract, nutmeg, cinnamon, allspice and ginger and stir well. Pour this into almond milk mix, stir and place over medium high heat. Cook for 4 minutes, transfer to dessert bowls and serve after you've chilled in the freezer for 2 hours. Enjoy!

Nutritional value: calories 246, fat 5.3, carbs 43, fiber 0.5, sugar 5, protein 6

Paleo Hazelnut Pancakes

These are perfect for dessert but also for breakfast!

Servings: 4
Preparation time: 15 minutes
Cooking time: 20 minutes

Ingredients:
- ¼ cup coconut milk
- 1 banana, peeled and mashed
- 4 eggs
- 1 teaspoon vanilla extract
- 1 and ½ cups hazelnut meal
- 2 tablespoons coconut flour
- ½ teaspoon baking soda
- Ghee for cooking

For the sauce:
- 2 tablespoons coconut oil
- 1 tablespoon lemon juice
- 2 blood oranges, peeled and sliced
- Juice from 1 blood orange
- 2 teaspoons honey
- 1 vanilla bean

Directions:
Heat up a pan with the coconut oil over medium heat, add orange juice, lemon juice, honey and vanilla bean, bring to a boil and simmer for 15 minutes stirring from time to time. In a bowl, mix eggs with vanilla extract and coconut milk and stir. Add mashed banana, coconut flour, baking soda and hazelnut meal and stir very well.
Heat up a pan with the ghee over medium heat, spoon ¼ cup pancake mix, spread a bit, cook for 3 minutes on one side, flip, cook for 1 more minute and transfer to a plate. Repeat this with the rest of the batter and serve pancakes with orange slices on the side and with the orange sauce on top. Enjoy!

Nutritional value: calories 90, fat 4.2, carbs 10, fiber 0.5, sugar 2.7, protein 2.4

Simple Paleo Cherry Jam

There are a lot of ways to make a good jam, but this recipe is one of the best!

Servings: 4
Preparation time: 10 minutes
Cooking time: 40 minutes

Ingredients:
- 1 cup raw honey
- 1 tablespoon lemon juice
- 6 cups cherries, pitted and roughly chopped

Directions:
Put cherries in a pan, add honey and leave aside for 10 minutes. Place pan over medium heat, bring to a simmer and mix with lemon juice. Cook for 30 minutes, stirring all the time, take off heat and serve in small dessert bowls. Keep the rest in the fridge. Enjoy!

Nutritional value: calories 50, fat 0, carbs 12, fiber 0, sugar 13, protein 0

Paleo Coconut Macaroons

It's a dessert with such an intense flavor! It's really good!

Servings: 4
Preparation time: 10 minutes
Cooking time: 40 minutes

Ingredients:
- 1 egg white
- 3 cups coconut flakes
- 2/3 cup almond milk
- ½ teaspoon vanilla extract
- 1 teaspoon lemon juice
- 1 teaspoon lemon zest

For the lemon curd:
- 5 tablespoons ghee, softened
- ½ cup raw honey
- 2 egg yolks
- 2 eggs
- 1 teaspoon lemon zest, grated
- 2/3 cup lemon juice

Directions:
In a bowl, mix honey with ghee and stir with a mixer for 3 minutes. Add 2 egg yolks and 2 eggs and mix again well. Add 2/3 cup lemon juice and mix 1 minute more. Transfer this to a pot, heat up over medium-low heat and cook for 15 minutes stirring often. Add 1 teaspoon lemon zest, stir, take off heat, transfer to a bowl and keep in the fridge for now. In a bowl, mix coconut flakes with almond milk, 1 egg white, vanilla extract, 1 teaspoon lemon juice, 1 teaspoon lemon zest and stir well. Shape small cookies, arrange them on a lined baking sheet, introduce in the oven at 325 degrees F and bake 20 minutes. Take cookies out of the oven, leave aside for 5 minutes and arrange them on a platter. Fill each macaroon with the lemon curd you've made and serve. Enjoy!

Nutritional value: calories 100, fat 4, carbs 11, fiber 2, sugar 9, protein 1

Spring Cheesecake

Think about how happy you'll make everyone with this Paleo dessert!

Preparation time: 2 hours and 10 minutes
Cooking time: 0 minutes
Servings: 4

Ingredients:
For the crust:
- ½ cup pecans
- ½ cup macadamia nuts
- ½ cup dates
- ½ cup walnuts

For the filling:
- 1 cup date paste
- 3 cups cashews, soaked for 3 hours
- ½ cup almond milk
- 2 cups strawberries
- ¾ cup coconut oil
- ¼ cup lime juice
- Sliced limes for serving
- Sliced strawberries for serving

Directions:
Put nuts, walnuts, dates and pecans in your food processor and blend well. Put 3 spoons of crust mix each part of a muffin tin, press well and leave aside for now. Put cashews, strawberries, date paste, lime juice, almond milk and coconut oil in your food processor and blend very well. Put 3 spoons of filling mix on top of crust mix, place in the freezer and keep for 2 hours. Transfer cheesecakes on a platter, top with strawberries and limes and serve. Enjoy!

Nutritional value: calories 140, fat 2, fiber 1, carbs 8, protein 2

Poached Rhubarb

It is so delicious!

Preparation time: 10 minutes
Cooking time: 5 minutes
Servings: 3

Ingredients:
- Juice of 1 lemon
- Some thin lemon zest strips
- 1 and ½ cup maple syrup
- 4 and ½ cups rhubarbs cut into medium pieces.
- 1 vanilla bean
- 1 and ½ cups water

Directions:
Put the water in a pan.
Add maple syrup, vanilla bean, lemon juice and lemon zest. Stir, bring to a boil and add rhubarb. Reduce heat, simmer for 5 minutes, take off heat and transfer rhubarb to a bowl. Allow liquid to cool down, discard vanilla bean and serve. Enjoy!

Nutritional value:: calories 108, fat 1, fiber 0, carbs 0, protein 1

Strawberry Cobbler

It's a delicate and elegant Paleo dessert!

Preparation time: 10 minutes
Cooking time: 30 minutes
Servings: 5

Ingredients:
- ¾ cup maple syrup
- 6 cups strawberries, halved
- 1/8 teaspoon baking powder
- 1 tablespoon lemon juice
- ½ cup coconut flour
- 1/8 teaspoon baking soda
- ½ cup water
- 3 and ½ tablespoons coconut oil
- A drizzle of avocado oil

Directions:
Grease a baking dish with a drizzle of avocado oil and leave aside. In a bowl, mix strawberries with maple syrup, sprinkle some flour and add lemon juice. Stir very well and pour into baking dish. In another bowl, mix flour with baking powder and soda and stir well. Add coconut and mix until the whole thing crumbles in your hands. Add ½ cup water and spread over strawberries. Place in the oven at 375 degrees F and bake for 30 minutes. Take cobbler out of the oven, leave aside for 10 minutes and then serve. Enjoy!

Nutritional value: calories 275, fat 9, fiber 4, carbs 9, protein 4

Avocado Pudding

You'll definitely want more!

Preparation time: 3 hours
Cooking time: 0 minutes
Servings: 4

Ingredients:
- 1 cup almond milk
- 2 avocados, peeled and pitted
- ¾ cup cocoa powder
- 1 teaspoon vanilla extract
- ¾ cup maple syrup
- ¼ teaspoon cinnamon
- Walnuts chopped for serving

Directions:
Put avocados in your kitchen blender and pulse well. Add cocoa powder, almond milk, maple syrup, cinnamon and vanilla extract and pulse well again. Pour into serving bowls, top with walnuts and keep in the fridge for 2-3 hours before you serve it. Enjoy!

Nutritional value: calories 231, fat 8, fiber 5, carbs 7, protein 2.9

Summer Sorbet

It's a Paleo dessert you should really try these days!

Preparation time: 2 hours
Cooking time: 0 minutes
Servings: 4

Ingredients:
- 1 cup dates, pitted and chopped
- 3 cups plums, chopped
- 2 and ½ cups water
- 1 teaspoon lemon juice

Directions:
Put dates and plums in your food processor t and blend well. Add water gradually and pulse a few more times. Add lemon juice, pulse for a few more seconds, transfer to a bowl and keep in the freezer for 2 hours. Scoop into dessert cups and serve right away! Enjoy!

Nutritional value: calories 85, fat 0, carbs 23, fiber 0, sugar 1, protein 1

Dessert Smoothie Bowl

It's easy and so delicious!

Preparation time: 6 minutes
Cooking time: 0 minutes
Servings: 4

Ingredients:
- ½ cup coconut water
- 1 and ½ cup avocado, chopped
- 2 tablespoons green tea powder
- 2 teaspoons lime zest
- 1 tablespoon honey
- Melted coconut butter for serving
- 1 mango thinly sliced for serving

Directions:
In your blender, mix water with avocado, green tea powder and lime zest and pulse well. Add honey and pulse again well. Transfer to a bowl, top with coconut butter spread all over and with sliced mango and serve. Enjoy!

Nutritional value: calories 337, fat 7, fiber 8, carbs 10, protein 10.4

Spring Ice Cream

It might be the best Paleo dessert!

Preparation time: 2 hours
Cooking time: 3 minutes
Servings: 8

Ingredients:
- 1 tablespoon arrowroot powder
- 2 cans coconut milk
- ¼ teaspoon vanilla beans
- 1 tablespoon water
- 1/3 cup pure maple syrup
- 1/3 cup coconut nectar

Directions:
Fill 1/3 of a bowl with ice cubes, place another bowl on top and leave aside for now. Pour coconut milk in a pot, reserve 2 tablespoons, put them in a bowl, mix with arrowroot starch and stir well. Add arrowroot mix of coconut milk to the pot and stir. Also add vanilla beans, maple syrup and coconut nectar, stir well, place on stove and heat up over medium heat. Stir well, bring to a boil, boil for 2 minutes, take off heat and pour into the bowl you've placed over the ice. Add water, stir well and leave aside for 1 hour and 30 minutes. Pour this into your ice cream machine and turn on. Pour into a container, place in the freezer and leave it there for 20 minutes. Serve right away! Enjoy!

Nutritional value: calories 136, fat 4, fiber 2, carbs 7, protein 2

Delicious Fruit Cream

It's the best spring Paleo combination of ingredients!

Preparation time: 6 hours and 10 minutes
Cooking time: 0 minutes
Servings: 6

Ingredients:
- 1 cup apples, chopped
- 1 cup pineapple, chopped
- 1 cup chickoo, chopped
- 1 cup melon, chopped
- 1 cup papaya, chopped
- ½ teaspoon vanilla powder
- ¾ cup cashews
- Stevia to the taste
- Some cold water

Directions:
Put cashews in a bowl, add some water on top, leave aside for 6 hours, drain them and put them in your food processor. Blend them well and add cold water to cover them. Also add stevia and vanilla, blend some more and keep in the fridge for now. In a bowl, arrange a layer of mixed apples with pineapples, melon, papaya and chickoo Add a layer of cold cashew paste, another layer of fruits, another one of cashew paste and to with a layer of fruits. Serve right away! Enjoy!

Nutritional value: calories 140, fat 1, fiber 1, carbs 3, protein 2

Chocolate Parfait

You won't believe this great taste!

Preparation time: 2 hours
Cooking time: 0 minutes
Servings: 4

Ingredients:
- 2 tablespoons cocoa powder
- 1 cup almond milk
- 1 tablespoon chia seeds
- A pinch of salt
- ½ teaspoon vanilla extract

Directions:
In a bowl, mix cocoa powder, almond milk, vanilla extract and chia seeds and stir well until they blend. Transfer to a dessert glass, place in the fridge for 2 hours and then serve. Enjoy!

Nutritional value: calories 130, fat 5, fiber 2, carbs 7, protein 16

Chocolate Butter Cups

They are incredible and delicious!

Preparation time: 40 minutes
Cooking time: 0 minutes
Servings: 4

Ingredients:
- 5 tablespoons almond flour
- ½ cup soft coconut butter
- 1 cup dark chocolate, chopped
- 1 teaspoon matcha powder+ some more for the topping
- 3 tablespoons maple syrup
- 1 teaspoon coconut oil
- Cocoa nibs

Directions:
In a bowl, mix coconut butter with almond flour, maple syrup and matcha powder, stir, cover and keep in the fridge for 10 minutes. Put dark chocolate in a bowl, place it over another bowl filled with boiling water, stir until it melts and mix with coconut oil. Spoon 2 teaspoons of this melted mix in a muffin liner. Repeat this with 7 other muffin liners. Take 1 tablespoon matcha mix and shape a ball, place in a muffin liner, press to flatten it and repeat this with the rest of the muffin liners. Top each with 1 tablespoon melted chocolate and spread evenly. Sprinkle some matcha powder all over muffins. Add cocoa nibs on top of each, introduce them in the freezer and keep there until they are solid. Take them out of the freezer, leave at room temperature for a few minutes and serve. Enjoy!

Nutritional value: calories 230, fat 2, fiber 1, carbs 9, protein 3

Caramel Ice Cream

It's different but amazing at the same time!

Preparation time: 10 minutes
Cooking time: 6 minutes
Servings: 6

Ingredients:
For the caramel sauce:
- ¾ cup stevia
- ½ cup coconut milk
- 2 tablespoons maple syrup
- 1 teaspoon vanilla extract

For the ice cream:
- 12 ounces firm almond cheese
- 1 can coconut milk
- 100 drops liquid stevia
- 2 teaspoons guar guar

Directions:
In a pan, heat up over medium high heat ½ cup coconut milk, ¾ cup stevia and maple syrup. Stir well, bring to a boil, reduce heat to low and simmer for 3-4 minutes. Take off heat, add vanilla extract, stir and leave in the fridge to cool down completely. In your food processor, mix canned coconut milk, almond cheese, a pinch of salt and the caramel and pulse well. Add guar guar and blend again well. Take mix from the fridge and transfer to an ice cream maker. When the ice cream is done, transfer to bowls and serve with caramel on top. Enjoy!

Nutritional value: calories 161, fat 7, fiber 1, carbs 10, protein 3.2

Chia Seeds Pudding

It's a very fresh and tasty Paleo dessert!

Preparation time: 1 hour and 20 minutes
Cooking time: 0 minutes
Servings: 4

Ingredients:
- 1 cup almond milk
- ½ cup pumpkin puree
- 2 tablespoons maple syrup
- ½ cup coconut milk
- ½ teaspoon cinnamon powder
- ½ teaspoon vanilla extract
- ¼ teaspoon ginger, grated
- ¼ cup chia seeds

Directions:
In a bowl, mix almond milk with coconut milk, pumpkin puree, cinnamon, maple syrup, vanilla and ginger and stir well. Add chia seeds, stir and leave aside for 20 minutes. Divide into 4 glasses, cover and keep in the fridge for 1 hour. Enjoy!

Nutritional value: calories 135, fat 7, fiber 7, carbs 10, protein 6.5

Summer Lemon Fudge

Sit back and enjoy this marvelous Paleo dessert!

Preparation time: 30 minutes
Cooking time: 0 minutes
Servings: 4

Ingredients:
- 1/3 cup natural cashew butter
- 1 and ½ tablespoons coconut oil
- 2 tablespoons coconut butter
- 5 tablespoons lemon juice
- ½ teaspoon lemon zest
- A pinch of salt
- 1 tablespoons maple syrup

Directions:
In a bowl, mix cashew butter with coconut one, coconut oil, lemon juice, lemon zest, a pinch of salt and maple syrup and stir until you obtain a creamy mix. Line a muffin tray with some parchment paper, scoop 1 tablespoon of lemon fudge mix in each of the 10 pieces, place in the freezer and keep the for a few hours. Take out of the fridge 20 minutes before you serve them. Enjoy!

Nutritional value: calories 72, fat 4, fiber 0, carbs 8, protein 1

Summer Energy Bars

They will give you so much energy!

Preparation time: 30 minutes
Cooking time: 0 minutes
Servings: 6

Ingredients:
- ¼ cup cocoa nibs
- 1 cup almonds, soaked for at least 3 hours
- 2 tablespoons cocoa powder
- ¼ cup hemp seeds
- ¼ cup goji berries
- ¼ cup coconut, shredded
- 8 dates, pitted and soaked

Directions:
Put almonds in your food processor and blend them well. Add hemp seeds, cocoa nibs, cocoa powder, goji, coconut and blend very well. Add dates gradually and blend some more. Transfer mix to a parchment paper, spread and press it. Cut in equal pieces and serve after you've kept them in the fridge for 30 minutes. Enjoy!

Nutritional value: calories 140, fat 6, fiber 3, carbs 7, protein 19

Delicious Pomegranate Fudge

It's so irresistible and delicious!

Preparation time: 2 hours
Cooking time: 5 minutes
Servings: 6

Ingredients:
- ½ cup coconut milk
- 1 teaspoon vanilla extract
- 1 and ½ cups dark chocolate, chopped
- ½ cup almonds, chopped
- ½ cup pomegranate seeds

Directions:
Put milk in a pan and heat up over medium low heat. Add chocolate and stir for 5 minutes. Take off heat, add vanilla extract, half of the pomegranate seeds and half the of the nuts and stir. Pour this into a lined baking pan, spread, sprinkle a pinch of salt, the rest of the pomegranate arils and nuts, cover and keep in the fridge for a few hours. Cut, arrange on a platter and serve. Enjoy!

Nutritional value: calories 68, fat 0.9, fiber 4, carbs 6, protein 0.2

Great and Intense Cheesecake

It's a good Paleo dessert!

Preparation time: 6 hours 10 minutes
Cooking time: 0 minutes
Servings: 4

Ingredients:

For the white layer:
- 6 tablespoons lemon juice
- 1 and ½ cups cashews, soaked overnight
- 6 tablespoons maple syrup
- 1 teaspoon vanilla extract
- 5 tablespoons coconut oil

For the yellow layer:
- ½ teaspoon cinnamon
- 1 and ½ teaspoon turmeric
- 1 cup mango chopped

For the orange layer:
- 1 and ½ carrots, chopped
- 1 cup dried apricots
- 1 tablespoon lemon juice
- 2 tablespoon coconut oil, melted
- 1 tablespoon maple syrup
- 1 teaspoon cinnamon
- A pinch of turmeric

Directions:
In your blender, mix 1 and ½ cups cashews with 6 tablespoons lemon juice, 6 tablespoons maple syrup, 5 tablespoons coconut oil and 1 teaspoon vanilla extract, blend very well, transfer to a bowl and leave aside. Clean your food processor and add 1 cup mango. Mix with turmeric and cinnamon, blend well, transfer to a bowl and also leave aside. Clean your food processor again and add apricots. Mix with carrots, 2 tablespoons coconut oil, 1 tablespoon lemon juice, 1 tablespoon maple syrup, 1 teaspoon cinnamon and a pinch of turmeric, blend well and transfer to a third bowl. Pour orange layer into a springform pan and spread evenly on the bottom. Pour the yellow layer on top and also spread well. End with the white layer, spread, keep cheese cake in the freezer for 6 hours, cut and serve it. Enjoy!

Nutritional value: calories 170, fat 6, fiber 4, carbs 6, protein 12

Pumpkin Custard

It's the perfect Paleo dessert for a cold winter day!

Preparation time: 10 minutes
Cooking time: 1 hour
Servings: 6

Ingredients:
- 1 and ½ cups pumpkin puree
- 2/3 cup maple syrup
- 1 cup coconut milk
- 2 tablespoons chia seeds ground and mixed with 5 tablespoons water
- 1 tablespoon baking powder
- 2 teaspoons pumpkin pie spice
- A pinch of salt
- 1 teaspoon cinnamon
- ½ teaspoon vanilla
- Pumpkin seeds for serving

Directions:
In a bowl, mix pumpkin puree with coconut milk, maple syrup, chia seeds mixed with water, baking powder, pumpkin pie spice, a pinch of salt, cinnamon and vanilla and stir well using your kitchen mixer. Pour this into small ramekins, arrange them on a baking tray filled half way with hot water, place in the oven at 325 degrees F and bake for 1 hour. Take custards out of the oven, leave them to cool down and serve with pumpkin seeds on top. Enjoy!

Nutritional value: calories 151, fat 2, fiber 2, carbs 6, protein 6

Berry and Cashew Cake

It's smooth and delicious!

Preparation time: 5 hours and 10 minutes
Cooking time: 0 minutes
Servings: 6

Ingredients:
For the crust:
- ½ cup dates, pitted
- 1 tablespoon water
- ½ teaspoon vanilla
- ½ cup almonds

For the cake:
- 2 and ½ cups cashews, soaked for 8 hours
- 1 cup blueberries
- ¾ cup maple syrup
- 1 tablespoon coconut oil

Directions:
In your food processor, mix dates with water, vanilla and almonds and pulse well. Transfer dough to a working surface and flatten it. Arrange into a lined round pan and leave aside for now. In your blender, mix maple syrup with coconut oil, cashews and blueberries and blend well. Spread evenly on the crust, introduce cake in the freezer for 5 hours, leave at room temperature for 15 minutes, then cut and serve it. Enjoy!

Nutritional value: calories 230, fat 0.5, fiber 5, carbs 12, protein 4

Fruit Jelly

Try it soon! It's really great!

Preparation time: 10 minutes
Cooking time: 0 minutes
Servings: 2

Ingredients:
- 1 pounds grapefruit jelly
- ½ pound coconut cream
- A handful fresh berries for serving
- A handful nuts, roughly chopped for serving

Directions:
In your food processor, combine grapefruit jelly with coconut cream and blend very well. Add berries and nuts, toss gently, transfer to dessert cups and serve right away! Enjoy!

Nutritional value: calories 70, fat 29, carbs 4.4, fiber 1, protein 3.5, sugar 1

Almond and Fig Dessert

This is one of the easiest winter Paleo desserts ever!

Preparation time: 10 minutes
Cooking time: 5 minutes
Servings: 4

Ingredients:
- 2 tablespoons coconut butter
- 12 figs cut in halves
- ¼ cup maple syrup
- 1 cup almonds, toasted and chopped

Directions:
Heat up a pot with the butter over medium high heat and stir until it melts. Add maple syrup and figs, stir well and cook for about 5 minutes. Add almonds, stir gently and take off heat. Transfer to dessert bowls and serve right away! Enjoy!

Nutritional value: calories 220, fat 6, fiber 8, carbs 9, protein 12

Great Tomato Cake

It's something really different and new!

Preparation time: 10 minutes
Cooking time: 30 minutes
Servings: 4

Ingredients:
- 1 and ½ cups coconut flour
- 1 teaspoon cinnamon
- 1 teaspoon baking powder
- 1 teaspoon baking soda
- ¾ cup maple syrup
- 1 cup tomatoes chopped
- ½ cup extra virgin olive oil
- 2 tablespoon apple cider vinegar

Directions:
In a bowl, mix flour with baking powder, baking soda, cinnamon and maple syrup and stir well. In another bowl, mix tomatoes with olive oil and vinegar and stir well. Combine the 2 mixtures, stir well and pour everything into a greased round pan. Introduce cake in the oven at 375 degrees F and bake for 30 minutes. Take cake out of the oven, leave aside to cool down, transfer to a platter, cut and serve it. Enjoy!

Nutritional value: calories 153, fat 3.2, carbs 28, fiber 0.8, sugar 11.5, protein 2.7

Green Apple Smoothie

This green smoothie is perfect for the cold season!

Preparation time: 10 minutes
Cooking time: 0 minutes
Servings: 3

Ingredients:
- 1 big green apple, cored and cut into medium cubes
- 1 cup baby spinach
- 1 tablespoon pure maple syrup
- A pinch of cardamom
- ½ teaspoon cinnamon
- ½ teaspoon vanilla extract

Directions:
Put apple cubes in your food processor. Add spinach, maple syrup, vanilla extract, cardamom and cinnamon and blend until you obtain a smooth cream. Pour into 2 glasses and serve right away! Enjoy!

Nutritional value: calories 145, fat 0.8, fiber 3, carbs 8, protein 4

Grapefruit Granita

It's a wonderful dessert idea for you and all your friends!

Preparation time: 4 hours and 20 minutes
Cooking time: 0 minutes
Servings: 6

Ingredients:
- 1 cup water
- 1 cup maple syrup
- ½ cup mint, chopped
- 64 ounces red grapefruit juice
- Mint leaves for serving

Directions:
Put 1 cup water in a pan, bring to a boil, add maple syrup, stir and take off heat. Add mint, cover and leave aside for 5 minutes. Strain into a plastic container, discard mint, add grapefruit juice, cover, place in the freezer for 4 hours. Take out of the freezer 15 minutes before you scrape with a fork and serve with mint leaves on top. Enjoy!

Nutritional value: 120, fat 0.3, carbs 2, fiber 0.2, protein 1

Mango Granita

It's a tropical dessert!

Preparation time: 6 hours
Cooking time: 10 minutes
Servings: 6

Ingredients:
- 4 cups mango, peeled and cubed
- 2 tablespoons lime juice
- 6 tablespoons maple syrup
- A pinch of salt
- A pinch of ground red pepper

Directions:
Put mango, lime juice, maple syrup, salt and red pepper in a pan, bring to a boil, stir, reduce heat to low and simmer for 10 minutes. Remove from heat, leave aside for 10 minutes, pour into your food processor, pulse a few times, strain into a bowl, discard solids, pour into a baking dish, place in the freezer and keep there for 6 hours scraping every hour. Scrape with a fork after 6 hours and serve! Enjoy!

Nutritional value: calories 127, fat 0.3, fiber 2, carbs 5, protein 0.7

Delicious Cherry Sorbet

It's different from any sorbets you had before!

Preparation time: 2 hours and 20 minutes
Cooking time: 0 minutes
Servings: 7

Ingredients:
- ½ cup dark cocoa powder
- ¾ cup Paleo red cherry jam
- ¼ cup maple syrup
- 2 cups water

For the compote:
- 2 tablespoons stevia
- 1 pound cherries, pitted and cut in halves

Directions:
In a pan, mix cherry jam with cocoa and maple syrup, stir, bring to a boil, gradually add the water, stir again, remove from heat, leave aside to cool down completely. Whisk this sorbet again, pour in a casserole and keep in the freezer for 1 hour. For the compote, mix in a bowl, stevia with cherries, toss to coat and leave aside for 1 hour. When the time has passed, serve this compote with the sorbet. Enjoy!

Nutritional value: calories 197, fat 1, fiber 4, carbs 9, protein 2

Fruits Mix and Vinaigrette

It's such a pleasure to share with you this amazing dessert idea!

Preparation time: 5 minutes
Cooking time: 15 minutes
Servings: 4

Ingredients:
- 2 tablespoons lemon juice
- 1 and ½ tablespoons maple syrup
- 1 and ½ tablespoons champagne vinegar
- 1 tablespoon olive oil
- 1 pound strawberries, halved
- 1 and ½ cups blueberries
- ¼ cup basil leaves, torn

Directions:
In a pot, mix lemon juice with maple syrup and vinegar, bring to a boil at a medium high temperature, simmer for 15 minutes, add oil, stir and leave aside for 2 minutes. In a bowl, mix blueberries with strawberries and lemon vinaigrette, toss to coat, sprinkle basil on top and serve! Enjoy!

Nutritional value: calories 163, fat 4, fiber 4, carbs 10, protein 2.1

Simple Passion Fruit Pudding

It's such a pleasure to teach you how to make this amazing Paleo dessert!

Preparation time: 10 minutes
Cooking time: 55 minutes
Servings: 6

Ingredients:
- 1 cup Paleo passion fruit curd
- 4 passion fruits, pulp and seeds
- 3 and ½ ounces maple syrup
- 3 eggs
- 2 ounces ghee, melted
- 3 and ½ ounces almond milk
- ½ cup almond flour
- ½ teaspoon baking powder

Directions:
Put half of the passion fruit curd in a bowl and leave aside. In another bowl, mix the rest of the curd with passion fruit seeds and pulp and stir. Divide this into 6 teacups. In a bowl, whisk eggs with maple syrup, ghee, the reserved curd, baking powder, milk and flour and stir well. Divide this into the 6 cups as well, put them in an oven pan, fill the pan halfway with water, place in the oven at 200 degrees F and bake for 50 minutes. Take puddings out of the oven, leave aside to cool down and serve! Enjoy!

Nutritional value: calories 430, fat 22, fiber 3, carbs 7, protein 8

Summer Carrot Cake

It looks so beautiful and it tastes wonderful!

Preparation time: 3 hours and 15 minutes
Cooking time: 0 minutes
Servings: 6

Ingredients:

For the cashew frosting:
- 2 tablespoons lemon juice
- 2 cups cashews, soaked
- 2 tablespoons coconut oil, melted
- 1/3 cup maple syrup
- Water

- 1 cup pineapple, dried and chopped
- 2 carrots, chopped
- 1 and ½ cups coconut flour
- 1 cup dates, pitted
- ½ cup dry coconut
- ½ teaspoon cinnamon

For the cake:

Directions:
In your blender, mix cashews with lemon juice, coconut oil, maple syrup and some apple, pulse very well, transfer to a bowl and leave aside for now. Put carrots in your food processor and pulse them a few times. Add flour, dates, pineapple, coconut and cinnamon and pulse very well again. Pour half of this mix into a springform pan and spread evenly. Add 1/3 of the frosting and also spread. Add the rest of the cake mix and the rest of the frosting. Place in the freezer and keep until it's hard enough. Cut and serve.

Nutritional value: calories 140, fat 3.7, fiber 4, carbs 8, protein 4.3

Carrot Cupcakes

We adore these cupcakes!

Preparation time: 1 hour and 10 minutes
Cooking time: 0 minutes
Servings: 6

Ingredients:
- 1 cup almonds
- 2 cups carrot pulp
- 1 cup dates, chopped
- ½ teaspoon ginger, grated
- 1 teaspoon cinnamon powder
- A pinch of nutmeg
- ¾ cup raisins

For the frosting:
- 1 cup cashews, soaked for 1 hour and drained
- A splash of water
- 1 teaspoon lemon juice
- 6 dates, pitted, soaked for 1 hour and drained

Directions:
In your food processor, mix 1 cup walnuts with 1 cup dates, carrot pulp, 1 teaspoon cinnamon, ginger, a pinch of nutmeg and the raisins and blend very well. Divide this between cupcakes tins and push it well. Clean your food processor, add 1 cup cashews, 6 dates, a splash of water and the lemon juice and blend these as well. Divide the frosting on the cupcakes, introduce them in the fridge and keep there for 1 hour. Enjoy!

Nutritional value: calories 150, fat 5, fiber 2, carbs 7, protein 1.4

Special Cupcakes

These will be done in no time and they are really great!

Preparation time: 1 hour and 10 minutes
Cooking time: 0 minutes
Servings: 6

Ingredients:
- 16 ounces mulberries, dried
- 1 teaspoon cinnamon, ground
- 16 ounces dates, pitted and chopped
- 3 ounces almond butter
- 3 ounces raw beet juice powder
- 3 ounces spirulina powder
- 8 ounces coconut water
- 1 and ½ cups raw cashews

Directions:
In your food processor, mix mulberries with dates, cinnamon and butter and blend very well. Scoop this mix into a cupcake pan and leave aside. Clean your food processor, mix spirulina powder with half of the cashews and half of the coconut water, blend well, transfer to a bowl and leave aside. Clean your blender again, add beet powder with the rest of the cashews and the coconut water and pulse well. Decorate half of the cupcakes with the beets frosting and the other half with the spirulina powder one. Keep cupcakes in the fridge for 1 hour and serve them. Enjoy!

Nutritional value: calories 340, fat 11, fiber 2, carbs 7, carbs 9, protein 15

Conclusion

How can you not love this great diet? How can you not be interested in following it?
All the wonderful recipes you've discovered earlier can help you make the best decision of your life: start a Paleo diet!

Go shopping, get all your ingredients and start making some of the best, most delicious and popular Paleo dishes. Make sure everyone around you will taste these special dishes! Your friends, loved ones and guests will be impressed for sure and they will end up following this Paleo diet in no time.

So what are you waiting for?
Get your Paleo cookbook right away and start your new life!
Have fun!

Recipe Index

A
African Stew, 73
Almond and Fig Dessert, 255
Amazing Bacon Waffles, 44
Amazing Beef and Spinach, 142
Amazing Beef Kabobs, 134
Amazing Beef Lasagna, 132
Amazing Butternut Squash Mix, 93
Amazing Cherry Mix, 192
Amazing Crab Cakes and Red Pepper Sauce, 164
Amazing Lamb Chops, 137
Amazing Lamb Chops and Mint Sauce, 139
Amazing Mahi Mahi Dish, 169
Amazing Paleo Potato Bites, 186
Amazing Paleo Shrimp Dish, 151
Amazing Party Meatballs, 108
Amazing Poached Kohlrabi Dish, 92
Amazing Pumpkin Muffins, 34
Amazing Roasted Beets, 84
Amazing Roasted Lamb, 139
Amazing Salmon and Chives, 173
Amazing Salmon and Spicy Slaw, 167
Amazing Salmon Tartar, 179
Amazing Seafood Soup, 58
Amazing Shrimp Dish, 163
Amazing Side Dish, 90
Amazing Slow-Cooked Beef, 138
Amazing Souvlaki, 131
Amazing Spicy Sweet Potatoes, 99
Amazing Squash Soup, 55
Amazing Taco Salad, 221
Amazing Turnips and Sauce, 87
Appetizer Salad, 105
Apple Omelet, 36
Artichokes and Tomatoes Dip, 208
Artichokes with Horseradish Sauce, 207
Asparagus and Mushrooms Side Dish, 79
Avocado Boats, 105
Avocado Pudding, 247
Avocado Salad, 227
Avocado Spread, 197
Awesome Avocado Muffins, 35

B
Bacon and Egg Breakfast Sandwich, 40
Bacon Muffins, 29
Baked Eggplant, 203
Baked Zucchini Chips, 107
Basil Zucchini Spaghetti, 96
Beef and Bok Choy, 147
Beef and Cabbage Delight, 141
Beef and Squash Skillet, 41
Beef and Sweet Potatoes Stew, 69
Beef and Tasty Veggies, 146
Beef Curry, 144
Beef in Amazing Tomato Marinade, 138
Beetroot Salad, 233
Bell Peppers Stuffed with Tuna, 202
Berry and Cashew Cake, 254
Breakfast Coconut Pancakes, 37
Breakfast Paleo Muffins, 15
Breakfast Sliders, 40
Breakfast Tomato and Eggs, 15
Broccoli and Carrots Salad, 231
Broccoli Salad, 225
Brussels Sprouts Salad, 215
Butternut Squash Bites, 106

C
Cabbage and Salmon Slaw, 225
Caramel Ice Cream, 251
Carne Asada, 137
Carrot Balls, 112
Carrot Cupcakes, 260
Carrots and Lime Delight, 209
Cauliflower Popcorn, 101
Cereal Bowl, 25
Chia Seeds Pudding, 251
Chicken Bites, 119
Chicken Salad and Raspberry Dressing, 230
Chicken Thighs with Tasty Butternut Squash, 121
Chocolate Butter Cups, 250
Chocolate Parfait, 250
Chorizo Breakfast Skillet, 42
Chorizo Salad, 234
Coconut and Almonds Granola, 26
Coconut and Zucchini Soup, 60
Cod and Herb Sauce, 175
Crazy Chicken Appetizer, 118
Crazy Oxtail Stew, 73
Creamy Mashed Pumpkin, 86
Crusted Snapper, 180
Cuban Radish Salad, 239
Cucumber and Tomato Salad, 236
Cucumber Noodles and Shrimp, 197
Cucumber Rolls, 117
Cucumber Wraps, 198

D
Delicious and Special Crackers, 111
Delicious Artichokes Dish, 207

Delicious Beef and Wonderful Gravy, 135
Delicious Beef Stew, 66
Delicious Braised Cabbage Side Dish, 96
Delicious Broccoli and Tasty Hazelnuts, 99
Delicious Cabbage Chips, 120
Delicious Cauliflower Cream, 60
Delicious Cauliflower Soup, 46
Delicious Cherry Sorbet, 258
Delicious Chicken Waffles, 44
Delicious Clam Soup, 63
Delicious Cucumber Soup, 64
Delicious Dinner Salad, 230
Delicious Eggplant and Mushrooms, 97
Delicious Eggplant Casserole, 204
Delicious Eggplant Dish, 203
Delicious Eggs and Artichokes, 27
Delicious Filet Mignon and Special Sauce, 133
Delicious Fruit Cream, 249
Delicious Gazpacho, 56
Delicious Grilled Oysters, 165
Delicious Hummus, 101
Delicious Kale Frittata, 29
Delicious Lamb Stew, 71
Delicious Lobster and Sauce, 170
Delicious Mashed Sweet Potatoes, 84
Delicious Mexican Steaks, 131
Delicious Mushroom Cream, 58
Delicious Mussels Mix, 169
Delicious Paleo Beef Casserole, 124
Delicious Paleo Salad, 219
Delicious Peppers Stuffed with Beef, 200
Delicious Pomegranate Fudge, 253
Delicious Pumpkin and Bok Choy, 85
Delicious Pumpkin Fries, 85
Delicious Purple Carrots, 210
Delicious Roasted Cauliflower, 91
Delicious Roasted Green Beans, 90
Delicious Roasted Okra, 83
Delicious Rosemary Lamb Chops, 148
Delicious Sausage Balls, 32
Delicious Sausage Frittata, 30
Delicious Scallops, 164
Delicious Shrimp and Cauliflower Rice, 166
Delicious Squid and Guacamole, 165
Delicious Steak, 134
Delicious Steak and Veggie Breakfast, 43
Delicious Stuffed Artichokes, 95
Delicious Stuffed Baby Peppers, 201
Delicious Stuffed Eggs, 104
Delicious Stuffed Peppers, 199
Delicious Summer Salad, 221
Delicious Thai Curry, 145
Delicious Turkey Casserole, 140
Delightful and Special Hummus, 102

Delightful Chicken Soup, 48
Delightful Pork Stew, 67
Delightful Salmon Dish, 163
Delightful Spaghetti Squash, 92
Delightful Wrapped Eggs, 33
Dessert Smoothie Bowl, 248
Different Beef Dish, 141
Different Breakfast Dish, 31
Different Grilled Steaks, 132
Dill Carrots, 100

E
Easy Asparagus Soup, 63
Egg Cups, 104
Eggplant and Garlic Sauce, 204
Eggplant Hash, 205
Eggplant Jam, 205
Exotic Beef Stew, 69

F
Figs and Cabbage Salad, 237
Flavored Taro Dish, 94
French Chicken Stew, 72
Fresh Salad, 228
Fried Peppers, 118
Fruit Jelly, 255
Fruits Mix and Vinaigrette, 258

G
Ginger Cauliflower Rice, 95
Glazed Salmon, 167
Grapefruit Granita, 257
Great and Intense Cheesecake, 253
Great Beef Teriyaki, 135
Great Carrot Hash, 209
Great Fennel Side Dish, 87
Great Onion Soup, 62
Great Steak Salad, 235
Great Stir Fried Side Dish, 94
Great Tomato Cake, 256
Great Winter Salad, 222
Greek Style Beef Bowls, 144
Green Apple and Shrimp Salad, 238
Green Apple Smoothie, 256
Grilled Artichokes, 208
Grilled Calamari, 171
Grilled Cherry Tomatoes, 194
Grilled Salmon and Avocado Sauce, 170
Grilled Salmon with Peaches, 159
Grilled Shrimp Salad, 238

H

Halibut and Tasty Salsa, 174
Ham and Mushroom Breakfast, 37
Hamburger Salad, 145
Hearty Chicken Salad, 228
Hearty Meat Stew, 68
Homemade Breakfast Granola, 25

I

Incredible Apple Pancakes, 38
Incredible Autumn Salad, 232
Incredible Beef and Basil, 143
Incredible Chard, 100
Incredible Chicken Strips, 108
Incredible Eggs and Ham, 28
Incredible Glazed Carrots, 210
Incredible Side Salad, 88
Incredible Swordfish, 180
Incredible Turkey Soup, 65
Incredibly Tasty Butternut Squash, 93
Indian Beef Patties, 140
Infused Clams, 162
Italian Breakfast Eggs, 28

K

Kale and Avocado Salad, 229
Kale and Carrots Salad, 222
Kale and Sausage Soup, 62
Kale Chips and Tasty Dip, 110
Kale, Mushrooms and Red Chard Side Dish, 98

L

Lamb and Eggplant Puree, 149
Lavender Lamb Chops, 149
Liver Stuffed Peppers, 202
Lovely Kale Dish, 98

M

Mango Granita, 257
Mexican Stew, 66
Mexican-Style Stuffed Peppers, 199
Moroccan Lamb, 148
Mushroom Boats, 115

N

Nettles Soup, 61
Noodles and Capers Sauce, 195

O

Orange and Dates Granola, 18
Orange and Vanilla Breakfast Delight, 26
Oyster Spread, 113

P

Paleo Almond Bars, 242
Paleo Asparagus Side Dish, 77
Paleo Baked Yuka with Tomato Sauce, 188
Paleo Banana Pancakes, 16
Paleo Barbeque Ribs, 128
Paleo Beef Soup, 47
Paleo Beef Stew, 50
Paleo Beef Stir Fry, 126
Paleo Beef Tenderloin with Special Sauce, 126
Paleo Blueberry Smoothie, 22
Paleo Breakfast Burger, 20
Paleo Breakfast Burrito, 18
Paleo Breakfast Sandwich, 21
Paleo Broccoli and Cauliflower Fritters, 189
Paleo Butternut Squash Side Dish, 77
Paleo Carrot and Cucumber Salad, 215
Paleo Cauliflower Pizza, 182
Paleo Celery Casserole, 190
Paleo Chard Side Dish, 78
Paleo Chicken Meatballs, 123
Paleo Chicken Salad, 213
Paleo Chicken Soup, 46
Paleo Chicken Stew, 52
Paleo Coconut Macaroons, 245
Paleo Cucumber Salsa, 186
Paleo Daikon Rolls, 181
Paleo Egg Salad, 211
Paleo Eggplant and Tomato Salad, 212
Paleo Eggplant French Toast, 17
Paleo Eggplant Stew, 54
Paleo Endive Bites, 182
Paleo Falafel, 181
Paleo Fish Tacos, 156
Paleo French Chicken Stew, 53
Paleo French Fries, 82
Paleo Glazed Salmon, 152
Paleo Green Smoothie, 22
Paleo Grilled Artichokes, 84
Paleo Grilled Calamari, 154
Paleo Grilled Lamb Chops, 124
Paleo Hazelnut Balls, 241
Paleo Hazelnut Pancakes, 244
Paleo Kohlrabi Dish, 187
Paleo Lamb and Coconut Stew, 52
Paleo Lamb Casserole, 125
Paleo Lamb Chops with Mint Sauce, 125
Paleo Lemon and Garlic Soup, 48
Paleo Lobster Salad, 216
Paleo Lobster with Sauce, 152
Paleo Maple Nut Porridge, 20

Paleo Mashed Carrots, 81
Paleo Mashed Cauliflower Dish, 76
Paleo Muffins, 242
Paleo Mushrooms and Thyme Side Dish, 80
Paleo Onion Rings, 188
Paleo Oxtail Stew, 54
Paleo Peach and Coconut Smoothie, 24
Paleo Pear Salad with Tasty Dressing, 211
Paleo Pomegranate Salad, 216
Paleo Pork Dish with Delicious Blueberry Sauce, 127
Paleo Pork Salad, 220
Paleo Pork Tenderloin with Carrot Puree, 129
Paleo Pork with Pear Salsa, 129
Paleo Pork with Strawberry Sauce, 130
Paleo Potato Salad, 213
Paleo Pumpkin Cookies, 241
Paleo Pumpkin Pudding, 244
Paleo Radish Salad, 214
Paleo Raspberry Popsicles, 243
Paleo Red Breakfast Smoothie, 23
Paleo Roasted Beets, 78
Paleo Roasted Bell Peppers, 82
Paleo Roasted Brussels Sprouts, 78
Paleo Roasted Cabbage Side Dish, 83
Paleo Roasted Carrots, 75
Paleo Roasted Cherry Tomatoes, 80
Paleo Roasted Cod, 157
Paleo Roasted Duck Dish, 123
Paleo Roasted Trout, 157
Paleo Salmon Pie, 153
Paleo Salmon Tartar, 158
Paleo Salmon with Avocado Sauce, 155
Paleo Sausage Casserole, 130
Paleo Sautéed Spinach Dish, 81
Paleo Scallops Tartar, 160
Paleo Scallops with Delicious Puree, 155
Paleo Seafood Salad, 220
Paleo Shrimp and Zucchini Noodles, 154
Paleo Shrimp Burgers, 159
Paleo Shrimp Salad, 212
Paleo Shrimp Skewers, 160
Paleo Slow Cooked Mushrooms, 76
Paleo Slow Cooker Stew, 50
Paleo Spinach and Mushroom Dish, 190
Paleo Steak Salad, 217
Paleo Steamed Clams, 153
Paleo Stuffed Apples, 243
Paleo Stuffed Eggplant, 185
Paleo Stuffed Mushrooms, 184
Paleo Stuffed Quail, 122
Paleo Summer Salad, 217
Paleo Surprise Dinner Dish, 189
Paleo Sweet Potato Waffles, 17
Paleo Sweet Potatoes and Cabbage Bake, 187

Paleo Sweet Potatoes Dish, 79
Paleo Tomato and Mushroom Skewers, 185
Paleo Turkey Breakfast Sandwich, 21
Paleo Turkey Casserole, 121
Paleo Veggie and Chorizo Stew, 51
Paleo Veggie Soup, 49
Paleo Veggie Stew, 53
Paleo Veggies Dish with Tasty Sauce, 183
Paleo Zucchini and Leeks Side Dish, 75
Paleo-Indian Pancakes, 183
Parsley and Pear Smoothie, 24
Plantain Fries, 88
Plantain Pancakes, 16
Poached Rhubarb, 246
Pork Skillet, 42
Pork Stuffed Bell Peppers, 201
Portobello Sandwich, 39
Pumpkin Custard, 254

Q
Quick and Tasty Salad, 227

R
Radish and Eggs Salad, 240
Red Cabbage Salad, 226
Rich Paleo Soup, 49
Rich Salad, 224
Roasted Broccoli, 88
Roasted Cod, 173
Roasted Eggplant Spread, 103
Roasted Veggie Stew, 72
Root Paleo Soup, 47
Rosemary Crackers, 110
Russian Salad, 235
Rutabaga Noodles and Cherry Tomatoes, 191

S
Salmon and Chili Sauce, 162
Salmon and Lemon Relish, 168
Salmon and Strawberry Salad, 231
Salmon and Tomato Pesto, 175
Salmon Delight, 176
Salmon Salad, 224
Salmon Skewers, 161
Scallops Bites, 120
Scallops Tartar, 177
Sheppard's Pie, 136
Shrimp and Chicken Soup, 59
Shrimp and Radish Salad, 234
Shrimp and Zucchini Noodles, 171
Shrimp Cocktail, 178
Shrimp with Mango and Avocado Mix, 176

Simple and Easy Pepperoni Bites, 107
Simple and Tasty Nuts Porridge, 39
Simple Beef and Brussels Sprouts, 142
Simple Beef Jerky, 109
Simple Breakfast Waffles, 43
Simple Broccoli Soup, 55
Simple Brussels Sprouts Side Dish, 89
Simple Burger, 32
Simple Chicken Salad, 223
Simple Chicken Skewers, 109
Simple Chicken Soup, 57
Simple Chicken Stew, 70
Simple Coconut Bars, 111
Simple Cucumber Salad, 239
Simple Garlic Tomatoes, 191
Simple Guacamole, 102
Simple Kale Dish, 85
Simple Nuts Snack, 112
Simple Paleo Cherry Jam, 245
Simple Passion Fruit Pudding, 259
Simple Pumpkin Salad, 86
Simple Roasted Tomatoes, 193
Simple Scallops Salad, 219
Simple Spinach Omelet, 35
Slow Cooked Delicious Stew, 70
Slow Cooked Lamb Shanks, 150
Smoked Salmon and Fresh Veggies, 156
Spaghetti Squash and Tomatoes, 195
Spanish Appetizer Cakes, 119
Special and Tasty Beef Stew, 67
Special Beef and Plantain Stew, 51
Special Blueberry Muffins, 33
Special Breakfast Pancakes, 31
Special Burrito, 27
Special Cauliflower Mini Hot Dogs, 116
Special Celery Soup, 65
Special Cupcakes, 260
Special Eggplant Stew, 74
Special Mint Zucchini, 98
Special Mixed Snack, 106
Special Mushroom and Broccoli Appetizer, 115
Special Paleo Beef Salad, 218
Special Paleo Chicken and Veggies Stir Fry, 122
Special Paleo Chicken Salad, 214
Special Paleo Fish Dish, 151
Special Paleo Pork Chops, 128
Special Paleo Soup, 45
Special Plantain Mash, 91
Special Salmon, 174
Special Stew, 71
Spicy Eggs, 30
Spicy Shrimp, 168
Spinach Frittata, 19
Spring Cheesecake, 246

Spring Ice Cream, 249
Squash Blossom Frittata, 19
Steak and Amazing Blueberry Sauce, 147
Steaks and Apricots, 133
Steaks and Scallops, 136
Strawberry and Kiwi Breakfast Smoothie, 23
Strawberry Cobbler, 247
Stuffed Calamari, 172
Stuffed Mushrooms, 114
Stuffed Poblanos, 200
Stuffed Portobello Mushrooms, 196
Stuffed Salmon Fillets, 166
Stuffed Zucchinis, 184
Summer Beef Skillet, 143
Summer Carrot Cake, 259
Summer Energy Bars, 252
Summer Lemon Fudge, 252
Summer Salad, 224
Summer Sorbet, 248
Sun Dried Tomatoes Spread, 103
Superb Tuna Dish, 158
Sweet Potato Breakfast, 41
Sweet Potato Salad, 223
Sweet Potato Soup, 61
Swiss Chard Salad, 236

T

Tapioca Root Fries, 89
Tasty Apricot Bites, 114
Tasty Brussels Sprouts Soup, 64
Tasty Cauliflower and Leeks, 97
Tasty Chorizo Stew, 68
Tasty Green Soup, 57
Tasty Kale and Beets, 99
Tasty Paleo Pulled Pork, 127
Tasty Porridge, 38
Tasty Sashimi Salad, 227
Tasty Shrimp Cobb Salad, 237
Tasty Squash and Cranberries, 100
Tasty Veggie Mix, 89
Tasty Veggie Soup, 56
Thai Lamb Chops, 150
Thai Shrimp Delight, 177
Tilapia Surprise, 178
Tomato and Basil Soup, 45
Tomato and Chicken Salad, 229
Tomato Quiche, 192
Tomato Salad, 225
Tuna and Chimichurri Sauce, 161
Tuna and Salsa, 179

V

Veal Rolls, 146

Veggie Mix and Tasty Scallops, 198
Veggie Omelet Cupcakes, 36
Veggies and Fish Mix, 194
Vietnamese Stew, 74

W
Warm Paleo Salad, 218
Warm Watercress Mix, 206
Watercress Soup, 206
Watermelon Salad, 226
Watermelon Wraps, 117
Wonderful Crusted Salmon, 172
Wrapped Olives, 113

Z
Zucchini and Chocolate Muffins, 34
Zucchini Noodles and Tasty Pesto, 196
Zucchini Noodles with Tomatoes and Spinach, 193
Zucchini Rolls, 116
Zucchini Soup, 59

Copyright 2017 by Jennifer Evans All rights reserved.

All rights Reserved. No part of this publication or the information in it may be quoted from or reproduced in any form by means such as printing, scanning, photocopying or otherwise without prior written permission of the copyright holder.

Disclaimer and Terms of Use: Effort has been made to ensure that the information in this book is accurate and complete, however, the author and the publisher do not warrant the accuracy of the information, text and graphics contained within the book due to the rapidly changing nature of science, research, known and unknown facts and internet. The Author and the publisher do not hold any responsibility for errors, omissions or contrary interpretation of the subject matter herein. This book is presented solely for motivational and informational purposes only.

Made in the USA
Columbia, SC
17 April 2018